Food Contamination and Safety

Food Contamination and Safety

Edited by
Emiliano Johnston

Larsen & Keller
www.larsen-keller.com

Food Contamination and Safety
Edited by Emiliano Johnston
ISBN: 978-1-63549-121-0 (Hardback)

Larsen & Keller
Published by Larsen and Keller Education,
5 Penn Plaza,
19th Floor,
New York, NY 10001, USA

Cataloging-in-Publication Data

Food contamination and safety / edited by Emiliano Johnston.
p. cm.
Includes bibliographical references and index.
ISBN 978-1-63549-121-0
1. Food contamination. 2. Food--Safety measures. 3. Food adulteration and inspection.
I. Johnston, Emiliano.
TX531 .F66 2017
363.192--dc23

Printed and bound in China.

For more information regarding Larsen and Keller Education and its products, please visit the publisher's website www.larsen-keller.com

Table of Contents

Preface

This book elucidates new techniques and the applications in the field of food contamination in a multidisciplinary approach. It elaborates on the different theories and concepts related to this area. Food contamination refers to the degradation of food because of harmful chemicals or bacteria that cause various diseases and infections. In order to ensure food quality, the finished product goes through a thorough quality check. In this text, effort has been made to present the explanation of various methods of food safety, easy and simple. It is designed specifically for students. The topics covered in this extensive textbook deal with the core subjects of food contamination and safety. It will serve as a valuable source of reference for those interested in this field.

To facilitate a deeper understanding of the contents of this book a short introduction of every chapter is written below:

Chapter 1- Contaminated food is food that has harmful chemicals and caused illness in consumers. Adulterated food is unsafe and is contaminated food. This chapter will provide an integrated understanding of adulterated food.

Chapter 2- Aflatoxins are chemicals that cause cancer; they are produced by certain molds that grow in the soil. The alternative natural toxins prions are aflatoxin B1, mycotoxin, prions, scrapie and bovine spongiform encephalopathy. The section serves as a source to understand the major natural toxins prions and carcinogens in food.

Chapter 3- Foodborne illnesses are illnesses that are caused because of contaminated food. Symptoms of food illness are fever, vomiting and aches. Bacterias that cause infection are pathogenic bacteria, bacillus cereus, staphylococcal enteritis and vibrio vulnificus. The section on food illness offers an insightful focus, keeping in mind the subject matter.

Chapter 4- Diseases that are related to food contamination are cholera, gastroenteritis, shigellosis, botulism, salmonellosis, Gerstmann-Straussler-Scheinker syndrome and kuru. Cholera is an infection caused by the bacterium vibrio cholera; the symptoms are vomiting and diarrhea. The section serves as a source to understand the diseases related to food contamination.

Chapter 5- The zoonotic diseases that spread through food are salmonellosis, bubonic plague, avian influenza, caliciviridae and trichinosis. Salmonellosis is an infection caused by bacterias, the symptoms of which vary from fever to abdominal cramps. The topics discussed in the chapter are of great importance to broaden the existing knowledge on zoonotic diseases.

Chapter 6- Food safety is the handling and storing of food in ways that helps in preventing foodborne illnesses. The aspects elucidated are food processing, food preservation, food storage and calcium propanoate. The major categories of food safety are dealt with great details in the chapter.

I would like to share the credit of this book with my editorial team who worked tirelessly on this book. I owe the completion of this book to the never-ending support of my family, who supported me throughout the project.

Editor

1

Understanding Food Contamination

Contaminated food is food that has harmful chemicals and caused illness in consumers. Adulterated food is unsafe and is contaminated food. This chapter will provide an integrated understanding of adulterated food.

Food Contaminant

Food contamination refers to the presence in food of harmful chemicals and microorganisms which can cause consumer illness. This article addresses the chemical contamination of foods, as opposed to microbiological contamination, which can be found under foodborne illness.

The impact of chemical contaminants on consumer health and well-being is often apparent only after many years of processing. Prolonged exposure at low levels (e.g., cancer). Chemical contaminants present in foods are often unaffected by thermal processing (unlike most microbiological agents). Chemical contaminants can be classified according to the source of contamination and the mechanism by which they enter the food product.

Agrochemicals

Agrochemicals are chemicals used in agricultural practices and animal husbandry with the intent to increase crops and reduce costs. Such agents include pesticides (e.g., insecticides, herbicides, rodenticides), plant growth regulators, veterinary drugs (e.g., nitrofuran, fluoroquinolones, malachite green, chloramphenicol), and bovine somatotropin (rBST).

Environmental Contaminants

Environmental contaminants are chemicals that are present in the environment in which the food is grown, harvested, transported, stored, packaged, processed, and consumed. The physical contact of the food with its environment results in its contamination. Possible sources of contamination include:

- Air: radionuclides (^{137}Caesium, ^{90}Strontium), polycyclic aromatic hydrocarbons (PAH)
- Water: arsenic, mercury
- Soil: cadmium, nitrates, perchlorates
- Polychlorinated biphenyls (PCB), dioxins, and polybrominated diphenyl ethers (PBDE) are ubiquitous chemicals
- Packaging materials: antimony, tin, lead, perfluorooctanoic acid (PFOA), semicarbazide,

benzophenone, isopropyl thioxanthone (ITX), bisphenol A

- Processing/cooking equipment: copper, or other metal chips, lubricants, cleaning, and sanitizing agents
- Naturally occurring toxins: mycotoxins, phytohaemagglutinin, pyrrolizidine alkaloids, grayanotoxin, mushroom toxins, scombrotoxin (histamine), ciguatera, shellfish toxins, tetrodotoxin, among many others.

Pesticides and Carcinogens

There are many cases of banned pesticides or carcinogens found in foods.

- Greenpeace exposed in 2006 in China that 25% of surveyed supermarkets agricultural products contained banned pesticides. Over 70% of tomatoes that tested were found to have the banned pesticide Lindane, and almost 40% of the samples had a mix of three or more types of pesticides. Fruits were also tested in this investigation. Tangerines, strawberries, and Kyofung grapes samples were found contaminated by banned pesticides, including the highly toxic Methamidophos. These fruits can also be found in Hong Kong market. Greenpeace says there exists no comprehensive monitoring on fruit produce in the Hong Kong as of 2006.
- In India, soft drinks were found contaminated with high levels of pesticides and insecticides, including lindane, DDT, malathion and chlorpyrifos.
- News of Formaldehyde, a carcinogen was found in Vietnamese national dish, Pho, broke in 2007 Vietnam food scare. Vegetables and fruits were also found to have banned pesticides. “Health agencies have known that Vietnamese soy sauce, the country’s second most popular sauce after fish sauce, has been chock full of cancer agents since at least 2001”, thundered the *Thanh Nien* daily. “Why didn’t anyone tell us?” The carcinogen in Asian sauces is 3-MCPD and its metabolite 1,3-DCP, which has been an ongoing problem before 2000 affecting multiple continents.
- 2005 Indonesia food scare, carcinogenic formaldehyde was added as a preservative to noodles, tofu, salted fish, and meatballs
- 2008 Chinese milk scandal

Hair in Food

There is a heavy stigma attached to the presence of hair in food in most societies. There is a risk that it may induce choking and vomiting, and also that it may be contaminated by toxic substances. Views differ as to the level of risk it poses to the inadvertent consumer.

In most countries, people working in the food industry are required to cover their hair because it will contaminate the food. When people are served food which contains hair in restaurants or cafés, it is usual for them to complain to the staff. Despite this, it is not a valid ground on which to sue the restaurant in the United States but in the United Kingdom it breaks the regulations of the UK Food Safety Act 1990, and people can sue over this.

There are a range of possible reasons for the objection to hair in food, ranging from cultural taboos to the simple fact that it is difficult to digest and unpleasant to eat. It may also be interpreted as a sign of more widespread problems with hygiene. The introduction of complete-capture hairnets is believed to have resulted in a decrease in incidents of contamination of this type.

Sometimes protein from human hair is used as a food ingredient, in bread and other such similar products. Such use of human hair in food is forbidden in Islam. Historically, in Judaism, finding hair in food was a sign of bad luck.

Processing Contaminants

Processing contaminants are generated during the processing of foods (e.g., heating, fermentation). They are absent in the raw materials, and are formed by chemical reactions between natural and/or added food constituents during processing. The presence of these contaminants in processed foods cannot be entirely avoided. Technological processes can be adjusted and/or optimized, however, in order to reduce the levels of formation of processing contaminants. Examples are: nitrosamines, polycyclic aromatic hydrocarbons (PAH), heterocyclic amines, histamine, acrylamide, furan, benzene, trans fat, 3-MCPD, semicarbazide, 4-hydroxynonenal (4-HNE), and ethyl carbamate. There is also the possibility of metal chips from the processing equipment contaminating food. These can be identified using metal detection equipment. In many conveyor lines, the line will be stopped, or when weighing the product with a Check weigher, the item can be rejected for being over- or underweight or because small pieces of metal are detected within it.

Emerging Food Contaminants

While many food contaminants have been known for decades, the formation and presence of certain chemicals in foods has been discovered relatively recently. These are the so-called emerging food contaminants like acrylamide, furan, benzene, perchlorate, perfluorooctanoic acid (PFOA), 3-monochloropropane-1,3-diol (3-MCPD), 4-hydroxynonenal, and (4-HNE).

Safety and Regulation

Acceptable Daily Intake (ADI) levels and tolerable concentrations of contaminants in individual foods are determined on the basis of the "No Observed Adverse Effect Level" (NOAEL) in animal experiments, by using a safety factor (usually 100). The maximum concentrations of contaminants allowed by legislation are often well below toxicological tolerance levels, because such levels can often be reasonably achieved by using good agricultural and manufacturing practices.

Regulatory officials, in order to combat the dangers associated with foodborne viruses, are pursuing various possible measures.

- The EFSA published a report in 2011 on "scientific opinion regarding an update of the present knowledge on the occurrence and control of foodborne viruses".
- This year, an expert working group created by the European Committee for Standardization (CEN), is expected to publish a standard method for the detection of norovirus and hepatitis A virus in food.

- The CODEX Committee on Food Hygiene (CCFH) is also working on a guideline which is now ready for final adoption.
- European Commission Regulation (EC) No 2073/2005 of 15 November 2005 indicates that "foodstuffs should not contain micro-organisms or their toxins or metabolites in quantities that present an unacceptable risk for human health", underlining that methods are required for foodborne virus detection.

Food Contaminant Testing

To maintain high quality of food and comply with health, safety and environmental regulatory standards it is best to rely on food contaminant testing through an independent third party such as laboratories, certification companies or similar. For manufacturers the testing for food contaminants can minimize the risk of noncompliance in relation to raw ingredients, semi-manufactured foods and final products. Also, food contaminant testing assures consumers safety and quality of purchased food products and can prevent foodborne diseases, and chemical, microbiological, or physical food hazards.

The establishment of ADIs for certain emerging food contaminants is currently an active area of research and regulatory debate.

Adulterated Food

Adulterated food is impure, unsafe, or unwholesome food. Incidents of food contamination have occurred because of poor harvesting or storage of grain, use of banned veterinary products, industrial discharges, human error and deliberate adulteration and fraud.

History of Incidents

Historians have recognized cases of food adulteration in Ancient Rome and the Middle Ages. Contemporary accounts of adulteration date from the 1850s to the present day .Now a days food are adulterated by chemicals such as plastic and so on This is a dangerous issue .Human beings are harmed by this adulterated food .Plastic is mixed up with certain food item such as chips ,rice etc .Drinking hot drinks in plastic cups glass is dangerous as the heat melts the plastic layer and the plastic mixes with the drink.

Legislative History

In the United States, the Food and Drug Administration (FDA), regulates and enforces laws on food safety as well as Food Defense. The FDA provides some technical definitions of adulterated food in various United States laws.

- 1906 (21 U.S.C. 601 et seq.)
- 1938 Federal Food, Drug, and Cosmetic Act (21 U.S.C. 321 et seq.)
- 1957 Poultry Products Inspection Act (21 U.S.C. 451 et seq.)

- 2011 Food Safety and Modernization Act

Definition

"Adulteration" is a legal term meaning that a food product fails to meet federal or state standards. Adulteration is an addition of another substance to a food item in order to increase the quantity of the food item in raw form or prepared form, which may result in the loss of actual quality of food item. These substances may be other available food items or non-food items. Among meat and meat products some of the items used to adulterate are water or ice, carcasses, or carcasses of animals other than the animal meant to be consumed.

Federal Food, Drug, and Cosmetic Act

The Federal Food, Drug, and Cosmetic (FD&C) Act 2888) provides that food is "adulterated" if it meets any one of the following criteria:

- (1) it bears or contains any "poisonous or deleterious substance" which may render it injurious to health;
- (2) it bears or contains any added poisonous or added deleterious substance (other than a pesticide residue, food additive, color additive, or new animal drug, which are covered by separate provisions) that is unsafe;
- (3) its container is composed, in whole or in part, of any poisonous or deleterious substance which may render the contents injurious to health;
- or (4) it bears or contains a pesticide chemical residue that is unsafe. (Note: The United States Environmental Protection Agency (EPA) establishes tolerances for pesticide residues in foods, which are enforced by the FDA.)

Food also meets the definition of adulteration if:

- (5) it is, or it bears or contains, an unsafe food additive;
- (6) it is, or it bears or contains, an unsafe new animal drug;
- (7) it is, or it bears or contains, an unsafe colour additive;
- (8) it consists, in whole or in part, of "any filthy, putrid, or decomposed substance" or is otherwise unfit for food;
- or (9) it has been prepared, packed, or held under unsanitary conditions (insect, rodent, or bird infestation) whereby it may have become contaminated with filth or rendered injurious to health.

Further, food is considered adulterated if:

- (10) it has been irradiated and the irradiation processing was not done in conformity with a regulation permitting irradiation of the food in question (the FDA has approved irradiation of a number of foods, including refrigerated or frozen uncooked meat, fresh or frozen uncooked poultry, and seeds for sprouting [21 C.F.R. Part 179].);

- (11) it contains a dietary ingredient that presents a significant or unreasonable risk of illness or injury under the conditions of use recommended in labelling (for example, foods or dietary supplements containing aristolochic acids, which have been linked to kidney failure, have been banned.);
- (12) a valuable constituent has been omitted in whole or in part or replaced with another substance; damage or inferiority has been concealed in any manner; or a substance has been added to increase the product's bulk or weight, reduce its quality or strength, or make it appear of greater value than it is (this is "economic adulteration");
- or (13) it is offered for import into the United States and is a food that has previously been refused admission, unless the person reoffering the food establishes that it is in compliance with U.S. law [21 U.S.C. § 342].

Federal Meat Inspection Act and the Poultry Products Inspection Act

The Federal Meat Inspection Act and the Poultry Products Inspection Act of 1957 contain similar provisions for meat and poultry products. [21 U.S.C. § 453(g), 601(m).

Poisonous or Deleterious Substances

Generally, if a food contains a poisonous or deleterious substance that may render it injurious to health, it is considered to be adulterated. For example, apple cider contaminated with E. coli O157:H7 and Brie cheese contaminated with Listeria monocytogenes are adulterated. There are two exceptions to this general rule. First, if the poisonous substance is inherent or naturally occurring and its quantity in the food does not ordinarily render it injurious to health, the food will not be considered adulterated. Thus, a food that contains a natural toxin at very low levels that would not ordinarily be harmful (for instance, small amounts of amygdalin in apricot kernels) is not adulterated.

Second, if the poisonous or deleterious substance is unavoidable and is within an established tolerance, regulatory limit, or action level, the food will not be deemed to be adulterated. Tolerances and regulatory limits are thresholds above which a food will be considered adulterated. They are binding on FDA, the food industry, and the courts. Action levels are limits at or above which FDA may regard food as adulterated. They are not binding on FDA. FDA has established numerous action levels (for example, one part per million methylmercury in fish), which are set forth in its booklet Action Levels for Poisonous or Deleterious Substances in Human Food and Animal Feed.

If a food contains a poisonous substance in excess of a tolerance, regulatory limit, or action level, mixing it with "clean" food to reduce the level of contamination is not allowed. The deliberate mixing of adulterated food with good food renders the finished product adulterated (FDA, Compliance Policy Guide [CPG § 555.200]).

Filth and Foreign Matter of Adulteration

Filth and extraneous material include any objectionable substances in foods, such as foreign matter (for example, glass, metal, plastic, wood, stones, sand, cigarette butts), undesirable parts of the raw plant material (such as stems, pits in pitted olives, pieces of shell in canned oysters), and filth (namely, mold, rot, insect and rodent parts, excreta, decomposition). Under a strict reading of the FD&C Act, any amount of filth in a food would render it adulterated. FDA regulations, however, authorize the agency to issue Defect Action Levels (DALs) for natural, unavoidable defects that at low levels do not pose a human health hazard [21 C.F.R. § 110.110]. These DALs are advisory only; they do not have the force of law and do not bind FDA. DALs are set forth in FDA's Compliance Policy Guides and are compiled in the FDA and Center for Food Safety and Applied Nutrition (CFSAN) Defect Action Level Handbook.

In most cases, DALs are food-specific and defect-specific. For example, the DAL for insect fragments in peanut butter is an average of thirty or more insect fragments per 100 grams (g) [CPG § 570.300]. In the case of hard or sharp foreign objects, the DAL, which is based on the size of the object and the likelihood it will pose a risk of choking or injury, applies to all foods.

Economic-Adulteration

A food is adulterated if it omits a valuable constituent or substitutes another substance, in whole or in part, for a valuable constituent (for instance, olive oil diluted with tea tree oil); conceals damage or inferiority in any manner (such as fresh fruit with food coloring on its surface to conceal defects); or any substance has been added to it or packed with it to increase its bulk or weight, reduce its quality or strength, or make it appear bigger or of greater value than it is (for example, scallops to which water has been added to make them heavier).

Microbiological Contamination and Adulteration of Food

The fact that a food is contaminated with pathogens (harmful microorganisms such as bacteria, viruses, or protozoa) may, or may not, render it adulterated. Generally, for ready-to-eat foods, the presence of pathogens will render the food adulterated. For example, the presence of Salmonella on fresh fruits or vegetables or in ready-to-eat meat or poultry products (such as luncheon meats) will render those products are adulterated.

For meat and poultry products, which are regulated by USDA, the rules are more complicated. Ready-to-eat meat and poultry products contaminated with pathogens, such as Salmonella or Listeria monocytogenes, are adulterated. (Note that hotdogs are considered ready-to-eat products.) For raw meat or poultry products, the presence of pathogens will not always render a product adulterated (because raw meat and poultry products are intended to be cooked, and proper cooking should kill pathogens). Raw poultry contaminated with Salmonella is not adulterated. However, USDA's Food Safety and Inspection Service (FSIS) has ruled that raw meat or poultry products contaminated with E. coli O157:H7 are adulterated. This is because normal cooking methods may not reduce E. coli O157:H7 below infectious levels. E. coli O157:H7 is the only pathogen that is considered an adulterant when present in raw meat or poultry products.

Enforcement Actions

If a food is adulterated, FDA and FSIS have a broad array of enforcement tools.They are of various types. These include seizing and condemning the product, detaining imported product, enjoining persons from manufacturing or distributing the product, or requesting a recall of the product.

Enforcement action is usually preceded by a Warning Letter from FDA to the manufacturer or distributor of the adulterated product. In the case of an adulterated meat or poultry product, FSIS has certain additional powers. FSIS may suspend or withdraw federal inspection of an official establishment. Without federal inspection, an establishment may not produce or process meat or poultry products, and therefore must cease operations. With the exception of infant formula, neither FDA nor FSIS has the authority to require a company to recall an adulterated food product. However, the ability to generate negative publicity gives them considerable powers of persuasion.

State regulators generally have similar enforcement tools at their disposal to prevent the manufacture and distribution of adulterated food. In addition, many states have the authority to immediately embargo adulterated food and to impose civil fines. Federal agencies often will coordinate with state or local authorities to remove unsafe food from the market as quickly as possible.

References

- Howard Schwartz (1991). Lilith's Cave: Jewish Tales of the Supernatural. ISBN 0-19-506726-6.
- Commission Regulation (EC) No 2073/2005, Official Journal of the European Union, 15 November 2005, Retrieved 7 April 2015

2

Natural Toxins, Prions and Carcinogens in Food

Aflatoxins are chemicals that cause cancer; they are produced by certain molds that grow in the soil. The alternative natural toxins prions are aflatoxin B1, mycotoxin, prions, scrapie and bovine spongiform encephalopathy. The section serves as a source to understand the major natural toxins prions and carcinogens in food.

Aflatoxin

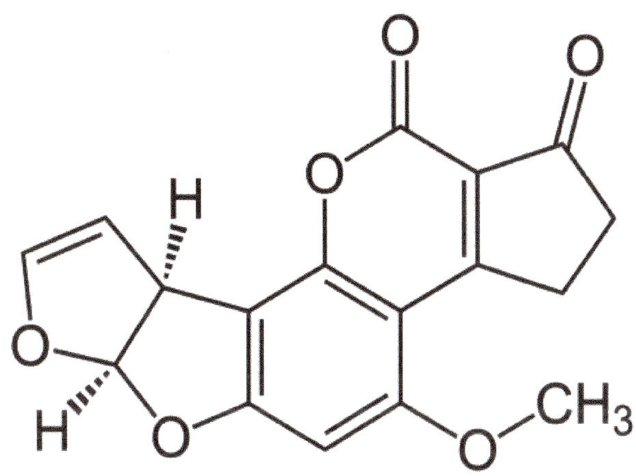

Chemical structure of aflatoxin B_1

Aflatoxins are poisonous and cancer-causing chemicals that are produced by certain molds (*Aspergillus flavus* and *Aspergillus parasiticus*) which grow in soil, decaying vegetation, hay, and grains. They are regularly found in improperly stored staple commodities such as cassava, chili peppers, corn, cotton seed, millet, peanuts, rice, sesame seeds, sorghum, sunflower seeds, tree nuts, wheat, and a variety of spices. When contaminated food is processed, aflatoxins enter the general food supply where they have been found in both pet and human foods, as well as in feedstocks for agricultural animals. Animals fed contaminated food can pass aflatoxin transformation products into eggs, milk products, and meat. For example, contaminated poultry feed is suspected in the findings of high percentages of samples of aflatoxin contaminated chicken meat and eggs in Pakistan.

Children are particularly affected by aflatoxin exposure, which leads to stunted growth, delayed development, liver damage, and liver cancer. Adults have a higher tolerance to exposure, but are also at risk. No animal species is immune. Aflatoxins are among the most carcinogenic substances known. After entering the body, aflatoxins may be metabolized by the liver to a reactive epoxide intermediate or hydroxylated to become the less harmful aflatoxin M_1.

Aflatoxins are most commonly ingested, but the most toxic type of aflatoxin, B_1, can permeate through the skin.

The United States Food and Drug Administration (FDA) action levels for aflatoxin present in food or feed is 20 to 300 ppb. The FDA has had occasion to declare both human and pet food recalls as a precautionary measure to prevent exposure.

The term "aflatoxin" is derived from the name of one of the molds that produce it, *Aspergillus flavus*. It was coined around 1960 after its discovery as the source of "Turkey X disease". Aflatoxins form one of the major groupings of mycotoxins.

Major Types and their Metabolites

At least 14 different aflatoxins are produced in nature. Aflatoxin B_1 is considered the most toxic and is produced by both *Aspergillus flavus* and *Aspergillus parasiticus*. Aflatoxin M_1 is present in the fermentation broth of *Aspergillus parasiticus*, but it and aflatoxin M_2 are also produced when an infected liver metabolizes aflatoxin B_1 and B_2.

- Aflatoxin B_1 and B_2, produced by *Aspergillus flavus* and *A. parasiticus*
- Aflatoxin G_1 and G_2, produced by some Group II *A. flavus* and *Aspergillus parasiticus*
- Aflatoxin M_1, metabolite of aflatoxin B_1 in humans and animals (exposure in ng levels may come from a mother's milk)
- Aflatoxin M_2, metabolite of aflatoxin B_2 in milk of cattle fed on contaminated foods
- Aflatoxicol
- Aflatoxin Q_1 (AFQ_1), major metabolite of AFB_1 in *in vitro* liver preparations of other higher vertebrates

Contamination Conditions

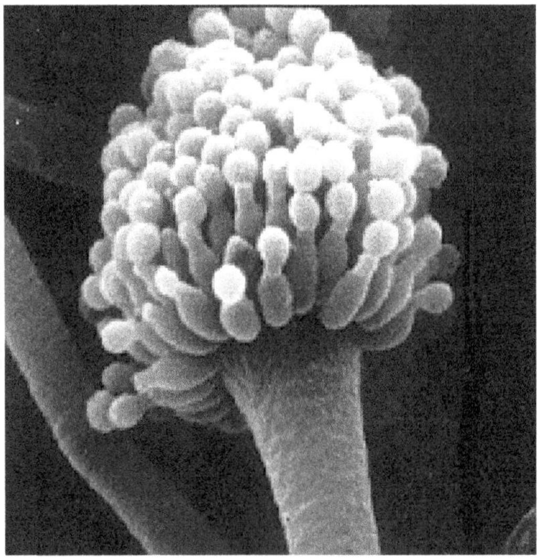

Aspergillus fumigatus as seen under an electron microscope

Aflatoxins are produced by both *Aspergillus flavus* and *Aspergillus parasiticus*, which are common forms of 'weedy' molds widespread in nature. The presence of those molds does not always indicate that harmful levels of aflatoxin are present, but does indicate a significant risk. The molds can colonize and contaminate food before harvest or during storage, especially following prolonged exposure to a high-humidity environment, or to stressful conditions such as drought.

The native habitat of *Aspergillus* is in soil, decaying vegetation, hay, and grains undergoing microbiological deterioration, but it invades all types of organic substrates whenever conditions are favorable for its growth. Favorable conditions include high moisture content (at least 7%) and high temperature. Aflatoxins have been isolated from all major cereal crops, and from sources as diverse as peanut butter and cannabis. The staple commodities regularly contaminated with aflatoxins include cassava, chillies, corn, cotton seed, millet, peanuts, rice, sorghum, sunflower seeds, tree nuts, wheat, and a variety of spices intended for human or animal consumption. Aflatoxin transformation products are sometimes found in eggs, milk products, and meat when animals are fed contaminated grains.

A study conducted in Kenya and Mali found that the predominant practices for drying and storage of maize were inadequate in minimizing exposure to aflatoxins.

Organic crops which are not treated with fungicides may be more susceptible to contamination with aflatoxins.

Pathology

No animal species is immune to the acute toxic effects of aflatoxins. Adult humans have a high tolerance for aflatoxin exposure and rarely succumb to acute aflatoxicosis, but children are particularly affected, and their exposure can lead to stunted growth and delayed development, in addition to all the symptoms mentioned below.

High-level aflatoxin exposure produces an acute hepatic necrosis, resulting later in cirrhosis or carcinoma of the liver. Acute liver failure is made manifest by bleeding, edema, alteration in digestion, changes to the absorption and/or metabolism of nutrients, and mental changes and/or coma.

Chronic exposure increases the risk of developing liver and gallbladder cancer, as aflatoxin metabolites may intercalate into DNA and alkylate the bases through epoxide moiety. This is thought to cause mutations in the *p53* gene, an important gene in preventing cell cycle progression when there are DNA mutations, or signaling apoptosis (programmed cell death). These mutations seem to affect some base pair locations more than others, for example, the third base of codon 249 of the p53 gene appears to be more susceptible to aflatoxin-mediated mutations than nearby bases.

Chronic, subclinical exposure does not lead to symptoms so dramatic as acute aflatoxicosis.

The expression of aflatoxin-related diseases is influenced by factors such as species, age, nutrition, sex, and the possibility of concurrent exposure to other toxins. The main target organ in mammals is the liver, so aflatoxicosis primarily is a hepatic disease. Conditions increasing the likelihood of aflatoxicosis in humans include limited availability of food, environmental conditions that favour mould growth on foodstuffs, and lack of regulatory systems for aflatoxin monitoring and control.

A regular diet including apiaceous vegetables, such as carrots, parsnips, celery, and parsley may reduce the carcinogenic effects of aflatoxin.

Aflatoxin B_1 can cause immune suppression, and exposure to it is associated with an increased viral load in HIV positive individuals.

There is no specific antidote for aflatoxicosis. Symptomatic and supportive care tailored to the severity of the liver disease may include intravenous fluids with dextrose, active vitamin K, B vitamins, and a restricted, but high-quality protein diet with adequate carbohydrate content.

Detection in Humans

There are two principal techniques that have been used most often to detect levels of aflatoxin in humans.

The first method is measuring the AFB_1-guanine adduct in the urine of subjects. The presence of this breakdown product indicates exposure to aflatoxin B_1 during the past 24 hours. This technique measures only recent exposure, however. Due to the half-life of this metabolite, the level of AFB_1-guanine measured may vary from day to day, based on diet, it is not ideal for assessing long-term exposure.

Another technique that has been used is a measurement of the AFB_1-albumin adduct level in the blood serum. This approach provides a more integrated measure of exposure over several weeks or months.

Animals

In dogs, aflatoxin has potential to lead to liver disease. Low levels of aflatoxin exposure require continuous consumption for several weeks to months in order for signs of liver dysfunction to appear. Some articles have suggested the toxic level in dog food is 100–300 ppb and requires continuous exposure or consumption for a few weeks to months to develop aflatoxicosis. No information is available to suggest that recovered dogs will later succumb to an aflatoxin-induced disease.

Turkeys are extremely susceptible to aflatoxicosis. Recent studies have revealed that this is due to the efficient cytochrome P450 mediated metabolism of aflatoxin B_1 in the liver of turkeys and deficient glutathione-S-transferase mediated detoxification.

Some studies on pregnant hamsters showed a significant relationship between exposure of aflatoxin B_1 (4 mg/kg, single dose) and the appearance of developmental anomalies in their offspring.

In 2005, Diamond Pet Foods discovered aflatoxin in a product manufactured at their facility in Gaston, South Carolina. In 23 states, Diamond voluntarily recalled 19 products formulated with corn and manufactured in the Gaston facility. Testing of more than 2,700 finished product samples conducted by laboratories confirmed that only two date codes of two adult dog formulas with the "Best By" dates of April 3, April 4, April 5, and April 11 had the potential to be toxic.

List of Outbreaks

International sources of commercial peanut butter, cooking oils (e.g. olive, peanut and sesame oil), and cosmetics have been identified as contaminated with aflatoxin. In some instances, liquid chromatography-tandem mass spectrometry (LC-MS/MS), and other analytical methods, revealed a range from 48% to 80% of selected product samples as containing detectable quantities of aflatoxin. In many of these contaminated food products, the aflatoxin exceeded the safe limits of the U.S. Food and Drug Administration (FDA), or other regulatory agency.

- 2003 Kenya: acute poisoning, 120 people died.
- February–March 2013: Romania, Serbia, Croatia imported into western Europe - 2013 aflatoxin contamination.
- February 2013: Iowa contamination.
- 2014 (ongoing): Nepal and Bangladesh, neonatal exposures, found in umbilical cord blood.

Aflatoxin B_1

Aflatoxin B_1 is an aflatoxin produced by *Aspergillus flavus* and *A. parasiticus*. It is arguably the most potent carcinogen known, and is up to twice as carcinogenic as an equitoxic dose of X-rays. Aflatoxin B_1 is a common contaminant in a variety of foods including peanuts, cottonseed meal, corn, and other grains; as well as animal feeds. Aflatoxin B_1 is considered the most toxic aflatoxin and it is highly implicated in hepatocellular carcinoma (HCC) in humans. In animals, aflatoxin B_1 has also been shown to be mutagenic, teratogenic, and to cause immunosuppression. Several sampling and analytical methods including thin-layer chromatography (TLC), high-performance liquid chromatography (HPLC), mass spectroscopy, and enzyme-linked immunosorbent assay (ELISA), among others, have been used to test for aflatoxin B_1 contamination in foods. According to the Food and Agriculture Organization (FAO), the worldwide maximum tolerated levels of aflatoxin B_1 was reported to be in the range of 1–20 μg/kg in food, and 5–50 μg/kg in dietary cattle feed in 2003.

Sources of Exposure

Aflatoxin B_1 is mostly found in contaminated food and humans are exposed to aflatoxin B_1 almost entirely through their diet. Occupational exposure to aflatoxin B_1 has also been reported in swine and poultry production.

Pathology

Aflatoxin B_1 can permeate through the skin. Dermal exposure to this aflatoxin in particular environmental conditions can lead to major health risks. The liver is the most susceptible organ to aflatoxin B_1 toxicity. In animal studies, pathological lesions associated with aflatoxin B_1 intoxication include reduction in weight of liver, vacuolation of hepatocytes, and hepatic carcinoma. Other liver lesions include enlargement of hepatic cells, fatty infiltration, necrosis, hemorrhage, fibrosis, regeneration of nodules, and bile duct proliferation/hyperplasia.

Biosynthetic Pathway

Aflatoxin B_1 is derived from both a dedicated fatty acid synthase (FAS) and a polyketide synthase

(PKS), together known as norsolorinic acid synthase. The biosynthesis begins with the synthesis of hexanoate by the FAS, which then becomes the starter unit for the iterative type I PKS. The PKS adds seven malonyl-CoA extenders to the hexanoate to form the C20 polyketide compound. The PKS folds the polyketide in a particular way to induce cyclization to form the anthraquinone norsolorinic acid. A reductase then catalyzes the reduction of the ketone on the norsolorinic acid side-chain to yield averantin. Averantin is converted to averufin via a two different enzymes, a hydroxylase and an alcohol dehydrogenase. This will oxygenate and cyclize averantin's side chain to form the ketal in averufin.

From this point on the biosynthetic pathway of aflatoxin B_1 becomes much more complicated, with several major skeletal changes. Most of the enzymes have not been characterized and there may be several more intermediates that are still unknown. However, what is known is that averufin is oxidized by a P450-oxidase, AvfA, in a Baeyer-Villiger oxidation. This opens the ether rings and upon rearrangement versiconal acetate is formed. Now an esterase, EstA, catalyzes the hydrolysis of the acetyl, forming the primary alcohol in versiconal. The acetal in versicolorin A is formed from the cyclization of the side-chain in versiconal, which is catalyzed by VERB synthase, and then VerB, a desaturase, reduces versicolorin B to form the dihydrobisfuran.

There are two more enzymes that catalyze the conversion of versicolorin A to demethylsterigmatocystin: AflN, an oxidase and AflM, a reductase. These enzymes use both molecular oxygen and two NADPH's to dehydrate one of the hydroxyl groups on the anthraquinone and open the quinine with the molecular oxygen. Upon forming the aldehyde in the ring opening step, it is oxidized to form the carboxylic acid and subsequently a decarboxylation event occurs to close the ring, forming the six-member ether ring system seen in demethylsterigmatocystin. The next two steps in the biosynthetic pathway is the methylation by *S*-adenosyl methionine (SAM) of the two hydroxyl groups on the xanthone part of demethysterigmatocystin by two different methyltransferases, OmtB and OmtA. This yields *O*-methylsterigmatocystin. In the final steps there is an oxidative cleavage of the aromatic ring and loss of one carbon in *O*-methylsterigmatocystin, which is catalyzed by OrdA, an oxidoreductase. Then a final recyclization occurs to form aflatoxin B_1.

Toxicity

Several aflatoxin B_1 toxicity studies have been conducted on various animal species.

Acute toxicity

The oral LD_{50} range of aflatoxin B_1 is estimated to be 0.3-17.9 mg/kg body weight for most animal species. For instance, the oral LD_{50} of aflatoxin B_1 is estimated to be 17.9 mg/kg body weight in female rats and 7.2 mg/kg body weight in male rats. Still in male rats, the intraperitoneal LD_{50} of aflatoxin B_1 is estimated to be 6.0 mg/kg body weight.

Subacute toxicity

Subacute toxicity studies of aflatoxin B_1 in animals showed moderate to severe liver damage. In monkeys for instance, subacute toxicity studies showed portal inflammation and fatty change.

Chronic toxicity

Chronic toxicity studies of aflatoxin B_1 in chicken showed decreased hepatic microsomal cytochrome P-450 concentration, reduction in feed consumption and decreased weight gain.

Subchronic toxicity

Subchronic toxicity studies of aflatoxin B_1 in fish showed fish to present with preneoplastic lesions, concurrently with changes in gill, pancreas, intestine and spleen.

Genotoxicity

Treatment of human liver cells with aflatoxin B_1 at doses that ranged from 3-5 μmol/l resulted in the formation of aflatoxin B_1-DNA adducts, 8-hydroxyguanine lesions and DNA damage.

Carcinogenicity

The carcinogenicity of aflatoxin B_1, which is characterized by the development of liver cell carcinoma, has been reported in rat studies.

Embryotoxicity

Embryonic death and impaired embryonic development of the bursa of Fabricius in chicken by aflatoxin B_1 has been reported.

Teratogenicity

The teratogenic effects of aflatoxin B_1 in rabbits have been reported to include reduced fetal weights, wrist drop, enlarged eye socket, agenesis of caudal vertebrae, micropthalmia, cardiac defects, and lenticular degeneration, among others.

Immunotoxicity

Studies in fish showed aflatoxin B_1 to have significant immunosuppressive effects including reduced serum total globulin and reduced bactericidal activities.

Risk Management and Regulations

Aflatoxin B_1 exposure is best managed by measures aimed at preventing contamination of crops in the field, post-harvest handling, and storage, or via measures aimed at detecting and decontaminating contaminated commodities or materials used in animal feed. For instance, biological decontamination involving the use of a single bacterial species, *Flavobacterium aurantiacum* has been used to remove aflatoxin B_1 from peanuts and corn.

Several countries around the world have rules and regulations governing aflatoxin B_1 in foods and these include the maximum permitted, or recommended levels of aflatoxin B_1 for certain foods.

United States (US)

US food safety regulations have set a maximum permitted level of 20 μg/kg for aflatoxin B_1, in combination with the other aflatoxins (B_2, G_1 and G_2) in all foods, with the exception of milk which has a maximum permitted level of 0.5 µg/kg. Higher levels of 100–300 µg/kg are tolerable for some animal feeds.

European Union (EU)

The EU has set maximum permitted levels for aflatoxin B_1 in nuts, dried fruits, cereals and spices to range from 2-12 µg/kg, while the maximum permitted level for aflatoxin B_1 in infant foods is set at 0.1 µg/kg. The maximum permitted levels for aflatoxin B_1 in animal feeds set by the EU range from 5-50 µg/kg and these levels are much lower than those set in the US.

Joint United Nations' Food and Agriculture Organization (FAO)/World Health Organization (WHO) Expert Committee on Food Additives (JECFA)

The FAO/WHO JECFA has set the maximum permitted levels of aflatoxin B_1 in combination with the other aflatoxins (B_2, G_1 and G_2) to be 15 µg/kg in raw peanuts and 10 µg/kg in processesd peanut; while the tolerance level of aflatoxin B_1 alone is 5 µg/kg for dairy cattle feed.

Mycotoxin

A mycotoxin is a toxic secondary metabolite produced by organisms of the fungus kingdom. The term 'mycotoxin' is usually reserved for the toxic chemical products produced by fungi that readily colonize crops. One mold species may produce many different mycotoxins, and several species may produce the same mycotoxin.

Production

Most fungi are aerobic (use oxygen) and are found almost everywhere in extremely small quantities due to the minute size of their spores. They consume organic matter wherever humidity and temperature are sufficient. Where conditions are right, fungi proliferate into colonies and mycotoxin levels become high. The reason for the production of mycotoxins is not yet known; they are not necessary for the growth or the development of the fungi. Because mycotoxins weaken the receiving host, the fungus may use them as a strategy to better the environment for further fungal proliferation. The production of toxins depends on the surrounding intrinsic and extrinsic environments and these substances vary greatly in their toxicity, depending on the organism infected and its susceptibility, metabolism, and defense mechanisms.

Major Groups

Aflatoxins are a type of mycotoxin produced by *Aspergillus* species of fungi, such as *A. flavus* and *A. parasiticus*. The umbrella term aflatoxin refers to four different types of mycotoxins produced, which are B_1, B_2, G_1, and G_2. Aflatoxin B_1, the most toxic, is a potent carcinogen and has been directly correlated to adverse health effects, such as liver cancer, in many animal species. Aflatoxins are largely associated with commodities produced in the tropics and subtropics, such as cotton, peanuts, spices, pistachios, and maize.

Ochratoxin is a mycotoxin that comes in three secondary metabolite forms, A, B, and C. All are produced by *Penicillium* and *Aspergillus* species. The three forms differ in that Ochratoxin B (OTB) is a nonchlorinated form of Ochratoxin A (OTA) and that Ochratoxin C (OTC) is an ethyl ester form Ochratoxin A. *Aspergillus ochraceus* is found as a contaminant of a wide range of commodities including beverages such as beer and wine. *Aspergillus carbonarius* is the main species found on vine fruit, which releases its toxin during the juice making process. OTA has been labeled as a carcinogen and a nephrotoxin, and has been linked to tumors in the human urinary tract, although research in humans is limited by confounding factors.

Citrinin is a toxin that was first isolated from *Penicillium citrinum*, but has been identified in over a dozen species of *Penicillium* and several species of *Aspergillus*. Some of these species are used to produce human foodstuffs such as cheese (*Penicillium camemberti*), sake, miso, and soy sauce (*Aspergillus oryzae*). Citrinin is associated with yellowed rice disease in Japan and acts as a nephrotoxin in all animal species tested. Although it is associated with many human foods (wheat, rice, corn, barley, oats, rye, and food colored with Monascus pigment) its full significance for human health is unknown. Citrinin can also act synergistically with Ochratoxin A to depress RNA synthesis in murine kidneys.

Ergot Alkaloids are compounds produced as a toxic mixture of alkaloids in the sclerotia of species of *Claviceps*, which are common pathogens of various grass species. The ingestion of ergot sclerotia from infected cereals, commonly in the form of bread produced from contaminated flour, cause ergotism the human disease historically known as St. Anthony's Fire. There are two forms of ergotism: gangrenous, affecting blood supply to extremities, and convulsive, affecting the central nervous system. Modern methods of grain cleaning have significantly reduced ergotism as a human disease, however it is still an important veterinary problem. Ergot alkaloids have been used pharmaceutically.

Patulin is a toxin produced by the *P. expansum*, *Aspergillus*, *Penicillium*, and *Paecilomyces* fungal species. *P. expansum* is especially associated with a range of moldy fruits and vegetables, in particular rotting apples and figs. It is destroyed by the fermentation process and so is not found in apple beverages, such as cider. Although patulin has not been shown to be carcinogenic, it has been reported to damage the immune system in animals. In 2004, the European Community set limits to the concentrations of patulin in food products. They currently stand at 50 μg/kg in all fruit juice concentrations, at 25 μg/kg in solid apple products used for direct consumption, and at 10 μg/kg for children's apple products, including apple juice.

Fusarium toxins are produced by over 50 species of *Fusarium* and have a history of infecting the grain of developing cereals such as wheat and maize. They include a range of mycotoxins, such as: the fumonisins, which affect the nervous systems of horses and may cause cancer in rodents; the trichothecenes, which are most strongly associated with chronic and fatal toxic effects in animals and humans; and zearalenone, which is not correlated to any fatal toxic effects in animals or humans. Some of the other major types of *Fusarium* toxins include: beauvercin and enniatins, butenolide, equisetin, and fusarins.

Occurrence

Although various wild mushrooms contain an assortment of poisons that are definitely fungal metabolites causing noteworthy health problems for humans, they are rather arbitrarily excluded from discussions of mycotoxicology. In such cases the distinction is based on the size of the producing fungus and human intention. Mycotoxin exposure is almost always accidental whereas with mushrooms improper identification and ingestion causing mushroom poisoning is commonly the case. Ingestion of misidentified mushrooms containing mycotoxins may result in hallucinations. The cyclopeptide-producing *Amanita phalloides* is well known for its toxic potential and is responsible for approximately 90% of all mushroom fatalities. The other primary mycotoxin groups found in mushrooms include: orellanine, monomethylhydrazine, disulfiram-like, hallucinogenic indoles, muscarinic, isoxazole, and gastrointestinal (GI)-specific irritants. The bulk of this article is about mycotoxins that are found in microfungi other than poisons from mushrooms or macroscopic fungi.

In Indoor Environments

Buildings are another source of mycotoxins and people living or working in areas with mold increase their chances of adverse health effects. Molds growing in buildings can be divided into three groups — primary, secondary, and tertiary colonizers. Each group is categorized by the ability to grow at a certain water activity requirement. It has become difficult to identify mycotoxin production by indoor molds for many variables, such as (i) they may be masked as derivatives (ii) they are poorly documented and (iii) the fact that they are likely to produce different metabolites on building materials. Some of the mycotoxins in the indoor environment are produced by *Alternaria*, *Aspergillus* (multiple forms), *Penicillium*, and *Stachybotrys*. *Stachybotrys chartarum* contains a higher number of mycotoxins than other molds grown in the indoor environment and has been associated with allergies and respiratory inflammation. The infestation of *S. chartarum* in buildings containing gypsum board, as well as on ceiling tiles, is very common and has recently become a more recognized problem. When gypsum board has been repeatedly introduced to moisture *S. chartarum* grows readily on its cellulose face. This stresses the importance of moisture controls and ventilation within residential homes and other buildings. The negative health effects of mycotoxins are a function of the concentration, the duration of exposure and the subject's sensitivities. The concentrations experienced in a normal home, office or school are often too low to trigger a health response in occupants.

In the 1990s, public concern over mycotoxins increased following multimillion-dollar toxic mold settlements. The lawsuits took place after a study by the Center for Disease Control (CDC) in Cleveland, Ohio reported an association between mycotoxins from *Stachybotrys* spores and pulmonary hemorrhage in infants. However, in 2000, based on internal and external reviews of their data, the CDC concluded that because of flaws in their methods, the association was not proven. *Stachybotrys* spores in animal studies have been shown to cause lung hemorrhaging, but only at very high concentrations.

One study by the Center of Integrative Toxicology at Michigan State University investigated the causes of Damp Building Related Illness (DBRI). They found that *Stachybotrys* is possibly an important contributing factor to DBRI. So far animal models indicate that airway exposure to *S. chartarum* can evoke allergic sensitization, inflammation, and cytotoxicity in the upper and lower respiratory tracts. Trichothecene toxicity appears to be an underlying cause of many of these adverse effects. Recent findings indicate that lower doses (studies usually involve high doses) can cause these symptoms.

Some toxicologists have used the Concentration of No Toxicological Concern (CoNTC) measure to represent the airborne concentration of mycotoxins that are expected to cause no hazard to humans (exposed continuously throughout a 70–yr lifetime). The resulting data of several studies have thus far demonstrated that common exposures to airborne mycotoxins in the built indoor environment are below the CoNTC, however agricultural environments have potential to produce levels greater than the CoNTC.

In food

Mycotoxins can appear in the food chain as a result of fungal infection of crops, either by being eaten directly by humans or by being used as livestock feed.

In 2004 in Kenya, 125 people died and nearly 200 others were treated after eating aflatoxin-contaminated maize. The deaths were mainly associated with homegrown maize that had not been treated with fungicides or properly dried before storage. Due to food shortages at the time, farmers may have been harvesting maize earlier than normal to prevent thefts from their fields, so that the grain had not fully matured and was more susceptible to infection.

Spices are susceptible substrate for growth of mycotoxigenic fungi and mycotoxin production. Red chilli, black pepper, and dry ginger were found to be the most contaminated spices.

In Animal Food

There were outbreaks of dog food containing aflatoxin in North America in late 2005 and early 2006, and again in late 2011.

Mycotoxins in animal fodder, particularly silage, can decrease the performance of farm animals and potentially kill them. Several mycotoxins reduce milk yield when ingested by dairy cattle.

In Dietary Supplements

Contamination of medicinal plants with mycotoxins can contribute to adverse human health problems and therefore represents a special hazard. Numerous natural occurrences of mycotoxins in medicinal plants and herbal medicines have been reported from various countries including Spain, China, Germany, India, Turkey and from the Middle East. In a 2015 analysis of plant-based dietary supplements, the highest mycotoxin concentrations were found in milk thistle-based supplements, at up to 37 mg/kg.

Health Effects

Some of the health effects found in animals and humans include death, identifiable diseases or health problems, weakened immune systems without specificity to a toxin, and as allergens or irritants. Some mycotoxins are harmful to other micro-organisms such as other fungi or even bacteria; penicillin is one example. It has been suggested that mycotoxins in stored animal feed are the cause of rare phenotypical sex changes in hens that causes them to look and act male.

In Humans

Mycotoxicosis is the term used for poisoning associated with exposures to mycotoxins. The symptoms of mycotoxicosis depend on the type of mycotoxin; the concentration and length of exposure; as well as age, health, and sex of the exposed individual. The synergistic effects associated with several other factors such as genetics, diet, and interactions with other toxins have been poorly studied. Therefore, it is possible that vitamin deficiency, caloric deprivation, alcohol abuse, and infectious disease status can all have compounded effects with mycotoxins. In turn, mycotoxins have the potential for both acute and chronic health effects via ingestion, skin contact, and inhalation. These toxins can enter the blood stream and lymphatic system; they inhibit protein synthesis, damage macrophage systems, inhibit particle clearance of the lung, and increase sensitivity to bacterial endotoxin.

Mitigation

Mycotoxins greatly resist decomposition or being broken down in digestion, so they remain in the food chain in meat and dairy products. Even temperature treatments, such as cooking and freezing, do not destroy some mycotoxins.

Removal

In the feed and food industry it has become common practice to add mycotoxin binding agents such as montmorillonite or bentonite clay in order to affectively adsorb the mycotoxins. To reverse the adverse effects of mycotoxins, the following criteria are used to evaluate the functionality of any binding additive:

- Efficacy of active component verified by scientific data
- A low effective inclusion rate
- Stability over a wide pH range
- High capacity to absorb high concentrations of mycotoxins
- High affinity to absorb low concentrations of mycotoxins
- Affirmation of chemical interaction between mycotoxin and adsorbent
- Proven *in vivo* data with all major mycotoxins
- Non-toxic, environmentally friendly component

Since not all mycotoxins can be bound to such agents, the latest approach to mycotoxin control is mycotoxin deactivation. By means of enzymes (esterase, de-epoxidase), yeast (*Trichosporon mycotoxinvorans*), or bacterial strains (Eubacterium BBSH 797), mycotoxins can be reduced during pre-harvesting contamination. Other removal methods include physical separation, washing, milling, nixtamalization, heat-treatment, radiation, extraction with solvents, and the use of chemical or biological agents. Irradiation methods have proven to be effective treatment against mold growth and toxin production.

Regulations

Many international agencies are trying to achieve universal standardization of regulatory limits for mycotoxins. Currently, over 100 countries have regulations regarding mycotoxins in the feed industry, in which 13 mycotoxins or groups of mycotoxins are of concern. The process of assessing a need for mycotoxin regulation includes a wide array of in-laboratory testing that includes extracting, clean-up and separation techniques. Most official regulations and control methods are based on high-performance liquid techniques (e.g., HPLC) through international bodies. It is implied that any regulations regarding these toxins will be in co-ordinance with any other countries with which a trade agreement exists. Many of the standards for the method performance analysis for mycotoxins is set by the European Committee for Standardization (CEN). However, one must take note that scientific risk assessment is commonly influenced by culture and politics, which, in turn, will affect trade regulations of mycotoxins.

Food-based mycotoxins were studied extensively worldwide throughout the 20th century. In Europe, statutory levels of a range of mycotoxins permitted in food and animal feed are set by a range of European directives and EC regulations. The U.S. Food and Drug Administration has regulated and enforced limits on concentrations of mycotoxins in foods and feed industries since 1985. It is through various compliance programs that the FDA monitors these industries to guarantee that mycotoxins are kept at a practical level. These compliance programs sample food products including peanuts and peanut products, tree nuts, corn and corn products, cottonseed, and milk. There is still a lack of sufficient surveillance data on some mycotoxins that occur in the U.S.

Use in Fiction

A fictional use of a mycotoxin occurs in William Gibson's seminal novel *Neuromancer* (1984). A "Russian war-time mycotoxin" is administered to Case, the novel's protagonist.

Mycotoxins are used as the basis for the infection in the 2013 video game *The Last of Us* for the PlayStation 3 and its remastering for PlayStation 4. A warning sign in one of the abandoned cities in the game reads "MYCOTOXINS" with fine print seeming to list the signs and symptoms of the game's fictional human infection. (In reality, biological toxins, while poisonous, do not cause an "infection".)

Fumonisin B1

Fumonisin B_1 is the most prevalent member of a family of toxins, known as fumonisins, produced by several species of *Fusarium* molds, such as *Fusarium verticillioides*, which occur mainly in maize (corn), wheat and other cereals. Fumonisin B1 contamination of maize has been reported worldwide at mg/kg levels. Human exposure occurs at levels of micrograms to milligrams per day and is greatest in regions where maize products are the dietary staple.

Fumonisin B_1 is hepatotoxic and nephrotoxic in all animal species tested. The earliest histological change to appear in either the liver or kidney of fumonisin-treated animals is increased apoptosis followed by regenerative cell proliferation. While the acute toxicity of fumonisin is low, it is the known cause of two diseases which occur in domestic animals with rapid onset: equine leukoencephalomalacia and porcine pulmonary oedema syndrome. Both of these diseases involve disturbed sphingolipid metabolism and cardiovascular dysfunction.

History

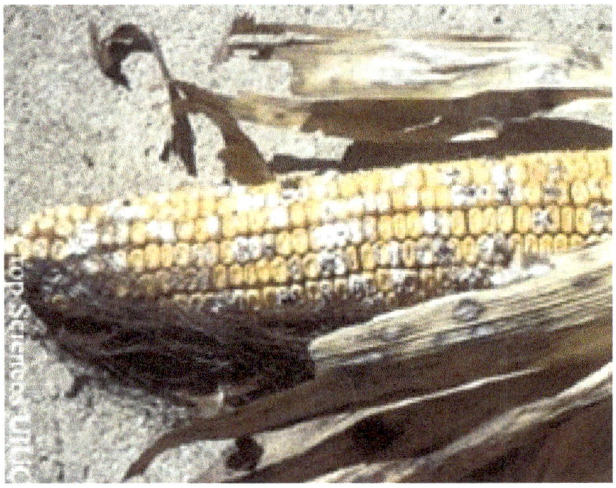

In 1970, an outbreak of leukoenchephalomalacia (ELEM) in horses in South Africa was associated with the contamination of corn with the fungus *Fusarium verticillioides*. It is one of the most prevalent seed-borne fungi associated with corn. Another study was done on the possible role of fungal toxins in the etiology of human esophageal cancer in a region in South Africa. The diet of the people living in this area was homegrown corn and F. verticillioides was the most prevalent fungus in the corn consumed by the people with high incidence of esophageal cancer. Further outbreaks of ELEM and people in certain regions with high incidence of esophageal cancer led to more research on F.verticillioides. Soon they found experimentally that F.verticillioides caused ELEM in horses and porcine pulmonary edema in pigs. It was found to be highly hepatotoxic and cardiotoxic in rats. In 1984 it was shown that the fungus was hepatocarcinogenic in rats. The chemical nature of the metabolite(s) causing all this had still not been discovered in 1984. After discovery of the carcinogenicity of the fungus, isolation and chemical characterization of the mycotoxin(s) and carcinogen(s) produced by F.verticillioides was urgent. It wasn't until 1988 that the chemical nature of the carcinogen was unraveled. Fumonisin B_1 and fumonisin B_2 were isolated from cultures of F.verticillioides at PROMEC (Programme on Mycotoxins and Experimental Carcinogenesis). The structures were elucidated in collaboration with the CSIR(Council for Scientific and Industrial Research). Now approximate 15 different fumonisins are discovered, the most important ones being fumonisin B_1, B_2 and B_3.

Toxicokinetics

Regarding toxicokinetics there are no human data available, but research on animals has been done.

Absorption

FB_1 is taken orally via food. Overall, FB_1 is poorly absorbed, less than 6%. Absorption of orally administered fumonisin B_1 (10 mg/kg body weight) to rats is low (3.5% of dose) but rapid (T_{max} = 1.02 h). FB_1 does not significantly permeate through the human skin and hence has no significant systemic health risk after dermal exposure.

Distribution

After absorption, some appears to be retained in liver and kidneys. For rats that were fed diets containing fumonisins for several weeks, the concentrations of the fumonisins in the kidneys were approximately 10-fold higher than in the liver.

Plasma distribution of the absorbed dose conformed to a two-compartment open model and the tissue (liver, kidney) concentration time results were consistent with a one-compartment open model.

Excretion

Elimination half-life in rats is 3.15 h for plasma, 4.07 h for liver, and 7.07 h for kidney. However, FB_1 is rapidly excreted mostly in its original form. Small amounts are excreted in urine; the most are excreted in feces.

Toxicodynamics

Because of their similarity, fumonisins are able to inhibit sphingosine-sphinganin-transferases and ceramide synthases and are therefore competitive inhibitors of sphingolipid biosynthesis and metabolism.

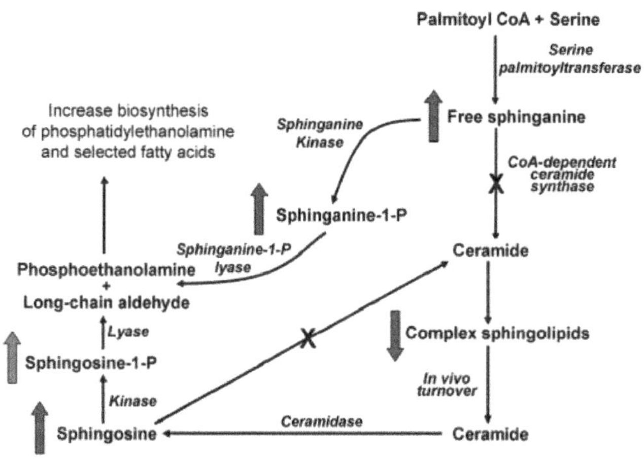

Figure 2: Sphingolipid metabolism showing the inhibition of ceramide synthase (x) by fumonisins and the changed concentrations of other compounds caused by this inhibition.

Figure 2 shows the sphingolipid metabolism (schematic) and the inhibition caused by fumonisins. Fumonisin B_1 inhibits the enzyme ceramide synthase (sphingosine *N*-acyltransferase), which acylates sphingoid bases. This blocks the formation of ceramide via two pathways. It inhibits de formation via de novo sphinganine and fatty acyl-CoA and via sphingosine produced by the breakdown of ceramide by ceramidase. The inhibition results in increased concentrations of sphinganine, sphingosine and their 1-phosphate metabolites and in decreased concentrations of complex sphingolipids. The accumulation of sphinganine and sphingosine is a primary cause of the toxicity of fumonisin B_1 Spinganine and sphingosine are cytotoxic, and have growth inhibitory effects. Also, these sphingoid bases induce apoptosis. Increased apoptosis seems to play an important role in the toxic effects including tumor induction. However, it should be mentioned that the reduced concentration of ceramide and the increased concentration of sphingosine-1-phosphate (as a result of FB_1 intake) cause an inhibition of apoptosis and promote mitosis and regeneration. The balance between the intracellular concentration of compounds that inhibit apoptosis and those that induce apoptosis will determine the cellular response. Also, the decreased concentrations of complex sphingolipids appear to play a role in the abnormal behavior and altered morphology of the affected cells.

Mechanism of Action

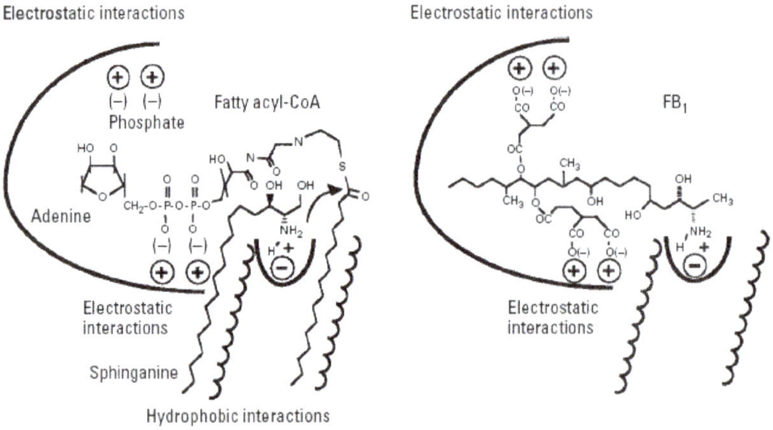

Figure 3: Proposed mechanism of action of ceramide synthase inhibition by FB_1; FB_1 mimics regions of the sphingoid base and the fatty acyl-CoA substrates. (Merrill et al., 2001)

The proposed mechanism of action is depicted in figure 3. Fumonisin B_1 occupies the space and electrostatic interactions of both sphinganine (or sphingosine) and fatty acyl-CoA in ceramide synthase. The part of FB_1 that has structural similarity with sphingoid bases (the aminopentol part) may interact with the sphinganine binding site, whereas the negatively charged tricarbyllic acid groups may interact with the fatty acyl-CoA binding site.

Because FB_1 also occupies the fatty acyl-CoA space, it isn't acylated, since acyl-CoA is necessary for the acylation; FB_1 only inhibits ceramide synthase. However, when the tricarbillic acid groups are removed from FB_1 by hydrolysis, the resulting product (aminopentol, AP1) doesn't only act as an inhibitor, but also as a substrate for ceramide synthase; aminopentol is acylated by ceramide synthase to form N-palmitoyl-AP1. This supports the suggestion that the aminopentol part of FB_1 occupies the space of sphinganine in the enzyme. N-palmitoyl-AP1 is an even more potent inhibitor of ceramide synthase and may therefore play a role in the toxicity of nixtamalized fumonisins.

Toxic Effects

The risks of fumonisin B1 have been evaluated by The World Health Organization's International Programme on Chemical Safety(IPCS) and the Scientific Committee on Food(SCF) of the European Commission. They determined a tolerable daily intake(TDI) for FB_1, FB_2, FB_3, alone or in combination of 2 µg/kg body weight. Until now, nothing about the kinetics and metabolism of fumonisin B_1 in humans have been reported. On other animals much research has been done, but it might not be comparable to humans. In mice the elimination of FB_1 is very rapid, but in humans it could be much slower considering their body weight. There are several possible pathways that cause toxic effects of Fumonisin B_1. Most toxic effects are due to altered sphingolipid metabolism by inhibition of ceramide synthase. Production of reactive oxygen species (ROS) could occur. This increases oxidative stress and induce lipid peroxidation and could damage cells. In agreement with this some studies showed decreased levels of glutathion(GSH) in liver, but other studies showed even elevated levels of GSH. Cytotoxic effects have also been reported. Another effect of exposure to FB_1 is apoptosis. This has been observed in a number of different cells and tissues. Inhibition of ceramide synthase is not responsible for this effect. The main factors could be DNA fragmentation and caspase-3 activation. FB_1 has also immunotoxic effects, but much more research is necessary to get a clear overview of the effects on the immune system.

Toxic effects in Humans

Neural tube Defects

Neural tube defect (NTD) are defects of the brain and spinal cord in the embryo resulting from failure of the neural tube to close. Epidemiological studies and clinical trials have pointed out folate deficiency as a major risk factor for NTD. FB_1 disrupts sphingolipid metabolism and therefore this could affect folate uptake and cause NTD. In 1990 and 1991 a sudden outbreak of neural tube defects occurred along the Texas-Mexico border. It is believed that this outbreak might have been due to high levels of FB_1 that were observed in corn during previous years. Also regions in China and South Africa with high corn consumption show a high prevalence of NTD.

Esophageal Cancer

It is thought that there is a relationship between the occurrence of F.verticillioides and human esophageal cancer. A low socioeconomic status and a less variated diet, that mainly exists of corn and wheat, is associated with the appearance of esophageal cancer. This derives from epidemiologic studies in various countries. Other studies show that a higher level of concentrations of FB_1, FB_2 and F. verticillioides are present in corn growing in regions with a high percentage of esophageal cancer. This in contrast with regions with low levels of F.verticillioides, FB_1 and FB_2 in corn. On top of this it seems that people with a high corn intake are at higher risk to develop esophageal cancer than people with low corn intake. This is observed by people in regions in Italy, Iran, Kenia, Zimbabwe, United States and Brazil with high incidence of esophageal cancer. Another study on the relationship between sphingolipid levels and cancer incidence didn't show any significant relationship between serum shpingolipids and risk of esophageal cancer. This is quite remarkable, because elevated levels of spingolipids shinganine and shingosine are believed to be biomarkers for exposure of FB_1.

Acute Mycotoxicosis

Acute mycotoxicosis is food poisoning by food products contaminated by fungi. In 1995 an outbreak of disease characterized by diarrhea and abdominal pain occurred in 27 villages in India. This was the result of consumption of moldy sorghum and corn due to rain damage. This outbreak was studied and the mycotoxicosis was connected to consumption of unleavened bread. Corn and sorghum samples were collected from the households and examined. The corn and sorghum were contaminated by Fusarium and Aspergillus and contained high levels of FB_1 compared with samples of unaffected households.

Toxic Effects in Animals

Much research has been done on toxic effects of FB_1 in animals. In vivo studies indicate that liver and kidneys are the main target organs. Fumonisins are poorly absorbed, rapidly eliminated and not metabolized in animals. In pigs and rats there is a wide distribution of FB_1 and small amounts have been found to accumulate only in liver and kidneys. In vervet monkeys, some FB_1 is partially hydrolyzed in the gut.

Carcinogenic Effects

In rats and mice that were exposed to FB_1 tumor formation occurred. Several studies on this subject have been done. Depending on the strain of mice being used different carcinomas were shown. FB_1 is shown to be nongenotoxic. Therefore, the mechanisms responsible for cancer development should lie elsewhere. Important mechanisms for cancer development due to fumonisin B_1 could be oxidative damage (ROS-production) and lipid peroxidation. Hepatic and renal tumors could also be due to apoptosis by FB_1. As a response to this there could be continuous regeneration of cells, causing cancer. It seems to be that disrupted sphingolipid metabolism is the causative factor for FB_1-induced carcinogenicity, as is the case with the toxic effects. Based on all these animal studies FB_1 is classified by The International Agency for Research on Cancer (IARC) as possibly carcinogenic to humans (Group 2B).

Porcine Pulmonary Edema

Porcine pulmonary edema due to FB_1 is intensively studied after the first report in 1981 of swine with pulmonary edema after exposure to corn contaminated with F.verticillioides. Alteration in sphingolipid biosynthesis are reported, especially in lung, heart, kindey and liver tissue. Lethal pulmonary edema was developed within 4–7 days after exposure to feed with concentrations of FB_1 >16 mg/kg body weight (>92 ppm). Doses of 10ppm developed a milder form of pulmonary edema.

Equine Leukoencephalomalacia

Leukoenchephalomalacia (ELEM) is a neurotoxic disease of horses. Outbreaks of this disease in the 20th century resulted in a number of studies. Apparently FB_1 was the cause for this disease. There were shown elevated levels of serum enzyme levels that indicate liver damage. They were normally observed by an elevation of the sphinganine/sphingosine ratio. FB_1 possibly induces cardiovascular function, because of the elevated sphinganine/sphingosine ratio. This could be one of the main factors that causes ELEM.

Toxicity in Laboratory Animals

Effects of feeding rats with FB_1 for up to 90 days were usually nephrotoxicity. Between different strains of rats, sensitivity to FB_1 varied. In the kidneys the main effect was apoptosis. Also tubular atrophy and regeneration as well as decreased kidney weight was reported. Histopathologic effects on rat liver were reported after both short- and long-term exposure. The main cause was apoptosis. Mice don't seem to be very sensitive to nephrotoxic effects in comparison with rats. In mouse kidneys little histological changes were seen by high dose exposure. The liver was also the main target organ in mice. Pathology is similar as in rats, with apoptosis and hepatocellular hyperplasia. Fumonisin B_1 is possibly embryotoxic if the dose is maternally toxic. A number of studies on genotoxicity inidicated no mutagenetic effects. Although fumonisin could damage DNA directly by production of reactive oxygen species(ROS). Mouse embryos were exposed to FB_1 and they showed inhibited sphingolipid synthesis and growth. It caused NTD. Folic acid uptake was dramatically inhibited. Treatment after exposure with folic acid reduced NTD by 50–65%.

Tolerable Daily Intake

The risks of fumonisin B1 have been evaluated by The World Health Organization's International Programme on Chemical Safety(IPCS) and the Scientific Committee on Food(SCF) of the European Commission. They determined a tolerable daily intake(TDI) for FB1, FB2, FB3, alone or in combination of 2 µg/kg body weight.

Detoxification

The inhibition of ceramide synthase by FB_1 is thought to be reversible, since the binding is formed by noncovalent interactions. Factors that will probably induce this reversibility are reduction of cellular FB_1-concentration and increasing of cellular concentrations of the substrates for ceramide synthase. Also, the rate of removal of the accumulated sphinganine and sphingosine will affect the detoxification. The information on metabolism and biotransformation of FB_1 is very sparse. However, metabolism most likely occurs in the gut since partially hydrolysed and fully hydrolysed FB_1 were recovered in faeces but not in bile of vervet monkeys. Bioavailability of FB_1 can be reduced by treating fumonisin-contaminated corn with glucomannans extracted from the cell wall of the yeast Saccharomyces cerevisiae. These polysaccharides are able to bind certain mycotoxins and have a 67% binding capacity for fumonisins.

Prion

A prion is an infectious agent composed entirely of protein material, called PrP (short for prion protein), that can fold in multiple, structurally distinct ways, at least one of which is transmissible to other prion proteins, leading to disease that is similar to viral infection. They are suspected to be the cause of transmissible spongiform encephalopathies (TSEs) among other diseases.

Prions were initially identified as the causative agent in animal TSEs such as bovine spongiform encephalopathy (BSE)—known popularly as "mad cow disease"—and scrapie in sheep. Human prion diseases include Creutzfeldt–Jakob disease (CJD) and its variant (vCJD), Gerstmann–Sträussler–Scheinker syndrome, fatal familial insomnia, and kuru. A 2015 study concluded that multiple system atrophy (MSA), a rare human neurodegenerative disease, is caused by a misfolded version of a protein called alpha-synuclein, and is therefore also classifiable as a prion disease. Several yeast proteins have been identified as having prionogenic properties as well.

A protein as a standalone infectious agent stands in contrast to all other known infectious agents such as viruses, bacteria, fungi, and parasites, all of which contain nucleic acids (DNA, RNA, or both). For this reason, a minority of researchers still consider the prion/TSE hypothesis unproven.

All known prion diseases in mammals affect the structure of the brain or other neural tissue; all are currently untreatable and universally fatal.

Prions may propagate by transmitting their misfolded protein state. When a prion enters a healthy organism, it induces existing, properly folded proteins to convert into the misfolded prion form. In this way, the prion acts as a template to guide the misfolding of more proteins into prion form. In yeast, this refolding is assisted by chaperone proteins such as Hsp104p. These refolded prions can then go on to convert more proteins themselves, leading to a chain reaction resulting in large amounts of the prion form. All known prions induce the formation of an amyloid fold, in which the protein polymerises into an aggregate consisting of tightly packed beta sheets. Amyloid aggregates are fibrils, growing at their ends, and replicate when breakage causes two growing ends to become four growing ends. The incubation period of prion diseases is determined by the exponential growth rate associated with prion replication, which is a balance between the linear growth and the breakage of aggregates. The propagation of the prion depends on the presence of normally folded protein in which the prion can induce misfolding; animals that do not express the normal form of the prion protein can neither develop nor transmit the disease.

Prion aggregates are extremely stable and accumulate in infected tissue, causing tissue damage and cell death. This structural stability means that prions are resistant to denaturation by chemical and physical agents, making disposal and containment of these particles difficult. Prion structure varies slightly between species, but nonetheless prion replication is subject to occasional epimutation and natural selection just like other forms of replication.

Prion Protein (PrP)

Discovery

During the 1960s, two London-based researchers, radiation biologist Tikvah Alper and biophysicist John Stanley Griffith, developed the hypothesis that some transmissible spongiform encephalopathies are caused by an infectious agent consisting solely of proteins. Earlier investigations by E. J. Field into scrapie and kuru had identified the transfer of pathologically inert polysaccharides that only become infectious in the host. Alper and Griffith wanted to account for the discovery that the mysterious infectious agent causing the diseases scrapie and Creutzfeldt–Jakob disease resisted ionizing radiation. (A single ionizing "hit" normally destroys an entire infectious particle, and the dose needed to hit half the particles depends on the size of the particles. The data suggested that the infectious agent was too small to be a virus.)

Francis Crick recognized the potential importance of the Griffith protein-only hypothesis for scrapie propagation in the second edition of his "Central dogma of molecular biology" (1970): While asserting that the flow of sequence information from protein to protein, or from protein to RNA and DNA was "precluded", he noted that Griffith's hypothesis was a potential contradiction (although it was not so promoted by Griffith). The revised hypothesis was later formulated, in part, to accommodate reverse transcription (which both Howard Temin and David Baltimore discovered in 1970).

In 1982, Stanley B. Prusiner of the University of California, San Francisco announced that his team had purified the hypothetical infectious prion, and that the infectious agent consisted mainly of a specific protein – though they did not manage to isolate the protein until two years after Prusiner's announcement. While the infectious agent was named a prion, the specific protein that the prion was composed of is also known as the Prion Protein (PrP), though this protein may occur both in infectious and non-infectious forms. Prusiner won the Nobel Prize in Physiology or Medicine in 1997 for his research into prions.

Structure

The protein that prions are made of (PrP) is found throughout the body, even in healthy people and animals. However, PrP found in infectious material has a different structure and is resistant to proteases, the enzymes in the body that can normally break down proteins. The normal form of the protein is called PrP^{C}, while the infectious form is called PrP^{Sc} — the *C* refers to 'cellular' PrP, while the *Sc* refers to 'scrapie', the prototypic prion disease, occurring in sheep. While PrP^{C} is structurally well-defined, PrP^{Sc} is certainly polydisperse and defined at a relatively poor level. PrP can be induced to fold into other more-or-less well-defined isoforms in vitro, and their relationship to the form(s) that are pathogenic in vivo is not yet clear.

PrP^{C}

PrP^{C} is a normal protein found on the membranes of cells. It has 209 amino acids (in humans), one disulfide bond, a molecular mass of 35–36 kDa and a mainly alpha-helical structure. Several topological forms exist; one cell surface form anchored via glycolipid and two transmembrane forms. The normal protein is not sedimentable; meaning that it cannot be separated by centrifuging techniques. Its function is a complex issue that continues to be investigated. PrP^{C} binds copper (II) ions with high affinity. The significance of this finding is not clear, but it is presumed to relate to PrP structure or function. PrP^{C} is readily digested by proteinase K and can be liberated from the cell surface in vitro by the enzyme phosphoinositide phospholipase C (PI-PLC), which cleaves the glycophosphatidylinositol (GPI) glycolipid anchor. PrP has been reported to play important roles in cell-cell adhesion and intracellular signaling *in vivo*, and may therefore be involved in cell-cell communication in the brain.

PrP^{res}

Protease-resistant PrP^{Sc}-like protein (PrP^{res}) is an isoform of PrP^{c} from which is structurally altered and converted into a misfolded proteinase K-resistant form *in vitro*. To model conversion of PrP^{C} to PrP^{Sc} in vitro, Saborio *et al.* rapidly converted PrP^{C} into a PrP^{res} by a procedure involving cyclic amplification of protein misfolding. The term "PrP^{res}" has been made to distinguish between PrP^{Sc}, which is isolated from infectious tissue and associated with the transmissible spongiform encephalopathy agent. For example, unlike PrP^{sc}, PrP^{res} may not necessarily be infectious.

PrP^{Sc}

The infectious isoform of PrP, known as PrP^{Sc}, is able to convert normal PrP^{C} proteins into the infectious isoform by changing their conformation, or shape; this, in turn, alters the way the proteins interconnect. PrP^{Sc} always causes prion disease. Although the exact 3D structure of PrP^{Sc} is not known, it has a higher proportion of β-sheet structure in place of the normal α-helix structure.

Aggregations of these abnormal isoforms form highly structured amyloid fibers, which accumulate to form plaques. It is unclear as to whether these aggregates are the cause of cell damage or are simply a side-effect of the underlying disease process. The end of each fiber acts as a template onto which free protein molecules may attach, allowing the fiber to grow. Under most circumstances, only PrP molecules with an identical amino acid sequence to the infectious PrP^{Sc} are incorporated into the growing fiber. However, rare cross-species transmission is also possible.

Function

The physiological function of the prion protein remains a controversial matter. While data from in vitro experiments suggest many dissimilar roles, studies on PrP knockout mice have provided only limited information because these animals exhibit only minor abnormalities. In research done in mice, it was found that the cleavage of PrP proteins in peripheral nerves causes the activation of myelin repair in Schwann Cells and that the lack of PrP proteins caused demyelination in those cells.

PrP and Long-term Memory

A review of evidence in 2005 suggested that PrP may have a normal function in maintenance of long-term memory. As well, a 2004 study found that mice lacking genes for normal cellular PrP protein show altered hippocampal long-term potentiation.

PrP and Stem Cell Renewal

A 2006 article from the Whitehead Institute for Biomedical Research indicates that PrP expression on stem cells is necessary for an organism's self-renewal of bone marrow. The study showed that all long-term hematopoietic stem cells express PrP on their cell membrane and that hematopoietic tissues with PrP-null stem cells exhibit increased sensitivity to cell depletion.

Prion Replication Mechanism

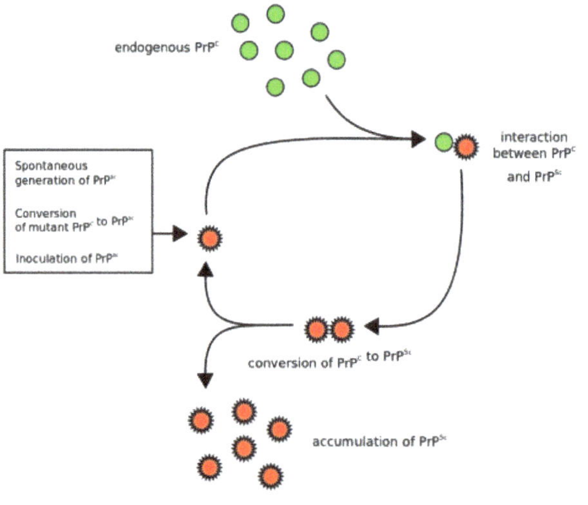

Heterodimer model of prion propagation

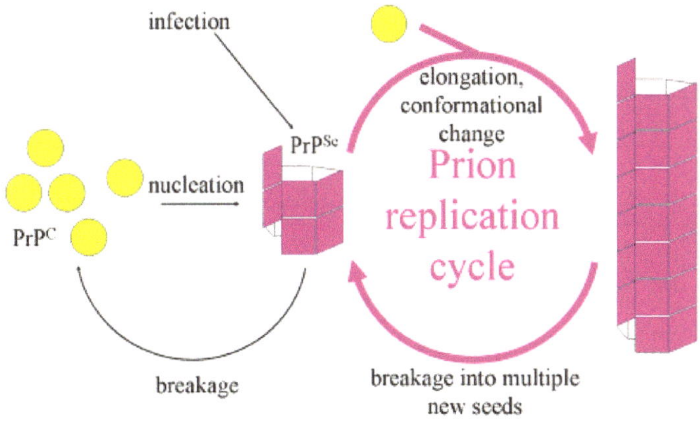

Fibril model of prion propagation.

The first hypothesis that tried to explain how prions replicate in a protein-only manner was the heterodimer model. This model assumed that a single PrP^{Sc} molecule binds to a single PrP^{C} molecule and catalyzes its conversion into PrP^{Sc}. The two PrP^{Sc} molecules then come apart and can go on to convert more PrP^{C}. However, a model of prion replication must explain both how prions propagate, and why their spontaneous appearance is so rare. Manfred Eigen showed that the heterodimer model requires PrP^{Sc} to be an extraordinarily effective catalyst, increasing the rate of the conversion reaction by a factor of around 10^{15}. This problem does not arise if PrP^{Sc} exists only in aggregated forms such as amyloid, where cooperativity may act as a barrier to spontaneous conversion. What is more, despite considerable effort, infectious monomeric PrP^{Sc} has never been isolated.

An alternative model assumes that PrP^{Sc} exists only as fibrils, and that fibril ends bind PrP^{C} and convert it into PrP^{Sc}. If this were all, then the quantity of prions would increase linearly, forming ever longer fibrils. But exponential growth of both PrP^{Sc} and of the quantity of infectious particles is observed during prion disease. This can be explained by taking into account fibril breakage. A mathematical solution for the exponential growth rate resulting from the combination of fibril growth and fibril breakage has been found. The exponential growth rate depends largely on the square root of the PrP^{C} concentration. The incubation period is determined by the exponential growth rate, and in vivo data on prion diseases in transgenic mice match this prediction. The same square root dependence is also seen in vitro in experiments with a variety of different amyloid proteins.

The mechanism of prion replication has implications for designing drugs. Since the incubation period of prion diseases is so long, an effective drug does not need to eliminate all prions, but simply needs to slow down the rate of exponential growth. Models predict that the most effective way to achieve this, using a drug with the lowest possible dose, is to find a drug that binds to fibril ends and blocks them from growing any further.

Prion Diseases and their Transmission Properties

Diseases caused by prions	
Affected animal(s)	**Disease**
sheep, goat	Scrapie
cattle	Bovine spongiform encephalopathy (BSE), mad cow disease
mink	Transmissible mink encephalopathy (TME)

white-tailed deer, elk, mule deer, moose	Chronic wasting disease (CWD)
cat	Feline spongiform encephalopathy (FSE)
nyala, oryx, greater kudu	Exotic ungulate encephalopathy (EUE)
ostrich	Spongiform encephalopathy (Has not been shown to be transmissible.)
human	Creutzfeldt–Jakob disease (CJD)
	Iatrogenic Creutzfeldt–Jakob disease (iCJD)
	Variant Creutzfeldt–Jakob disease (vCJD)
	Familial Creutzfeldt–Jakob disease (fCJD)
	Sporadic Creutzfeldt–Jakob disease (sCJD)
	Gerstmann–Sträussler–Scheinker syndrome (GSS)
	Fatal familial insomnia (FFI)
	Kuru
	Familial spongiform encephalopathy
	Multiple System Atrophy (MSA): Not a TSE and is not by typical prions Prp/PrP^{Sc} but by a misfolded α-Synuclein.

Until 2015, all known mammalian prion diseases were caused by the so-called prion protein, PrP, when Multiple System Atrophy was found to be likely caused by a new prion called Alpha-synuclein, The endogenous, properly folded form is denoted PrP^{C} (for *Common* or *Cellular*), whereas the disease-linked, misfolded form is denoted PrP^{Sc} (for *Scrapie*, after one of the diseases first linked to prions and neurodegeneration.) The precise structure of the prion is not known, though they can be formed by combining PrP^{C}, polyadenylic acid, and lipids in a Protein Misfolding Cyclic Amplification (PMCA) reaction. Proteins showing prion-type behavior are also found in some fungi, which has been useful in helping to understand mammalian prions. Fungal prions do not appear to cause disease in their hosts.

Prions cause neurodegenerative disease by aggregating extracellularly within the central nervous system to form plaques known as amyloid, which disrupt the normal tissue structure. This disruption is characterized by "holes" in the tissue with resultant spongy architecture due to the vacuole formation in the neurons. Other histological changes include astrogliosis and the absence of an inflammatory reaction. While the incubation period for prion diseases is relatively long (5 to 20 years), once symptoms appear the disease progresses rapidly, leading to brain damage and death. Neurodegenerative symptoms can include convulsions, dementia, ataxia (balance and coordination dysfunction), and behavioural or personality changes.

All known prion diseases, collectively called *transmissible spongiform encephalopathies* (TSEs), are untreatable and fatal. However, a vaccine developed in mice may provide insight into providing a vaccine to resist prion infections in humans. Additionally, in 2006 scientists announced that they had genetically engineered cattle lacking a necessary gene for prion production – thus theoretically making them immune to BSE, building on research indicating that mice lacking normally occurring prion protein are resistant to infection by scrapie prion protein. In 2013, a study revealed that 1 in 2,000 people in the United Kingdom might harbour the infectious prion protein that causes vCJD.

Many different mammalian species can be affected by prion diseases, as the prion protein (PrP) is very similar in all mammals. Due to small differences in PrP between different species it is unusual for a prion disease to transmit from one species to another. The human prion disease variant Creutzfeldt–Jakob disease, however, is believed to be caused by a prion that typically infects cattle, causing Bovine spongiform encephalopathy and is transmitted through infected meat.

Transmission

It has been recognized that prion diseases can arise in three different ways: acquired, familial, or sporadic. It is often assumed that the diseased form directly interacts with the normal form to make it rearrange its structure. One idea, the "Protein X" hypothesis, is that an as-yet unidentified cellular protein (Protein X) enables the conversion of PrP^{C} to PrP^{Sc} by bringing a molecule of each of the two together into a complex.

Current research suggests that the primary method of infection in animals is through ingestion. It is thought that prions may be deposited in the environment through the remains of dead animals and via urine, saliva, and other body fluids. They may then linger in the soil by binding to clay and other minerals.

A University of California research team, led by Nobel Prize winner Stanley Prusiner, has provided evidence for the theory that infection can occur from prions in manure. And, since manure is present in many areas surrounding water reservoirs, as well as used on many crop fields, it raises the possibility of widespread transmission. It was reported in January 2011 that researchers had discovered prions spreading through airborne transmission on aerosol particles, in an animal testing experiment focusing on scrapie infection in laboratory mice. Preliminary evidence supporting the notion that prions can be transmitted through use of urine-derived human menopausal gonadotropin, administered for the treatment of infertility, was published in 2011.

Prions in Plants

In 2015, researchers at The University of Texas Health Science Center at Houston found that plants can be a vector for prions. When researchers fed hamsters grass that grew on ground where a deer that died with chronic wasting disease (CWD) was buried, the hamsters became ill with CWD, suggesting that prions can bind to plants, which then take them up into the leaf and stem structure, where they can be eaten by herbivores, thus completing the cycle. It is thus possible that there is a progressively accumulating number of prions in the environment.

Sterilization

Infectious particles possessing nucleic acid are dependent upon it to direct their continued replication. Prions, however, are infectious by their effect on normal versions of the protein. Sterilizing prions, therefore, requires the denaturation of the protein to a state in which the molecule is no longer able to induce the abnormal folding of normal proteins. In general, prions are quite resistant to proteases, heat, ionizing radiation, and formaldehyde treatments, although their infectivity can be reduced by such treatments. Effective prion decontamination relies upon protein hydrolysis or reduction or destruction of protein tertiary structure. Examples include sodium hypochlorite, sodium hydroxide, and strongly acidic detergents such as LpH. 134 °C (274 °F) for 18 minutes in a pressurized steam autoclave has been found to be somewhat effective in deactivating the agent of disease. Ozone sterilization is currently being studied as a potential method for prion denaturation and deactivation. Renaturation of a completely denatured prion to infectious status has not yet been achieved; however, partially denatured prions can be renatured to an infective status under certain artificial conditions.

The World Health Organization recommends any of the following three procedures for the sterilization of all heat-resistant surgical instruments to ensure that they are not contaminated with prions:

1. Immerse in 1N sodium hydroxide and place in a gravity-displacement autoclave at 121 °C for 30 minutes; clean; rinse in water; and then perform routine sterilization processes.
2. Immerse in 1N sodium hypochlorite (20,000 parts per million available chlorine) for 1 hour; transfer instruments to water; heat in a gravity-displacement autoclave at 121 °C for 1 hour; clean; and then perform routine sterilization processes.
3. Immerse in 1N sodium hydroxide or sodium hypochlorite (20,000 parts per million available chlorine) for 1 hour; remove and rinse in water, then transfer to an open pan and heat in a gravity-displacement (121 °C) or in a porous-load (134 °C) autoclave for 1 hour; clean; and then perform routine sterilization processes.

Prion-like Domains

While PrP is considered the only mammalian prion, prion-like domains have been found in a variety of other mammalian proteins. Some of these proteins have been implicated in the ontogeny of age-related neurodegenerative disorders such as amyotrophic lateral sclerosis (ALS, known as Motor Neurone Disease outside the US), frontotemporal lobar degeneration with ubiquitin-positive inclusions (FTLD-U), Alzheimer's disease, and Huntington's disease, as well as some forms of Systemic Amyloidosis including AA (Secondary) Amyloidosis that develops in humans and animals with inflammatory and infectious diseases such as Tuberculosis, Crohn's disease, Rheumatoid arthritis, and HIV AIDS. AA amyloidosis, like prion disease, may be transmissible. This has given rise to the 'prion paradigm', where otherwise harmless proteins can be converted to a pathogenic form by a small number of misfolded, nucleating proteins.

The definition of a prion-like domain arises from the study of fungal prions. In yeast, prionogenic proteins have a portable prion domain that is both necessary and sufficient for self-templating and protein aggregation. This has been shown by attaching the prion domain to a reporter protein, which then aggregates like a known prion. Similarly, removing the prion domain from a fungal prion protein inhibits prionogenesis. This modular view of prion behaviour has led to the hypothesis that similar prion domains are present in animal proteins, in addition to PrP. These fungal prion domains have several characteristic sequence features. They are typically enriched in asparagine, glutamine, tyrosine and glycine residues, with an asparagine bias being particularly conducive to the aggregative property of prions. Historically, prionogenesis has been seen as independent of sequence and only dependent on relative residue content. However, this has been shown to be false, with the spacing of prolines and charged residues having been shown to be critical in amyloid formation.

Bioinformatic screens have predicted that over 250 human proteins contain prion-like domains (PrLD). These domains are hypothesized to have the same transmissible, amyloidogenic properties of PrP and known fungal proteins. As in yeast, proteins involved in gene expression and RNA binding seem to be particularly enriched in PrLD's, compared to other classes of protein. In particular, 29 of the known 210 proteins with an RNA recognition motif also have a putative prion domain. Meanwhile, several of these RNA-binding proteins have been independently identified as pathogenic in cases of ALS, FTLD-U, Alzheimer's disease, and Huntington's disease.

Role in Neurodegenerative Disease

The pathogenicity of prions and proteins with prion-like domains arises from their self-templating ability and the resulting exponential growth of amyloid fibrils. The presence of amyloid fibrils in patients with degenerative diseases has been well documented. These amyloid fibrils are seen as the result of pathogenic proteins that self-propagate and form highly stable, non-functional aggregates. While this does not necessarily imply a causal relationship between amyloid and degenerative diseases, the toxicity of certain amyloid forms and the overproduction of amyloid in familial cases of degenerative disorders supports the idea that amyloid formation is generally toxic.

Specifically, aggregation of TDP-43, an RNA-binding protein, has been found in ALS/MND patients, and mutations in the genes coding for these proteins have been identified in familial cases of ALS/MND. These mutations promote the misfolding of the proteins into a prion-like conformation. The misfolded form of TDP-43 forms cytoplasmic inclusions in afflicted neurons, and is found depleted in the nucleus. In addition to ALS/MND and FTLD-U, TDP-43 pathology is a feature of many cases of Alzheimer's disease, Parkinson's disease and Huntington's disease. The misfolding of TDP-43 is largely directed by its prion-like domain. This domain is inherently prone to misfolding, while pathological mutations in TDP-43 have been found to increase this propensity to misfold, explaining the presence of these mutations in familial cases of ALS/MND. As in yeast, the prion-like domain of TDP-43 has been shown to be both necessary and sufficient for protein misfolding and aggregation.

Similarly, pathogenic mutations have been identified in the prion-like domains of heterogeneous nuclear riboproteins hnRNPA2B1 and hnRNPA1 in familial cases of muscle, brain, bone and motor neuron degeneration. The wild-type form of all of these proteins show a tendency to self-assemble into amyloid fibrils, while the pathogenic mutations exacerbate this behaviour and lead to excess accumulation.

Fungi

Fungal proteins exhibiting templated conformational change were discovered in the yeast *Saccharomyces cerevisiae* by Reed Wickner in the early 1990s. For their mechanistic similarity to mammalian prions, they were termed yeast prions. Subsequent to this, a prion has also been found in the fungus *Podospora anserina*. These prions behave similarly to PrP, but, in general, are nontoxic to their hosts. Susan Lindquist's group at the Whitehead Institute has argued some of the fungal prions are not associated with any disease state, but may have a useful role; however, researchers at the NIH have also provided arguments suggesting that fungal prions could be considered a diseased state. There is mounting evidence that fungal proteins have evolved specific functions that are beneficial to the microorganism that enhance their ability to adapt to their diverse environments.

As of 2012 , there are eight known prion proteins in fungi, seven in *Saccharomyces cerevisiae* (Sup35, Rnq1, Ure2, Swi1, Mot3, Cyc8, and Mod5) and one in *Podospora anserina* (HET-s). The article that reported the discovery of a prion form, the Mca1 protein, was retracted due to the fact that the data could not be reproduced. Notably, most of the fungal prions are based on glutamine/asparagine-rich sequences, with the exception of HET-s and Mod5.

Research into fungal prions has given strong support to the protein-only concept, since purified protein extracted from cells with a prion state has been demonstrated to convert the normal form of the protein into a misfolded form *in vitro*, and in the process, preserve the information corresponding to different strains of the prion state. It has also shed some light on prion domains, which are regions in a protein that promote the conversion into a prion. Fungal prions have helped to suggest mechanisms of conversion that may apply to all prions, though fungal prions appear distinct from infectious mammalian prions in the lack of cofactor required for propagation. The characteristic prion domains may vary between species—e.g., characteristic fungal prion domains are not found in mammalian prions.

Fungal prions					
Protein	**Natural host**	**Normal function**	**Prion state**	**Prion phenotype**	**Year identified**
Ure2p	*Saccharomyces cerevisiae*	Nitrogen catabolite repressor	[URE3]	Growth on poor nitrogen sources	1994
Sup35p	*S. cerevisiae*	Translation termination factor	[PSI+]	Increased levels of nonsense suppression	1994
HET-S	*Podospora anserina*	Regulates heterokaryon incompatibility	[Het-s]	Heterokaryon formation between incompatible strains	
Rnq1p	*S. cerevisiae*	Protein template factor	[RNQ+],[PIN+]	Promotes aggregation of other prions	
Mca1	*S. cerevisiae*	Putative yeast caspase	[MCA+]	Unknown	2008
Swi1	*S. cerevisiae*	Chromatin remodeling	[SWI+]	Poor growth on some carbon sources	2008
Cyc8	*S. cerevisiae*	Transcriptional repressor	[OCT+]	Transcriptional derepression of multiple genes	2009
Mot3	*S. cerevisiae*	Nuclear transcription factor	[MOT3+]	Transcriptional derepression of anaerobic genes	2009
Sfp1	*S. cerevisiae*	Putative transcription factor	[ISP+]	Antisuppression	2010

Research

Potential Treatments and Diagnosis

Advancements in computer modeling have allowed scientists to identify compounds that can treat prion-caused diseases, such as one compound found to bind a cavity in the PrP^{C} and stabilize the conformation, reducing the amount of harmful PrP^{Sc}.

Antiprion antibodies capable of crossing the blood-brain-barrier and targeting cytosolic prion protein (an otherwise major obstacle in prion therapeutics) have been described.

In the last decade, some progress dealing with ultra-high-pressure inactivation of prion infectivity in processed meat has been reported.

In 2011, it was discovered that prions could be degraded by lichens.

There continues to be a very practical problem with diagnosis of prion diseases, including BSE and CJD. They have an incubation period of months to decades, during which there are no symptoms, even though the pathway of converting the normal brain PrP protein into the toxic, disease-related PrP^{Sc} form has started. At present, there is virtually no way to detect PrP^{Sc} reliably except by examining the brain using neuropathological and immunohistochemical methods after death. Accumulation of the abnormally folded PrP^{Sc} form of the PrP protein is a characteristic of the disease, but it is present at very low levels in easily accessible body fluids like blood or urine. Researchers have tried to develop methods to measure PrP^{Sc}, but there are still no fully accepted methods for use in materials such as blood.

In 2010, a team from New York described detection of PrP^{Sc} even when initially present at only one part in a hundred billion (10^{-11}) in brain tissue. The method combines amplification with a novel technology called Surround Optical Fiber Immunoassay (SOFIA) and some specific antibodies against PrP^{Sc}. After amplifying and then concentrating any PrP^{Sc}, the samples are labelled with a fluorescent dye using an antibody for specificity and then finally loaded into a micro-capillary tube. This tube is placed in a specially constructed apparatus so that it is totally surrounded by optical fibres to capture all light emitted once the dye is excited using a laser.

The RT-QuIC assay, a microplate reader-based prion detection method which uses as reagents normally folded prions, fluorescently labelled so that they "light up" when they are misfolded; samples suspected of containing misfolded prions are added and misfolded reagents can be detected by standard fluorescence detection methods.

Astemizole has been found to have anti-prion activity.

Another chemical that may be effective against prion infection are luminescent conjugated polythiophenes, fluorescent compounds that are often used to stain tissue samples. In a 2015 study, led by Adriano Aguzzi, professor of neurobiology at the University of Zurich, found that when they injected mice with a prion disease and then with polythiophenes, the mice survived eighty percent longer than the control mice that were only injected with the prion disease.

Causal Hypotheses

Whether prions cause disease or are merely a symptom caused by a different agent is still debated by a minority of researchers. The following sections describe several hypotheses: Some pertain to the composition of the infectious agent (protein-only, protein with other components, virus, or other), while others pertain to its mechanism of reproduction.

Protein-only Hypothesis

Prior to the discovery of prions, it was thought that all pathogens used nucleic acids to direct their replication. The "protein-only hypothesis" states that a protein structure can replicate without the use of nucleic acids. This was initially controversial as it contradicts the central dogma of molecular biology, which describes nucleic acid as the central form of replicative information.

Evidence in favor of a protein-only hypothesis includes:

- Infectivity titre in TSEs roughly correlates with prion amyloid (PrP^{Sc}) titre, however, prion amyloid is absent in approximately 10% of CJD cases.
- No virus particles, bacteria, or fungi have been conclusively associated with prion diseases, although virus-like particles and Spiroplasma-like inclusions can be detected in some TSE cases, but not in controls (uninfected individuals).
- No nucleic acid has been conclusively associated with infectivity; agent is resistant to ultraviolet radiation and nucleases, although in 2016, studies have suggested that the agent can be destroyed by nucleases under certain situations and that part of the resistance to nucleases and radiation may be that byproducts from degenerating neurons may help protect a nucleic acid.
- No immune or inflammatory response to infection.
- PrP^{Sc} experimentally transmitted between one species and another results in PrP^{Sc} with the amino-acid sequence of the recipient species, suggesting that nucleic acid-mediated replication of the donor agent does not occur.
- Familial prion disease occurs in families with a mutation in the PrP gene, and mice with PrP mutations develop prion disease despite controlled conditions where transmission is prevented. These mice can then transmit the disease to healthy, wild type mice, suggesting that mice with PrP mutations spontaneously generate infectivity.
- Animals lacking PrP^C do not contract prion disease.

Genetic Factors

A gene for the normal protein has been identified: the *PRNP* gene. In all inherited cases of prion disease, there is a mutation in the *PRNP* gene. Many different *PRNP* mutations have been identified and these proteins are more likely to fold into abnormal prion. Although this discovery puts a hole in the general prion hypothesis, that prions can aggregate only proteins of identical amino acid make-up. These mutations can occur throughout the gene. Some mutations involve expansion of the octapeptide repeat region at the N-terminal of PrP. Other mutations that have been identified as a cause of inherited prion disease occur at positions 102, 117 & 198 (GSS), 178, 200, 210 & 232 (CJD) and 178 (Fatal Familial Insomnia, FFI). The cause of prion disease can be sporadic, genetic, or infectious, or a combination of these factors. For example, to have scrapie, both an infectious agent and a susceptible genotype must be present.

Multi-component Hypothesis

Despite much effort, significant titers of prion infectivity have never been produced by refolding pure PrP molecules, raising doubt about the validity of the "protein only" hypothesis. In addition the "protein only" hypothesis fails to provide a molecular explanation for the ability of prion strains to target specific areas of the brain in distinct patterns. These shortcomings, along with additional experimental data, have given rise to the "multi-component" or "cofactor variation" hypothesis.

In 2007, biochemist Surachai Supattapone and his colleagues at Dartmouth College produced purified infectious prions *de novo* from defined components (PrP^C, co-purified lipids, and a synthetic polyanionic molecule). These researchers also showed that the polyanionic molecule required for prion formation was selectively incorporated into high-affinity complexes with PrP molecules, leading them to hypothesize that infectious prions may be composed of multiple host components, including PrP, lipid, and polyanionic molecules, rather than PrP^{Sc} alone.

In 2010, Jiyan Ma and colleagues at The Ohio State University produced infectious prions from a recipe of bacterially expressed recombinant PrP, POPG phospholipid, and RNA, further supporting the multi-component hypothesis. This finding is in contrast to studies that found minimally infectious prions produced from recombinant PrP alone.

In 2012, Supattapone and colleagues purified the membrane lipid phosphatidylethanolamine as a solitary endogenous cofactor capable of facilitating the formation of high-titer recombinant prions derived from multiple prion strains. They also reported that the cofactor is essential for maintaining the infectious conformation of PrP^{Sc}, and that cofactor molecules dictate the strain properties of infectious prions.

Heavy Metal Poisoning Hypothesis

Reports suggest that imbalance of brain metal homeostasis may be a cause of PrP^{Sc}-associated neurotoxicity, though the underlying mechanisms are difficult to explain based on existing information. Proposed hypotheses include a functional role for PrP^C in metal metabolism, and loss of this function due to aggregation to the disease-associated PrP^{Sc} form as the cause of brain metal imbalance. Other views suggest gain of toxic function by PrP^{Sc} due to sequestration of PrP^C-associated metals within the aggregates, resulting in the generation of redox-active PrP^{Sc} complexes. The physiological implications of some PrP^C-metal interactions are known, while others are still unclear. The pathological implications of PrP^C-metal interaction include metal-induced oxidative damage, and in some instances conversion of PrP^C to a PrP^{Sc}-like form.

Viral Hypothesis

The protein-only hypothesis has been criticised by those maintaining that the simplest explanation of the evidence to date is viral. For more than a decade, Yale University neuropathologist Laura Manuelidis has been proposing that prion diseases are caused instead by an unidentified slow virus. In January 2007, she and her colleagues published an article reporting to have found a virus in 10%, or less, of their scrapie-infected cells in culture.

Evidence in favor of a viral hypothesis includes:

- Strain variation: differences in prion infectivity, incubation, symptomology, and progression among species resembles that seen between viruses, especially RNA viruses
- The long incubation and rapid onset of symptoms resembles lentiviruses, such as HIV-induced AIDS
- Viral-like particles that do not appear to be composed of PrP have been found in some of the cells of scrapie- or CJD-infected cell lines.
- Many viruses, including HIV which needs CD4 and CXCR4, need a receptor to attach to and enter into host cells. The host prion, PrP^c may be a receptor protein for an as yet undiscovered TSE virus, explaining why animals lacking host prion do not become infected with experimental prion disease.
- A prion like protein, called MAVS, has been shown to misfold as part of the innate immune response against pathogenic viruses, similarly the cellular prion, PrP^C has been shown to have anti HIV properties, and it is hypothesized that the misfolding of the prion in TSEs may be an antiviral response against an unknown virus.
- In 2016, studies have demonstrated susceptibility to nucleases under certain situations: >99% of infectivty was destroyed, but there was no reduction of prion protein, suggesting the presence of a nucleic acid.

Studies propagating TSE infectivity in cell-free reactions and in purified component chemical reactions is thought to strongly suggest against TSE viral nature. However, some viruses, such as Poliovirus, have the ability to replicate in cell-free reactions.

Using a similar defined recipe of multiple components (PrP, POPG lipid, RNA), Jiyan Ma and colleagues generated infectious prions from recombinant PrP expressed from *E. coli*, casting further doubt on the viral hypothesis. However, the infectivity reported in Ma et al. experiments could be explained by contamination, as infectious material from scrapie infected mice was used earlier in the same laboratory prior to working with recombinant PrP.

Virino Hypothesis

The 'virino hypothesis' postulates that the TSE agent is a foreign, self replicating nucleic acid or nucleic acid fragment bound to PrP.

Spiroplasma Hypothesis

Spiroplasma is a cell wall–deficient bacteria related to *Mycoplasma*, which some think may be the cause of the TSEs. The lack of a cell wall means they are not susceptible to conventional antibiotics such as penicillin, which target cell wall synthesis. Frank O. Bastian of Louisiana State University first discovered *Spiroplasma*-like inclusions in the brain of a CJD patient during an autopsy in 1979 and has hypothesized that this bacterium could possibly be the cause of the TSEs.

However, as of 2015 , with the exception of *Spiroplasma mirum* strain SMCA causing spongiform microcystic encephalitis in suckling rats, other researchers have been unable to duplicate these findings, casting doubt on the *Spiroplasma* hypothesis. In defense of the *Spiroplasma* hypothesis,

Bastian pointed out that *Spiroplasma* is hard to culture and that strain variation makes it hard to detect certain strains using PCR and other techniques, thus giving a false negative.

Acinetobacter-autoimmunity Hypothesis

Acinetobacter is a bacterium which some think is the cause of the TSEs.

Etymology and Pronunciation

The word *prion*, coined in 1982 by Stanley B. Prusiner, is a portmanteau derived from protein and infection, hence prion, and is short for "proteinaceous infectious particle", in reference to its ability to self-propagate and transmit its conformation to other proteins.

Scrapie

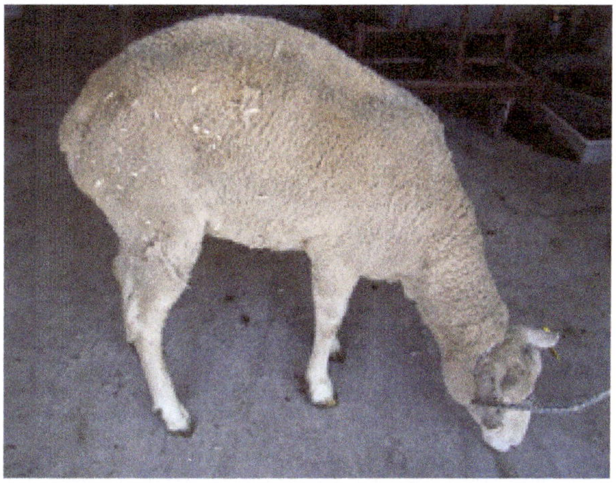

Ewe with scrapie with weight loss and hunched appearance

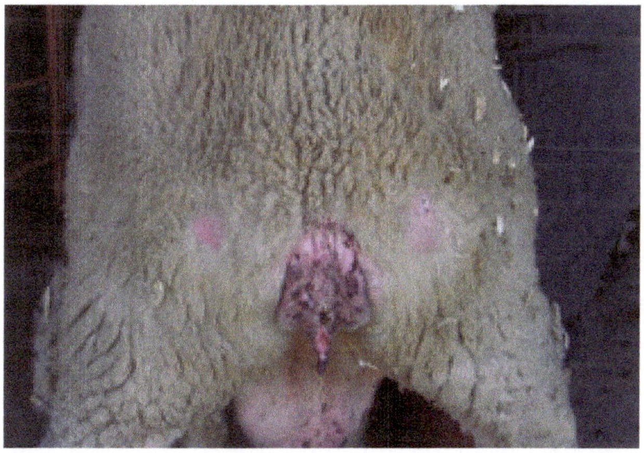

Same ewe as above with bare patches on rear end from scraping

Scrapie is a fatal, degenerative disease that affects the nervous systems of sheep and goats. It is one of several transmissible spongiform encephalopathies (TSEs), which are related to bovine spongiform encephalopathy (BSE or "mad cow disease") and chronic wasting disease of deer. Like other spongiform encephalopathies, scrapie is caused by a prion. Scrapie has been known since 1732, and does not appear to be transmissible to humans.

The name scrapie is derived from one of the clinical signs of the condition, wherein affected animals will compulsively scrape off their fleeces against rocks, trees, or fences. The disease apparently causes an itching sensation in the animals. Other clinical signs include excessive lip smacking, altered gaits, and convulsive collapse.

Scrapie is infectious and transmissible among conspecifics, so one of the most common ways to contain it (since it is incurable) is to quarantine and destroy those affected. However, scrapie tends to persist in flocks and can also arise apparently spontaneously in flocks that have not previously had cases of the disease. The mechanism of transmission between animals and other aspects of the biology of the disease are only poorly understood, and these are active areas of research. Recent studies suggest prions may be spread through urine and persist in the environment for decades.

Scrapie usually affects sheep around three to five years of age. The potential for transmission at birth and from contact with placental tissues is apparent. No evidence indicates scrapie is infectious to humans.

Uptake of Prions

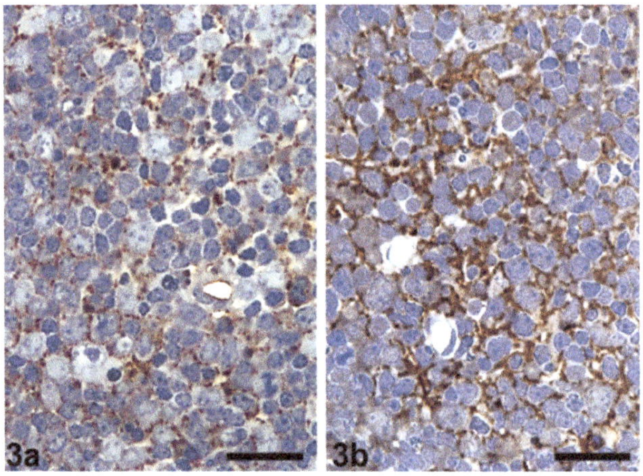

Lymph nodes from (a) healthy and (b) infected sheep - colouring with antibodies shows clear sign of scrapie prions in the tissue of the infected sheep

The protein enters through the intestines or through cuts in the skin. The prions cause normal proteins of the sheep to fold into the wrong shape. These proteins are gradually accumulated in the body, especially in nerve cells, which subsequently die. When the prions are absorbed through the intestines, they first appear in the lymph nodes, especially in Peyer's patches at the small intestine.

An experiment has shown lambs risk being infected through milk from infected ewes, but the lambs in the experiment also infected each other, making the risk of infection difficult to assess. The experiment did not continue long enough to show if the lambs developed symptoms, but merely that the prion was present in their bodies.

Clinical Signs and Diagnosis

Changes are mild at first; slight behavioural changes and an increase in chewing movements may occur. Ataxia and neurological signs then develop, and affected sheep struggle to keep up with the flock.

Some sheep scratch excessively and show patches of wool loss and lesions on the skin. Scratching sheep over the rump area may lead to a nibbling reflex, which is characteristic for the condition.

Signs of a chronic systemic disease appear later, with weight loss, anorexia, lethargy, and death.

Post mortem examination is important for the diagnosis of scrapie. Histology of tissues shows accumulation of prions in the central nervous system, and immunohistochemical staining and ELISA can also be used to demonstrate the protein.

Treatment and Preventive Action

No treatment is available for affected sheep.

A test performed by sampling a small amount of lymphatic tissue from the third eyelid is now available.

In the United Kingdom, the government has put in place a National Scrapie Plan, which encourages breeding from sheep that are genetically more resistant to scrapie. This is intended to eventually reduce the incidence of the disease in the UK sheep population. Scrapie occurs in Europe and North America, but to date, Australia and New Zealand (both major sheep-producing countries) are scrapie-free.

Breeds such as Cheviot and Suffolk are more susceptible to scrapie than other breeds. Specifically, this is determined by the genes coding for the naturally occurring prion proteins. The most resistant sheep have a double set of *ARR* alleles, while sheep with the *VRQ* allele are the most susceptible. A simple blood test reveals the allele of the sheep, and many countries are actively breeding away the *VRQ* allele.

Out of fear of BSE, many European countries banned some traditional sheep or goat products made without removing the spinal cord, such as smalahove and smokie.

In 2010, a team from New York described detection of PrP^{Sc} even when initially present at only one part in a hundred billion (10^{-11}) in brain tissue. The method combines amplification with a novel technology called surround optical fiber immunoassay and some specific antibodies against PrP^{Sc}. The technique allowed detection of PrP^{Sc} after many fewer cycles of conversion than others have achieved, substantially reducing the possibility of artefacts, as well as speeding up the assay. The researchers also tested their method on blood samples from apparently healthy sheep that went on to develop scrapie. The animals' brains were analysed once any symptoms became apparent. They could therefore compare results from brain tissue and blood taken once the animals exhibited symptoms of the diseases, with blood obtained earlier in the animals' lives, and from uninfected animals. The results showed very clearly that PrP^{Sc} could be detected in the blood of animals long before the symptoms appeared. After further development and testing, this method could be of great value in surveillance as a blood- or urine-based screening test for scrapie.

Transmission/exposure Pathways

Various studies have indicated prions (PrP^{SC}) that infect sheep and goats with the fatal transmissible encephalopathy known as scrapie, are able to persist in soil for years without losing their pathogenic activity. Dissemination of prions into the environment can occur from several sources: mainly, infectious placenta or amniotic fluid of sheep and possibly environmental contamination by saliva or excrement.

Confirmatory testing for scrapie can only be achieved by applying immunohistochemistry of disease-associated prion protein (PrP^{SC}) to tissues collected *post mortem*, including obex (a brainstem structure), retropharyngeal lymph node and palatine tonsil. A live animal diagnostic, not confirmatory, test was approved in 2008 for immunochemistry testing on rectal biopsy-derived lymphoid tissue by USDA.

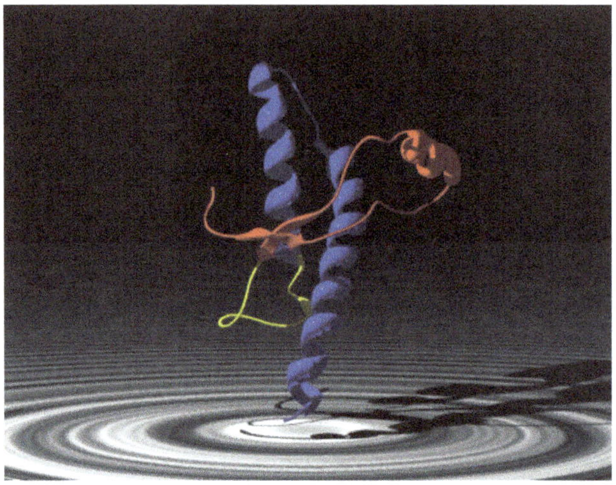

Human prion protein, residues 125-228, created from protein database (PDB) entry 1QM3. The coloring illustrates the subdomains, that are proposed to initiate the conversion from the normal cellular to the scrapie form by slow motions.

Natural transmission of scrapie in the field seems to occur via the alimentary tract in the majority of cases, and scrapie-free sheep flocks can become infected on pastures where outbreaks of scrapie had been observed before. These findings point to a sustained contagion in the environment, notably in the soil.

Prion concentration in birth fluids does not alter the infectivity of the prions. Naturally or experimentally infected does and ewes transmit the infection to the kids, even when placentas have little PrP^{SC}. PrP^{SC} is shed at a higher percentage in sheep placentas (52%-72%) than in goat placenta (5-10%) in study trials at the USDA Agricultural Research Service.

Detectable PrP^{SC} has been reported in the feces of sheep both in the terminal and the early preclinical stages of the disease, suggesting the prions are likely to be shed into the environment throughout the course of the disease. Several sources of prions in feces could be postulated, including environmental ingestion and swallowing infected saliva; however, the most likely source is shedding from the gut-associated lymphoid tissue. Ruminant animals have specialized Peyer's patches that, throughout the length of the ileum, amount to about 100,000 follicles, and all of these could be infected and shedding prions into the lumen. Scrapie prions have been found in the Peyer's patches of naturally infected asymptomatic lambs as young as four months of age.

Exposure Through Contaminated Soil

Ingestion of soil by grazing sheep has been measured in two soil types, at two stocking rates, and over two grazing seasons. Animals ingested up to 400 g soil per kg of body weight between May and November. Rainfall and stocking rate emerged as factors influencing ingestion. The effect of soil type and vegetation type was less evident.

The average weight of an adult sheep is around 250 pounds. If an adult sheep ate 400g/kg of soil as predicted by D. McGrath *et al.*, then the average sheep would ingest about 45,000 g over six months, or 251 g per day. Assuming the soil was contaminated with prions (PrP^{SC}) from feces or birth fluids, then potentially the sheep would become infected. The concentration of the prions in the soil is uncertain, and concentration is not directly proportional to infectivity. Factors affecting prion infectivity in the soil have been shown to include the length of time in the soil and the binding abilities of the soil.

For a detailed risk assessment of scrapie-contaminated soil, it was of major importance to analyze whether the detectable PrP^{Sc} in the soil extracts still exhibited oral infectivity after incubation times up to 29 months. A bioassay with Syrian hamsters was performed by feeding the animals with contaminated soil or aqueous soil extracts that had been collected after soil incubation for 26 and 29 months, respectively. Hamsters fed with contaminated soil exhibited their first scrapie-associated symptoms at two weeks to six months (95% CI) after the first feeding. The hamsters reached the terminal stage of scrapie at five to 21 months (95% CI) after the first feeding. This indicated substantial amounts of persistent infectivity in soil that had been incubated for 26 and 29 months. In Iceland in 1978, a program was implemented to eradicate scrapie, and affected flocks were culled, premises were disinfected, and sheep houses were burnt; after two to three years, the premises were restocked with lambs from scrapie-free areas. Between 1978 and 2004, scrapie recurred on 33 farms. Nine recurrences occurred 14–21 years after culling as a result of persistent environmental contamination with PrP^{Sc}.

The binding abilities of different soil types have been shown to enhance disease penetrance into a population. Soil containing the common clay mineral montmorillonite (Mte) and kaolinite (Kte) binds more effectively with the prions than soil containing quartz. Enhanced transmissibility of soil-bound prions may explain the environmental spread of scrapie despite low levels shed into the environment. The mechanism by which Mte or other soil components enhances the transmissibility of particle bound prions remains to be clarified. Prion binding to Mte or other soil components may partially protect PrP^{SC} from denaturation or proteolysis in the digestive tract, allowing more disease agent to be taken up from the gut. Adsorption of PrP^{Sc} soil may alter the aggregation state of the protein, shifting the size distribution toward more infectious prion protein particles, thereby increasing the infectious units. For prion disease to be transmitted via ingestion of prion contaminated soil, prions must also remain infectious by the oral route of exposure. Researchers at the University of Wisconsin investigated the oral infectivity of Mte-bound and soil-bound prions. The effects of prion source (via infected brain homogenate and purified PrP^{Sc}) and dose on penetrance (proportion of animals eventually exhibiting clinical signs of scrapie) and incubation period (time to onset of clinical symptoms) was evaluated. About 38% of animals receiving orally 200 ng of unbound, clarified PrP^{Sc} derived from soil exhibited clinical symptoms, with an incubation period for infected animals of 203 to 633 days. All animals orally dosed with an equivalent amount of Mte-bound PrP^{Sc} manifested disease symptoms in 195 to 637 days. By contrast, animals orally receiving Mte soil alone or one-tenth as much unbound clarified PrP^{Sc} (20 ng) remained asymptomatic throughout the course of the experiment. These data established that Mte-bound prions remain infectious via the oral route of exposure, and that the binding agent Mte increases disease penetrance, enhancing the efficiency of oral transmission.

Transmission Summary

Prions (PrP^{Sc}) are shed from sheep and goats in birth fluids, feces and other excrement. The concentration of the prions is uncertain, but is not directly proportional to infectivity. Sheep ingest a considerable amount of soil, so soil represents a plausible environmental reservoir of scrapie prions, which can persist in the environment for years. Longevity of the prions and the attachment of soil particles likely influences the persistence and infectivity of prions in the environment.

Effective methods of inactivating prions in the soil are currently lacking, and the effects of natural degradation mechanisms on prion infectivity are largely unknown. An improved understanding of the processes affecting the mobility, persistence and bioavailability of prions in soil is needed for the management of prion-contaminated environments. A system for estimating the prion-binding capacity of soil on farms using simple soil analysis may allow an estimate of the prion risk in the environment, and whether altering prion binding by the use of soil amendments may help to mitigate the infectious prions. Lichens, specifically, *Parmelia sulcata*, *Cladonia rangiferina* and *Lobaria pulmonaria*, may have potential for reducing the number of prions because some lichen species contain proteases that show promise in breaking down the prion. Further work to clone and characterize the proteases, assess their effects on prion infectivity, and determine which component organism or organisms present in lichens produce or influence the protease activity is warranted and is currently under investigation.

Bovine Spongiform Encephalopathy

Bovine spongiform encephalopathy (BSE), commonly known as mad cow disease, is a fatal neurodegenerative disease (encephalopathy) in cattle that causes a spongy degeneration of the brain and spinal cord. BSE has a long incubation period, of 2.5 to 5 years, usually affecting adult cattle at a peak age onset of four to five years. BSE is caused by a misfolded protein—a prion. In the United Kingdom, the country worst affected by an epidemic in 1986–1998, more than 180,000 cattle were infected and 4.4 million slaughtered during the eradication program.

The disease may be most easily transmitted to humans by eating food contaminated with the brain, spinal cord or digestive tract of infected carcasses. However, the infectious agent, although most highly concentrated in nervous tissue, can be found in virtually all tissues throughout the body, including blood. In humans, it is known as new variant Creutzfeldt–Jakob disease (vCJD or nvCJD), and by June 2014 it had killed 177 people in the United Kingdom, and 52 elsewhere, primarily in western Europe in countries supplied with beef or beef products from the UK. Between 460,000 and 482,000 BSE-infected animals had entered the human food chain before controls on high-risk offal were introduced in 1989.

A British and Irish inquiry into BSE concluded the epizootic was caused by cattle, which are normally herbivores, being fed the remains of other cattle in the form of meat and bone meal (MBM), a protein supplement in concentrated feeds. Since dairy calves are generally fed concentrated feed after they are weaned, they usually develop this disease more often then beef cattle

The cause of BSE may be from the contamination of MBM from sheep with scrapie that were processed in the same slaughterhouse. The epidemic was probably accelerated by the recycling of infected bovine tissues prior to the recognition of BSE. The origin of the disease itself remains unknown. The infectious agent is distinctive for the high temperatures at which it remains viable, over 600 °C (about 1100 °F). This contributed to the spread of the disease in the United Kingdom, which had reduced the temperatures used during its rendering process. Another contributory factor was the feeding of infected protein supplements to very young calves.

Pathogenesis

The pathogenesis of BSE is not well understood or documented like other diseases of this nature. Even though BSE is disease that results in neurological defects, its pathogenesis occurs in areas that reside outside of the nervous system. There was a strong deposition of PrP^{Sc} initially located in the Ileal Peyer's patches of the small intestine. The lymphatic system has been identified in the pathogenesis of scrapies, it has not, however, been determined to be an essential part of the pathogenesis of BSE. The Ileal Peyer's patches have been the only organ from this system that has been found to play a major role in the pathogenesis. Infectivity of the Ileal Peyer's patches has been observed as early as 4 months after inoculation. PrP^{Sc} accumulation was found to occur mostly in tangible body macrophages of the Ileal Peyer's patches. Tangible body macrophages involved in PrP^{Sc} clearance are thought to play a role in in PrP^{Sc} accumulation in the Peyer's patches. Accumulation of PrP^{Sc} was also found in follicular dendritic cells; however, it was of a lesser degree. Six months after inoculation, there was no infectivity in any tissues, only that of the ileum. This led researchers to believe that the disease agent replicates here. In naturally confirmed cases, there have been no reports of infectivity in the Ileal Peyer's patches. Generally, in clinical experiments, high doses of the disease are administered. In natural cases, it was hypothesized that low doses of the agent were present, and therefore, infectivity could not be observed.

Signs and Symptoms

Symptoms are not seen immediately in cattle due to the diseases' extremely long incubation period. Some cattle have been observed to have an abnormal gait, changes in behavior, tremors and hyperresponsiveness to certain stimuli. Hindlimb ataxia affects the animal's gait and occurs when muscle control is lost. This results in poor balance and coordination. Behavioural changes may include aggression, anxiety relating to certain situations, nervousness, frenzy or an overall change in temperament. Some rare but previously observed symptoms also include persistent pacing, rubbing or licking. Additionally, nonspecific symptoms have also been observed which include weight loss, decreased milk production, lameness, ear infections and teeth grinding due to pain. Some animals may show a combination of these symptoms, while others may only be observed demonstrating one of the many reported. Once clinical symptoms arise, they typically get worse over the upcoming weeks and months, eventually leading to recumbency, coma and death.

Cause

The infectious agent in BSE is believed to be a specific type of misfolded protein called a prion. Other theories state that the agent is a virus, virino, *Spiroplasma* species, or *Acinetobacter* species. Prions are not destroyed even if the beef or material containing them is cooked or heat-treated. Prion proteins carry the disease between individuals and cause deterioration of the brain. BSE is a type of transmissible spongiform encephalopathy (TSE). TSEs can arise in animals that carry an allele which causes previously normal protein molecules to contort by themselves from an alpha helical arrangement to a beta pleated sheet, which is the disease-causing shape for the particular protein. Transmission can occur when healthy animals come in contact with tainted tissues from others with the disease. In the brain, these proteins cause native cellular prion protein to deform into the infectious state, which then goes on to deform further prion protein in an exponential cascade. This results in protein aggregates, which then form dense plaque fibers leading to the microscopic appearance of "holes" in the brain, degeneration of physical and mental abilities, and ultimately death.

Different hypotheses exist for the origin of prion proteins in cattle. Two leading hypotheses suggest it may have jumped species from the disease scrapie in sheep, or that it evolved from a spontaneous form of "mad cow disease" that has been seen occasionally in cattle for many centuries. In the fifth century BC, Hippocrates described a similar illness in cattle and sheep, which he believed also occurred in man. Publius Flavius Vegetius Renatus recorded cases of a disease with similar characteristics in the fourth and fifth centuries AD. The British Government enquiry took the view the cause was not scrapie, as had originally been postulated, but was some event in the 1970s that was not possible to identify.

Research in 2008 suggested that mad cow disease also is caused by a genetic mutation within the prion protein gene. The research showed, for the first time, that a 10-year-old cow from Alabama with an atypical form of bovine spongiform encephalopathy had the same type of prion protein gene mutation as found in human patients with the genetic form of Creutzfeldt–Jakob disease (genetic CJD). This form of Creutzfeldt–Jakob disease is called variant CJD.

Diagnosis

Diagnosis of BSE continues to be a practical problem. It has an incubation period of months to years, during which no symptoms are noticed, though the pathway of converting the normal brain prion protein (PrP) into the toxic, disease-related PrP^{Sc} form has started. At present, virtually no way is known to detect PrP^{Sc} reliably except by examining *post mortem* brain tissue using neuropathological and immunohistochemical methods. Accumulation of the abnormally folded PrP^{Sc} form of PrP is a characteristic of the disease, but it is present at very low levels in easily accessible body fluids such as blood or urine. Researchers have tried to develop methods to measure PrP^{Sc}, but no methods for use in materials such as blood have been accepted fully.

The traditional method of diagnosis relies on histopathological examination of the medulla oblongata of the brain, and other tissues, *post mortem*. Immunohistochemistry can be used to demonstrate prion protein accumulation.

In 2010, a team from New York described detection of PrP^{Sc} even when initially present at only one part in a hundred billion (10^{-11}) in brain tissue. The method combines amplification with a novel technology called surround optical fiber immunoassay and some specific antibodies against PrP^{Sc}. After amplifying and then concentrating any PrP^{Sc}, the samples are labelled with a fluorescent dye using an antibody for specificity and then finally loaded into a microcapillary tube. This tube is placed in a specially constructed apparatus so it is totally surrounded by optical fibres to capture all light emitted once the dye is excited using a laser. The technique allowed detection of PrP^{Sc} after many fewer cycles of conversion than others have achieved, substantially reducing the possibility of artifacts, as well as speeding up the assay. The researchers also tested their method on blood samples from apparently healthy sheep that went on to develop scrapie. The animals' brains were analysed once any symptoms became apparent. The researchers could, therefore, compare results from brain tissue and blood taken once the animals exhibited symptoms of the diseases, with blood obtained earlier in the animals' lives, and from uninfected animals. The results showed very clearly that PrP^{Sc} could be detected in the blood of animals long before the symptoms appeared. After further development and testing, this method could be of great value in surveillance as a blood- or urine-based screening test for BSE.

Prevention

A ban on feeding meat and bone meal to cattle has resulted in a strong reduction in cases in countries where the disease was present. In disease-free countries, control relies on import control, feeding regulations, and surveillance measures.

In UK and US slaughterhouses, the brain, spinal cord, trigeminal ganglia, intestines, eyes, and tonsils from cattle are classified as specified risk materials, and must be disposed of appropriately.

An enhanced BSE-related feed ban is in effect in both the United States and Canada to help improve prevention and elimination of BSE.

Epidemiology

Country	BSE cases	vCJD cases
Austria	5	0
Belgium	133	0
Canada	17	2
Czech Republic	28	0
Denmark	14	0
Falkland Islands	1	0
Finland	1	0
France	900	27
Germany	312	0
Greece	1	0
Hong Kong	2	0
Republic of Ireland	1353	4
Israel	1	0
Italy	138	2

Country	BSE cases	vCJD cases
Japan	26	1
Liechtenstein	2	0
Luxembourg	2	1
Netherlands	85	3
Oman	2	0
Poland	21	0
Portugal	875	2
Saudi Arabia	0	1
Slovakia	15	0
Slovenia	7	0
Spain	412	5
Sweden	1	0
Switzerland	453	0
Thailand		2
United Kingdom	183841	176
United States	4	3
Total	**188,652**	**229**

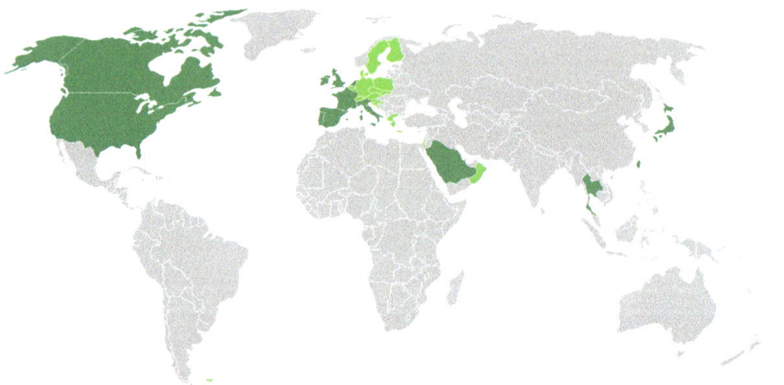

Dark green areas are countries with confirmed human cases of vCJD; light green shows countries which have reported cases of only BSE.

The table to the right summarizes reported cases of BSE and of vCJD by country. (The vCJD column is by country of residence of patient at time of diagnosis and not suspected origin of beef.) BSE is the disease in cattle, while vCJD is the disease in people.

The tests used for detecting BSE vary considerably, as do the regulations in various jurisdictions for when, and which cattle, must be tested. For instance in the EU, the cattle tested are older (30 months or older), while many cattle are slaughtered younger than that. At the opposite end of the scale, Japan tests all cattle at the time of slaughter. Tests are also difficult, as the altered prion protein has very low levels in blood or urine, and no other signal has been found. Newer tests[specify] are faster, more sensitive, and cheaper, so future figures possibly may be more comprehensive. Even so, currently the only reliable test is examination of tissues during a necropsy.

As for vCJD in humans, autopsy tests are not always done, so those figures, too, are likely to be too low, but probably by a lesser fraction. In the United Kingdom, anyone with possible vCJD symptoms must be reported to the Creutzfeldt–Jakob Disease Surveillance Unit. In the United States, the CDC has refused to impose a national requirement that physicians and hospitals report cases of the disease. Instead, the agency relies on other methods, including death certificates and urging physicians to send suspicious cases to the National Prion Disease Pathology Surveillance Center (NPDPSC) at Case Western Reserve University in Cleveland, which is funded by the CDC.

To control potential transmission of vCJD within the United States, the American Red Cross has established strict restrictions on individuals' eligibility to donate blood. Individuals who have spent a cumulative time of 3 months or more in the United Kingdom between 1980 and 1996, or a cumulative time of 5 years or more from 1980 to present in any combination of countries in Europe, are prohibited from donating blood.

North America

The first reported case in North America was in December 1993 from Alberta, Canada. Another Canadian case was reported in May 2003. The first known U.S. occurrence came in December of the same year, though it was later confirmed to be a cow of Canadian origin imported to the U.S. Canada announced two additional cases of BSE from Alberta in early 2005. In June 2005, John R. Clifford, chief veterinary officer for the United States Department of Agriculture animal health inspection service, confirmed a fully domestic case of BSE in Texas.

Practices in the United States Relating to BSE

Soybean meal is cheap and plentiful in the United States. Cottonseed meal, 1.5 million tons of which are produced in the U.S. every year, none of which is suitable for humans or any other simple-stomach animals, is even cheaper than soybean meal. Historically, meat and bone meal, blood meal, and meat scraps have almost always commanded a higher price as a feed additive than oilseed meals in the U.S., so not much incentive existed to use animal products to feed ruminants. As a result, the use of animal byproduct feeds was never common, as it was in Europe. However, U.S. regulations only partially prohibited the use of animal byproducts in feed. In 1997, regulations prohibited the feeding of mammalian byproducts to ruminants such as cattle and goats. However, the byproducts of ruminants can still be legally fed to pets or other livestock, including pigs and poultry. In addition, it is legal for ruminants to be fed byproducts from some of these animals. Because of this, some authors have suggested that under certain conditions, it is still possible for BSE incidence to increase in U.S. cattle. A proposal to end the use of cattle blood, restaurant scraps, and poultry litter (fecal matter, feathers, bedding material) in January 2004 has yet to be implemented.

In February 2001, the US Government Accountability Office reported the FDA, which is responsible for regulating feed, had not adequately enforced the various bans. Compliance with the regulations was shown to be extremely poor before the discovery of a cow in Washington infected with BSE in 2003, but industry representatives report that compliance is now total. Even so, critics call the partial prohibitions insufficient. Indeed, US meat producer Creekstone Farms was forcibly prevented from conducting BSE testing by the USDA, which under an obscure 1913 law had the authority to restrict sales of BSE testing kits, allegedly to protect other producers from being forced to conduct the same tests to stay competitive.

The USDA has issued recalls of beef supplies that involved introduction of downer cows into the food supply. Hallmark/Westland Meat Packing Company was found to have used electric shocks to prod downer cows into the slaughtering system in 2007. Possibly due to pressure from large agribusiness, the United States has drastically cut back on the number of cows inspected for BSE.

Effect on the US Beef Industry

Japan was the top importer of US beef, buying 240,000 tons valued at $1.4 billion in 2003. After the discovery of the first case of BSE in the US on 23 December 2003, Japan halted US beef imports. In December 2005, Japan once again allowed imports of US beef, but reinstated its ban in January 2006 after a violation of the US-Japan beef import agreement: a vertebral column, which should have been removed prior to shipment, was included in a shipment of veal.

Tokyo yielded to US pressure to resume imports, ignoring consumer worries about the safety of US beef, said Japanese consumer groups. Michiko Kamiyama from Food Safety Citizen Watch and Yoko Tomiyama from Consumers Union of Japan said about this: "The government has put priority on the political schedule between the two countries, not on food safety or human health."

Sixty-five nations implemented full or partial restrictions on importing US beef products because of concerns that US testing lacked sufficient rigor. As a result, exports of US beef declined from 1,300,000 metric tons in 2003, (before the first mad cow was detected in the US) to 322,000 metric tons in 2004. This has increased since then to 771,000 metric tons in 2007.

On 31 December 2006, Hematech, Inc, a biotechnology company based in Sioux Falls, South Dakota, announced it had used genetic engineering and cloning technology to produce cattle that lacked a necessary gene for prion production – thus theoretically making them immune to BSE.

In April 2012, some South Korean retailers ceased importing beef from the United States after a case of BSE was reported. Indonesia also suspended imports of beef from the US after a dairy cow with mad cow disease was discovered in California.

Japan

With 36 confirmed cases, Japan experienced one of the largest number of cases of BSE outside Europe. It was the only country outside Europe and the Americas to report non-imported cases. Reformation of food safety in the light of the BSE cases resulted in the establishment of a governmental Food Safety Commission in 2003.

Britain

Cattle are naturally herbivores, eating grasses. In modern industrial cattle-farming, though, various commercial feeds are used, which may contain ingredients including antibiotics, hormones, pesticides, fertilizers, and protein supplements. The use of meat and bone meal, produced from the ground and cooked leftovers of the slaughtering process, as well as from the carcasses of sick and injured animals such as cattle or sheep, as a protein supplement in cattle feed was widespread in Europe prior to about 1987. Worldwide, soybean meal is the primary plant-based protein supplement fed to cattle. However, soybeans do not grow well in Europe, so cattle raisers throughout Europe turned to the cheaper animal byproduct feeds as an alternative. The British Inquiry dismissed suggestions that changes to processing might have increased the infectious agents in cattle feed, saying, "changes in process could not have been solely responsible for the emergence of BSE, and changes in regulation were not a factor at all." (The prion causing BSE is not destroyed by heat treatment.)

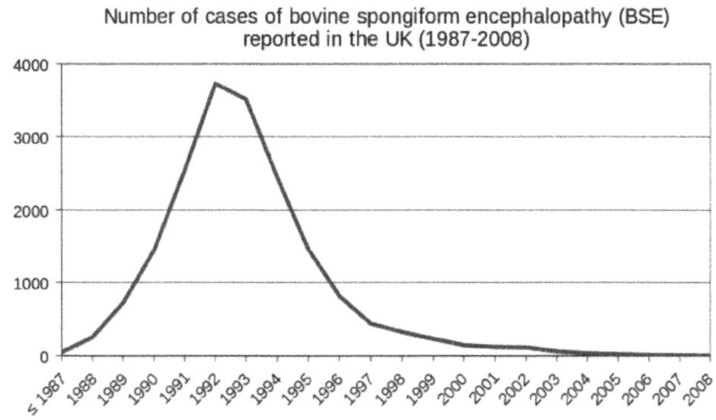

Evolution of the Bovine spongiform encephalopathy (BSE) in UK.

The first confirmed instance in which an animal fell ill with the disease occurred in 1986 in the United Kingdom, and lab tests the following year indicated the presence of BSE; by November 1987, the British Ministry of Agriculture accepted it had a new disease on its hands. Subsequently, 177 people (as of June 2014) contracted and died of a disease with similar neurological symptoms subsequently called (new) variant Creutzfeldt–Jakob disease (vCJD). This is a separate disease from 'classical' Creutzfeldt–Jakob disease, which is not related to BSE and has been known about since the early 1900s. Three cases of vCJD occurred in people who had lived in or visited the UK – one each in the Republic of Ireland, Canada, and the United States of America. Also, some concern existed about those who work with (and therefore inhale) cattle meat and bone meal, such as horticulturists, who use it as fertilizer. Up-to-date statistics on all types of CJD are published by the National Creutzfeldt–Jakob Disease Surveillance Unit in Edinburgh, Scotland.

For many of the vCJD patients, direct evidence exists that they had consumed tainted beef, and this is assumed to be the mechanism by which all affected individuals contracted it. Disease incidence also appears to correlate with slaughtering practices that led to the mixture of nervous system tissue with ground meat (mince) and other beef. An estimated 400,000 cattle infected with BSE entered the human food chain in the 1980s. Although the BSE epizootic was eventually brought under control by culling all suspect cattle populations, people are still being diagnosed with vCJD each year (though the number of new cases currently has dropped to fewer than five per year). This is attributed to the long incubation period for prion diseases, which is typically measured in years or decades. As a result, the full extent of the human vCJD outbreak is still not known.

The scientific consensus is that infectious BSE prion material is not destroyed through cooking procedures, meaning that even contaminated beef foodstuffs prepared "well done" may remain infectious. In fact the infectious agent remains viable over 600 °C (about 1100 °F).

Alan Colchester, a professor of neurology at the University of Kent, and Nancy Colchester, writing in the 3 September 2005 issue of the medical journal *The Lancet*, proposed a theory that the most likely initial origin of BSE in the United Kingdom was the importation from the Indian Subcontinent of bone meal which contained CJD-infected human remains. The government of India vehemently responded to the research, calling it "misleading, highly mischievous; a figment of imagination; absurd," further adding that India maintained constant surveillance and had not had a single case of either BSE or vCJD. The authors responded in the 22 January 2006 issue of *The Lancet* that their theory is unprovable only in the same sense as all other BSE origin theories are and that the theory warrants further investigation.

During the course of the investigation into the BSE epizootic, an enquiry was also made into the activities of the Department of Health Medicines Control Agency (MCA). On 7 May 1999, David Osborne Hagger, a retired civil servant who worked in the Medicines Division of the Department of Health between 1984 and 1994, produced a written statement to the BSE Inquiry in which he gave an account of his professional experience of BSE.

In February 1989, the MCA had been asked to "identify relevant manufacturers and obtain information about the bovine material contained in children's vaccines, the stocks of these vaccines and how long it would take to switch to other products." In July, "[the] use of bovine insulin in a small group of mainly elderly patients was noted and it was recognised that alternative products for this group were not considered satisfactory." In September, the BSE Working Party of the Committee on the Safety of Medicines (CSM) recommended that "no licensing action is required at present in regard to products produced from bovine material or using prepared bovine brain in nutrient media and sourced from outside the United Kingdom, the Channel Isles and the Republic of Ireland provided that the country of origin is known to be free of BSE, has competent veterinary advisers and is known to practise good animal husbandry."

In 1990, the British Diabetic Association became concerned regarding the safety of bovine insulin. The CSM assured them "[that] there was no insulin sourced from cattle in the UK or Ireland and that the situation in other countries was being monitored."

In 1991, the European Commission "[expressed] concerns about the possible transmission of the BSE/scrapie agent to man through use of certain cosmetic treatments."

In 1992, sources in France reported to the MCA "that BSE had now been reported in France and there were some licensed surgical sutures derived from French bovine material." Concerns were also raised at a CSM meeting "regarding a possible risk of transmission of the BSE agent in gelatin products."

The Ban on British Beef

The BSE crisis led to the European Union banning exports of British beef with effect from March 1996; the ban lasted for 10 years before it was finally lifted on 1 May 2006 despite attempts in May 1996 by British prime minister John Major to get the ban lifted. The ban resulted in trade controversies between the UK and other EU states, dubbed "beef war" by media. Restrictions remained for beef containing "vertebral material" and for beef sold on the bone.

Russia was proceeding to lift the ban sometime after November 2012 after 16 years; the announcement was made during a visit by the UK's chief veterinary officer Nigel Gibbens.

It was successfully negotiated that beef from Wales was allowed to be exported to the Dutch market, which had formerly been an important market for Northern Irish beef. Of two approved export establishments in the United Kingdom in 1999, one was in Scotland – an establishment to which live beef was supplied from Northern Ireland. As the incidence of BSE was very low in Northern Ireland – only six cases of BSE by 1999 – partly due to the early adoption of an advanced herd tagging and computerization system in the region, calls were made to remove the EU ban on exports with regard to Northern Irish beef.

References

- Dewick, P.M. (2009). Medicinal Natural Products: A Biosynthetic Approach (3rd ed.). Wiley. pp. 122–4. ISBN 0470742798.
- Godish, Thad (2001). Indoor environmental quality. Chelsea, Mich: Lewis Publishers. pp. 183–4. ISBN 1-56670-402-2.
- Krull IS, Nunnally BK (2004). Prions and mad cow disease. New York, N.Y: Marcel Dekker. p. 6. ISBN 0-8247-4083-1.
- Robbins SL, Cotran RS, Kumar V, et al., eds. (1999). Robbins pathologic basis of disease. Philadelphia: Saunders. ISBN 0-7216-7335-X.
- Groschup MH, Kretzschmar HA, eds. (2001). Prion Diseases Diagnosis and Pathogeneis. Archives of Virology. Suppl 16. New York: Springer. ISBN 978-3-211-83530-2.
- Singh N, Das D, Singh A, Mohan ML (2010). "Prion Protein and Metal Interaction: Physiological and Pathological Implications". In Tatzelt J. The Prion Protein. Savanna Press. ISBN 978-0-9543335-2-2.
- Eddie Straiton, "Sheep Ailments - recognition and treatment", 7th edition (2001) ISBN 1-86126-397-X
- Synnøve Vatn, Lisbeth Hektoen, Ola Nafstad "Helse og Velferd hos sau" 1. utgave, Tun Forlag (2008) ISBN 978-82-529-3180-8
- Rampton, Sheldon; Stauber, John (2004). Mad Cow USA (1st ed.). Monroe, Maine: Common Courage Press. ISBN 978-1-56751-110-9.
- Beecher, Coockson (June 1, 2015). "Surprising' Discovery Made About Chronic Wasting Disease". Food Safety News. Retrieved 2016-04-08.
- Botsios S.; Manuelidis L. (2016). "CJD and Scrapie Require Agent-Associated Nucleic Acids for Infection". Journal of Cellular Biochemistry. doi:10.1002/jcb.25495. PMID 26773845.
- Botsios, Sotirios; Manuelidis, Laura (2016). "CJD and Scrapie Require Agent-Associated Nucleic Acids for Infection". Journal of Cellular Biochemistry. doi:10.1002/jcb.25495. PMID 26773845.
- "Bovine Spongiform Encephalopathy" (PDF). The Center for Food Security & Public Health. The Center for Food Security & Public Health. August 2016. Retrieved October 30, 2016.
- "Ataxias and Cerebellar or Spinocerebellar Degeneration Information Page: National Institute of Neurological Disorders and Stroke (NINDS)". www.ninds.nih.gov. Retrieved 2016-12-01.
- "Feed Bans BSE (Bovine Spongiform Encephalopathy) | Prion Diseases | CDC". www.cdc.gov. Retrieved 2016-09-30.
- Pritzkow, Sandra; Morales, Rodrigo; Moda, Fabio; et al. (May 26, 2015). "Grass Plants Bind, Retain, Uptake, and Transport Infectious Prions". Cell. 11 (8): 1168–1175. doi:10.1016/j.celrep.2015.04.036.
- Haley NJ, Hoover EA (2015). "Chronic wasting disease of cervids: current knowledge and future perspectives". Annu Rev Anim Biosci. 3: 305–25. doi:10.1146/annurev-animal-022114-111001. PMID 25387112.
- "Mad Cow in Canada: The science and the story". CBC News. 24 August 2006. Retrieved 20 January 2015.
- Murakami, T.; Ishiguro, N.; Higuchi, K. (2014). "Transmission of Systemic AA Amyloidosis in Animals". Veterinary Pathology. 51 (2): 363–71. doi:10.1177/0300985813511128. PMID 24280941.

- Bastian F (3 August 2014). "Striking a Nerve: Prions Not the Last Word in TSEs". MedPageToday.
- Xu H, He X, Zheng H, Huang LJ, Hou F, Yu Z, de la Cruz MJ, Borkowski B, Zhang X, Chen ZJ, Jiang QX (2014). "Structural basis for the prion-like MAVS filaments in antiviral innate immunity". eLife. 3: e01489. PMID 24569476.

3

Foodborne Disease and Related Pathogens

Foodborne illnesses are illnesses that are caused because of contaminated food. Symptoms of food illness are fever, vomiting and aches. Bacterias that cause infection are pathogenic bacteria, bacillus cereus, staphylococcal enteritis and vibrio vulnificus. The section on food illness offers an insightful focus, keeping in mind the subject matter.

Foodborne Illness

Foodborne illness (also foodborne disease and colloquially referred to as food poisoning) is any illness resulting from the food spoilage of contaminated food, pathogenic bacteria, viruses, or parasites that contaminate food, as well as chemical or natural toxins such as poisonous mushrooms and various species of beans that have not been boiled for at least 10 minutes.

Symptoms vary depending on the cause, and are described below in this section. A few broad generalizations can be made, e.g.: The incubation period ranges from hours to days, depending on the cause and on how much was consumed. The incubation period tends to cause sufferers to not associate the symptoms with the item consumed, and so to cause sufferers to attribute the symptoms to gastroenteritis for example. Symptoms often include vomiting, fever, and aches, and may include diarrhea. Bouts of vomiting can be repeated with an extended delay in between, because even if infected food was eliminated from the stomach in the first bout, microbes (if applicable) can pass through the stomach into the intestine via cells lining the intestinal walls and begin to multiply. Some types of microbes stay in the intestine, some produce a toxin that is absorbed into the bloodstream, and some can directly invade deeper body tissues.

Causes

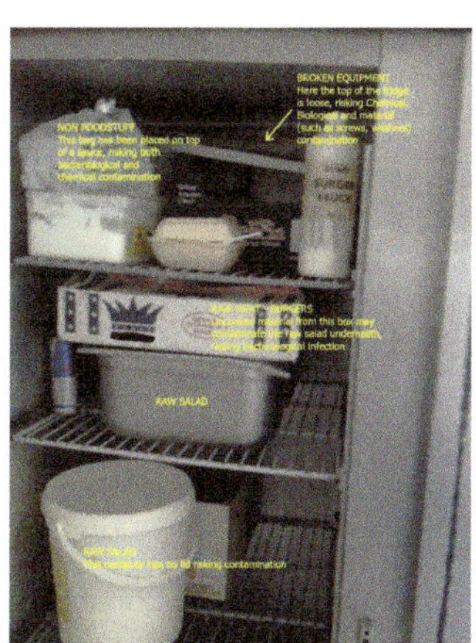

Poorly stored food in a refrigerator

Foodborne illness usually arises from improper handling, preparation, or food storage. Good hygiene practices before, during, and after food preparation can reduce the chances of contracting an illness. There is a consensus in the public health community that regular hand-washing is one of the most effective defenses against the spread of foodborne illness. The action of monitoring food to ensure that it will not cause foodborne illness is known as food safety. Foodborne disease can also be caused by a large variety of toxins that affect the environment.

Foodborne illness can also be caused by pesticides or medicines in food and naturally toxic substances such as poisonous mushrooms or reef fish.

Bacteria

Bacteria are a common cause of foodborne illness. In the United Kingdom during 2000, the individual bacteria involved were the following: *Campylobacter jejuni* 77.3%, *Salmonella* 20.9%, *Escherichia coli* O157:H7 1.4%, and all others less than 0.56%. In the past, bacterial infections were thought to be more prevalent because few places had the capability to test for norovirus and no active surveillance was being done for this particular agent. Toxins from bacterial infections are delayed because the bacteria need time to multiply. As a result, symptoms associated with intoxication are usually not seen until 12–72 hours or more after eating contaminated food. However, in some cases, such as Staphylococcal food poisoning, the onset of illness can be as soon as 30 minutes after ingesting contaminated food.

Most common bacterial foodborne pathogens are:

- *Campylobacter jejuni* which can lead to secondary Guillain–Barré syndrome and periodontitis
- *Clostridium perfringens*, the "cafeteria germ"
- *Salmonella* spp. – its *S. typhimurium* infection is caused by consumption of eggs or poultry that are not adequately cooked or by other interactive human-animal pathogens

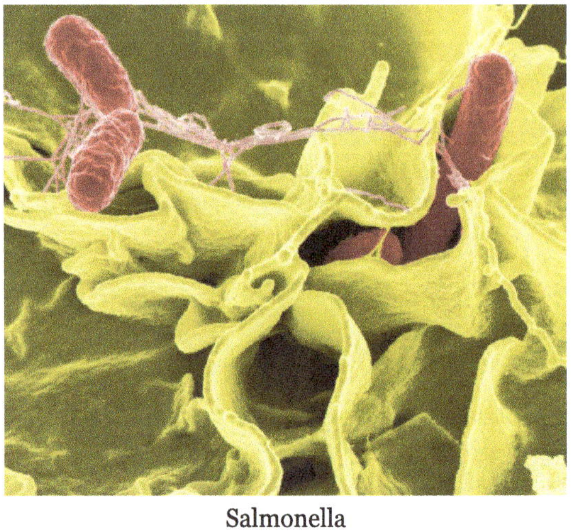

Salmonella

- *Escherichia coli O157:H7* enterohemorrhagic (EHEC) which can cause hemolytic-uremic syndrome

Other common bacterial foodborne pathogens are:

- *Bacillus cereus*
- *Escherichia coli*, other virulence properties, such as enteroinvasive (EIEC), enteropathogenic (EPEC), enterotoxigenic (ETEC), enteroaggregative (EAEC or EAgEC)
- *Listeria monocytogenes*
- *Shigella* spp.
- *Staphylococcus aureus*
- *Staphylococcal enteritis*
- *Streptococcus*
- *Vibrio cholerae*, including O1 and non-O1
- *Vibrio parahaemolyticus*
- *Vibrio vulnificus*
- *Yersinia enterocolitica* and *Yersinia pseudotuberculosis*

Less common bacterial agents:

- *Brucella* spp.
- *Corynebacterium ulcerans*
- *Coxiella burnetii* or Q fever
- *Plesiomonas shigelloides*

Enterotoxins

In addition to disease caused by direct bacterial infection, some foodborne illnesses are caused by enterotoxins (exotoxins targeting the intestines). Enterotoxins can produce illness even when the microbes that produced them have been killed. Symptom appearance varies with the toxin but may be rapid in onset, as in the case of enterotoxins of *Staphylococcus aureus* in which symptoms appear in one to six hours. This causes intense vomiting including or not including diarrhea (resulting in staphylococcal enteritis), and staphylococcal enterotoxins (most commonly staphylococcal enterotoxin A but also including staphylococcal enterotoxin B) are the most commonly reported enterotoxins although cases of poisoning are likely underestimated. It occurs mainly in cooked and processed foods due to competition with other biota in raw foods, and humans are the main cause of contamination as a substantial percentage of humans are persistent carriers of *S. aureus*. The CDC has estimated about 240,000 cases per year in the United States.

- *Clostridium botulinum*
- *Clostridium perfringens*
- *Bacillus cereus*

The rare but potentially deadly disease botulism occurs when the anaerobic bacterium *Clostridium botulinum* grows in improperly canned low-acid foods and produces botulin, a powerful paralytic toxin.

Pseudoalteromonas tetraodonis, certain species of Pseudomonas and Vibrio, and some other bacteria, produce the lethal tetrodotoxin, which is present in the tissues of some living animal species rather than being a product of decomposition.

Emerging Foodborne Pathogens

Many foodborne illnesses remain poorly understood.

- *Aeromonas hydrophila, Aeromonas caviae, Aeromonas sobria*

Preventing Bacterial Food Poisoning

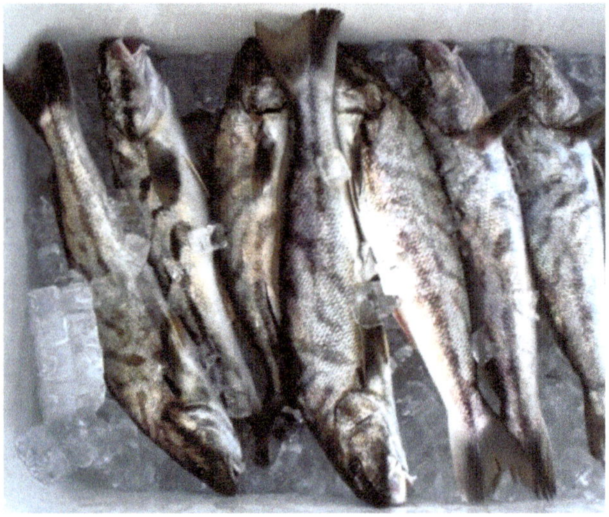

Proper storage and refrigeration of food help in the prevention of food poisoning

Prevention is mainly the role of the state, through the definition of strict rules of hygiene and a public services of veterinary surveying of animal products in the food chain, from farming to the transformation industry and delivery (shops and restaurants). This regulation includes:

- traceability: in a final product, it must be possible to know the origin of the ingredients (originating farm, identification of the harvesting or of the animal) and where and when it was processed; the origin of the illness can thus be tracked and solved (and possibly penalized), and the final products can be removed from the sale if a problem is detected;
- enforcement of hygiene procedures such as HACCP and the "cold chain";
- power of control and of law enforcement of veterinarians.

In August 2006, the United States Food and Drug Administration approved Phage therapy which involves spraying meat with viruses that infect bacteria, and thus preventing infection. This has raised concerns, because without mandatory labelling consumers would not be aware that meat and poultry products have been treated with the spray.

At home, prevention mainly consists of good food safety practices. Many forms of bacterial poisoning can be prevented by cooking it sufficiently, and either eating it quickly or refrigerating it effectively. Many toxins, however, are not destroyed by heat treatment.

Techniques that help prevent food borne illness in the kitchen are hand washing, rinsing produce, preventing cross-contamination, proper storage, and maintaining cooking temperatures. In general, freezing or refrigerating prevents virtually all bacteria from growing, and heating food sufficiently kills parasites, viruses, and most bacteria. Bacteria grow most rapidly at the range of temperatures between 40 °F and 140 °F, called the "danger zone". Storing food below or above the "danger zone" can effectively limit the production of toxins. For storing leftovers, the food must be put in shallow containers for quick cooling and must be refrigerated within two hours. When food is reheated, it must reach an internal temperature of 165 °F (74 °C) or until hot or steaming to kill bacteria.

Mycotoxins and Alimentary Mycotoxicoses

The term alimentary mycotoxicoses refers to the effect of poisoning by Mycotoxins (The term 'mycotoxin' is usually reserved for the toxic chemical products produced by fungi that readily colonize crops) through food consumption. Mycotoxins sometimes have important effects on human and animal health. For example, an outbreak which occurred in the UK in 1960 caused the death of 100,000 turkeys which had consumed aflatoxin-contaminated peanut meal. In the USSR in World War II, 5,000 people died due to Alimentary Toxic Aleukia (ALA). The common foodborne Mycotoxins include:

- Aflatoxins – originated from Aspergillus parasiticus and Aspergillus flavus. They are frequently found in tree nuts, peanuts, maize, sorghum and other oilseeds, including corn and cottonseeds. The pronounced forms of Aflatoxins are those of B1, B2, G1, and G2, amongst which Aflatoxin B1 predominantly targets the liver, which will result in necrosis, cirrhosis, and carcinoma. In the US, the acceptable level of total aflatoxins in foods is less than 20 μg/kg, except for Aflatoxin M1 in milk, which should be less than 0.5 μg/kg. The official document can be found at FDA's website.
- Altertoxins – are those of Alternariol (AOH), Alternariol methyl ether (AME), Altenuene (ALT), Altertoxin-1 (ATX-1), Tenuazonic acid (TeA) and Radicinin (RAD), originated from Alternaria spp. Some of the toxins can be present in sorghum, ragi, wheat and tomatoes. Some research has shown that the toxins can be easily cross-contaminated between grain commodities, suggesting that manufacturing and storage of grain commodities is a critical practice.
- Citrinin
- Citreoviridin
- Cyclopiazonic acid
- Cytochalasins
- Ergot alkaloids / Ergopeptine alkaloids – Ergotamine
- Fumonisins – Crop corn can be easily contaminated by the fungi Fusarium moniliforme,

and its Fumonisin B1 will cause Leukoencephalomalacia (LEM) in horses, Pulmonary edema syndrome (PES) in pigs, liver cancer in rats and Esophageal cancer in humans. For human and animal health, both the FDA and the EC have regulated the content levels of toxins in food and animal feed.

- Fusaric acid
- Fusarochromanone
- Kojic acid
- Lolitrem alkaloids
- Moniliformin
- 3-Nitropropionic acid
- Nivalenol
- Ochratoxins – In Australia, The Limit of Reporting (LOR) level for Ochratoxin A (OTA) analyses in 20th Australian Total Diet Survey was 1 μg/kg, whereas the EC restricts the content of OTA to 5 μg/kg in cereal commodities, 3 μg/kg in processed products and 10 μg/kg in dried vine fruits.
- Oosporeine
- Patulin – Currently, this toxin has been advisably regulated on fruit products. The EC and the FDA have limited it to under 50 μg/kg for fruit juice and fruit nectar, while limits of 25 μg/kg for solid-contained fruit products and 10 μg/kg for baby foods were specified by the EC.
- Phomopsins
- Sporidesmin A
- Sterigmatocystin
- Tremorgenic mycotoxins – Five of them have been reported to be associated with molds found in fermented meats. These are Fumitremorgen B, Paxilline, Penitrem A, Verrucosidin, and Verruculogen.
- Trichothecenes – sourced from Cephalosporium, Fusarium, Myrothecium, Stachybotrys and Trichoderma. The toxins are usually found in molded maize, wheat, corn, peanuts and rice, or animal feed of hay and straw. Four trichothecenes, T-2 toxin, HT-2 toxin, diacetoxyscirpenol (DAS) and deoxynivalenol (DON) have been most commonly encountered by humans and animals. The consequences of oral intake of, or dermal exposure to, the toxins will result in Alimentary toxic aleukia, neutropenia, aplastic anemia, thrombocytopenia and/or skin irritation. In 1993, the FDA issued a document for the content limits of DON in food and animal feed at an advisory level. In 2003, US published a patent that is very promising for farmers to produce a trichothecene-resistant crop.
- Zearalenone

- Zearalenols

Viruses

Viral infections make up perhaps one third of cases of food poisoning in developed countries. In the US, more than 50% of cases are viral and noroviruses are the most common foodborne illness, causing 57% of outbreaks in 2004. Foodborne viral infection are usually of intermediate (1–3 days) incubation period, causing illnesses which are self-limited in otherwise healthy individuals; they are similar to the bacterial forms described above.

- Enterovirus
- Hepatitis A is distinguished from other viral causes by its prolonged (2–6 week) incubation period and its ability to spread beyond the stomach and intestines into the liver. It often results in jaundice, or yellowing of the skin, but rarely leads to chronic liver dysfunction. The virus has been found to cause infection due to the consumption of fresh-cut produce which has fecal contamination.
- Hepatitis E
- Norovirus
- Rotavirus

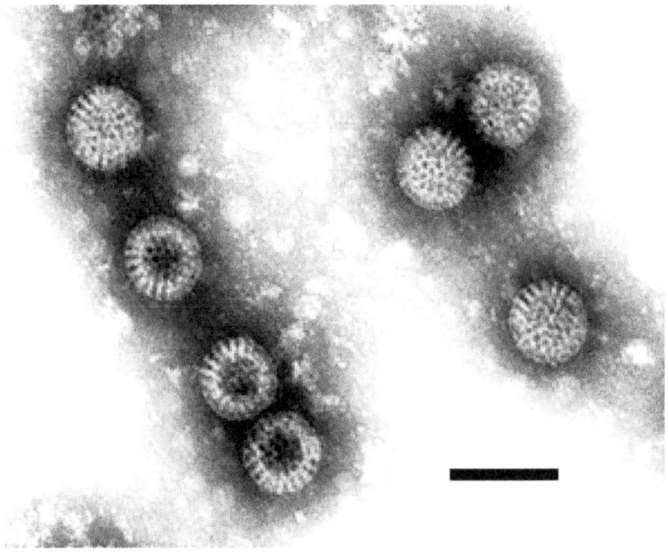

Rotavirus

Parasites

Most foodborne parasites are zoonoses.

- Platyhelminthes:
  - *Diphyllobothrium* sp.
  - *Nanophyetus* sp.

  - *Taenia saginata*
  - *Taenia solium*
  - *Fasciola hepatica*
- Nematode:
  - *Anisakis* sp.
  - *Ascaris lumbricoides*
  - *Eustrongylides* sp.
  - *Trichinella spiralis*
  - *Trichuris trichiura*
- Protozoa:
  - *Acanthamoeba* and other free-living amoebae
  - *Cryptosporidium parvum*
  - *Cyclospora cayetanensis*
  - *Entamoeba histolytica*
  - *Giardia lamblia*

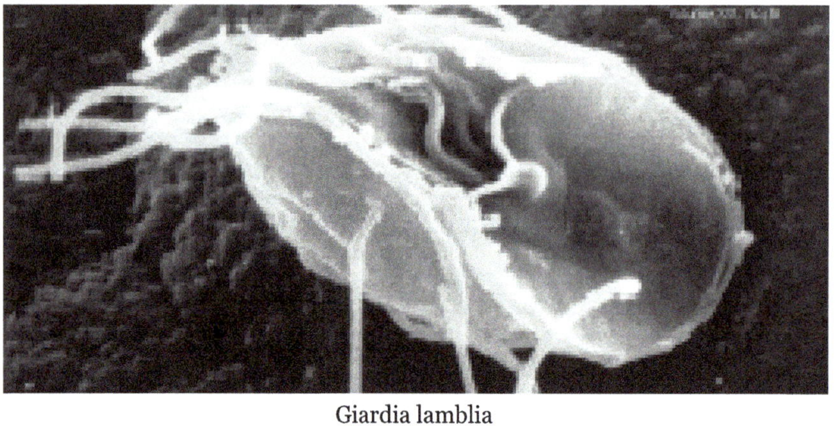

Giardia lamblia

  - *Sarcocystis hominis*
  - *Sarcocystis suihominis*
  - *Toxoplasma gondii*

Natural Toxins

Several foods can naturally contain toxins, many of which are not produced by bacteria. Plants in particular may be toxic; animals which are naturally poisonous to eat are rare. In evolutionary terms, animals can escape being eaten by fleeing; plants can use only passive defenses such as poisons and distasteful substances, for example capsaicin in chili peppers and pungent sulfur compounds in garlic and onions. Most animal poisons are not synthesised by the animal, but acquired by eating poisonous plants to which the animal is immune, or by bacterial action.

- Alkaloids
- Ciguatera poisoning
- Grayanotoxin (honey intoxication)
- Mushroom toxins
- Phytohaemagglutinin (red kidney bean poisoning; destroyed by boiling)
- Pyrrolizidine alkaloids
- Shellfish toxin, including paralytic shellfish poisoning, diarrhetic shellfish poisoning, neurotoxic shellfish poisoning, amnesic shellfish poisoning and ciguatera fish poisoning
- Scombrotoxin
- Tetrodotoxin (fugu fish poisoning)

Some plants contain substances which are toxic in large doses, but have therapeutic properties in appropriate dosages.

- Foxglove contains cardiac glycosides.
- Poisonous hemlock (conium) has medicinal uses.

Other Pathogenic Agents

- Prions, resulting in Creutzfeldt–Jakob disease

"Ptomaine Poisoning"

In 1883, the Italian professor Salmi, of Bologna, introduced the generic name *ptomaine* for alkaloids found in decaying animal and vegetable matter, especially (as reflected in their names) putrescine and cadaverine. The 1892 *Merck's Bulletin* stated, "We name such products of bacterial origin ptomaines; and the special alkaloid produced by the comma bacillus is variously named Cadaverine, Putrescine, etc." While *The Lancet* stated, "The chemical ferments produced in the system, the...ptomaines which may exercise so disastrous an influence." It is now known that the "disastrous...influence" is due to the direct action of bacteria and only slightly to the alkaloids. Thus, the use of the phrase "ptomaine poisoning" is now obsolete.

Tainted potato salad sickening hundreds at a Communist political convention in Massillon, Ohio, and aboard a Washington DC cruise boat in separate incidents during a single week in 1932 drew national attention to the dangers of so-called "ptomaine poisoning" in the pages of the American news weekly, *Time*. Another newspaper article from 1944 told of more than 150 persons being hospitalized in Chicago with ptomaine poisoning apparently from rice pudding served by a chain of restaurants.

Mechanism

Incubation Period

The delay between consumption of a contaminated food and appearance of the first symptoms of illness is called the incubation period. This ranges from hours to days (and rarely months or even years, such as in the case of listeriosis or bovine spongiform encephalopathy), depending on the agent, and on how much was consumed. If symptoms occur within one to six hours after eating the food, it suggests that it is caused by a bacterial toxin or a chemical rather than live bacteria.

The long incubation period of many foodborne illnesses tends to cause sufferers to attribute their symptoms to gastroenteritis.

During the incubation period, microbes pass through the stomach into the intestine, attach to the cells lining the intestinal walls, and begin to multiply there. Some types of microbes stay in the intestine, some produce a toxin that is absorbed into the bloodstream, and some can directly invade the deeper body tissues. The symptoms produced depend on the type of microbe.

Infectious Dose

The infectious dose is the amount of agent that must be consumed to give rise to symptoms of foodborne illness, and varies according to the agent and the consumer's age and overall health. Pathogens vary in minimum infectious dose; for example, *Shigella sonnei* has a low estimated minimum dose of < 500 colony-forming units (CFU) while *Staphylococcus aureus* has a relatively high estimate.

In the case of *Salmonella* a relatively large inoculum of 1 million to 1 billion organisms is necessary to produce symptoms in healthy human volunteers, as *Salmonellae* are very sensitive to acid. An unusually high stomach pH level (low acidity) greatly reduces the number of bacteria required to cause symptoms by a factor of between 10 and 100.

Epidemiology

Asymptomatic subclinical infection may help spread these diseases, particularly *Staphylococcus aureus, Campylobacter, Salmonella, Shigella, V. cholerae,* and *Yersini*. For example, as of 1984 it was estimated that in the United States, 200,000 people were asymptomatic carriers of Salmonella.

United States

In the United States, using FoodNet data from 2000–2007, the CDCP estimated there were 47.8 million foodborne illnesses per year (16,000 cases for 100,000 inhabitants) with 9.4 million of these caused by 31 known identified pathogens.

- 127,839 were hospitalized (43 per 100,000 inhabitants per year).
- 3,037 people died (1.0 per 100,000 inhabitants per year).

Causes of foodborne illness in U. S.			
	Cause	**Annual cases**	**Rate (per 100,000 inhabitants)**
1	*Norovirus*	5,461,731 cases	X
2	*Salmonella*	1,027,561 cases	X
3	*Clostridium perfringens*	965,958 cases	X
4	Campylobacter	845,024 cases	X

Causes of death by foodborne illness in U. S.			
	Cause	**Annual deaths**	**Rate (per 100,000 inhabitants)**
1	*Salmonella*	378 cases	0.126
2	*Toxoplasma gondii*	327 cases	0.109
3	*Listeria*	255 cases	0.085
4	*Norovirus*	149 cases	0.050

France

This data pertains to reported medical cases of 23 specific pathogens, as opposed to total population estimates of all food-borne illness for the United States.

In France, for 750,000 cases (1210 per 100,000 inhabitants):

- 70,000 people consulted in the emergency department of an hospital (113 per 100,000 inhabitants.);
- 113,000 people were hospitalized (182 per 100,000 inhabitants);
- 460 people died (0.75 per 100,000 inhabitants).

Causes of foodborne illness in France			
	Cause	**Annual hospitalizations**	**Rate (per 100,000 inhabitants)**
1	*Salmonella*	~8,000 cases	13
2	*Campylobacter*	~3,000 cases	4.8
3	Parasites incl. Toxoplasma	~500 cases ~400 cases	0.8 0.65
4	*Listeria*	~300 cases	0.5
5	Hepatitis A	~60 cases	0.1

Causes of death by foodborne illness in France			
	Cause	**Annual**	**Rate (per 100,000 inhabitants)**
1	*Salmonella*	~300 cases	0.5
2	*Listeria*	~80 cases	0.13
3	Parasites	~37 cases	0.06 (95% due to toxoplasma)
4	*Campylobacter*	~15 cases	0.02
5	Hepatitis A	~2 cases	0.003

Australia

A study by the Australian National University, published in November 2014, found in 2010 that there were an estimated 4.1 million cases of foodborne gastroenteritis acquired in Australia on average each year, along with 5,140 cases of non-gastrointestinal illness. The study was funded by the Australian Department of Health, Food Standards Australia New Zealand and the NSW Food Authority.

The main causes were Norovirus, pathogenic Escherichia coli, Campylobacter spp. and non-typhoidal Salmonella spp., although the causes of approximately 80% of illnesses were unknown. Approximately 25% (90% CrI: 13%–42%) of the 15.9 million episodes of gastroenteritis that occur in Australia were estimated to be transmitted by contaminated food. This equates to an average of approximately one episode of foodborne gastroenteritis every five years per person. Data on the number of hospitalisations and deaths represent the occurrence of serious foodborne illness. Including gastroenteritis, non-gastroenteritis and sequelae, there were an estimated annual 31,920 (90% CrI: 29,500–35,500) hospitalisations due to foodborne illness and 86 (90% CrI: 70–105) deaths due to foodborne illness circa 2010. This study concludes that these rates are similar to recent estimates in the US and Canada.

A main aim of this study was to compare if foodborne illness incidence had increased over time. In this study, similar methods of assessment were applied to data from circa 2000, which showed that the rate of foodborne gastroenteritis had not changed significantly over time. Two key estimates were the total number of gastroenteritis episodes each year, and the proportion considered foodborne. In circa 2010, it was estimated that 25% of all episodes of gastroenteritis were foodborne. By applying this proportion of episodes due to food to the incidence of gastroenteritis circa 2000, there were an estimated 4.3 million (90% CrI: 2.2–7.3 million) episodes of foodborne gastroenteritis circa 2000, although credible intervals overlap with 2010. Taking into account changes in population size, applying these equivalent methods suggests a 17% decrease in the rate of foodborne gastroenteritis between 2000 and 2010, with considerable overlap of the 90% credible intervals.

This study replaces a previous estimate of 5.4 million cases of food-borne illness in Australia every year, causing:

- 18,000 hospitalizations
- 120 deaths (0.5 deaths per 100,000 inhabitants)
- 2.1 million lost days off work
- 1.2 million doctor consultations
- 300,000 prescriptions for antibiotics.

Most foodborne disease outbreaks in Australia have been linked to raw or minimally cooked eggs or poultry. The Australian Food Safety Information Council estimates that one third of cases of food poisoning occur in the home

Comparison between Countries

Country	Annual deaths per 100,000 inhabitants	Annual hospitalization per 100,000 inhabitants
USA	1.0	43
France	0.75	182
Australia	0.5	82

Outbreaks

The vast majority of reported cases of foodborne illness occur as individual or sporadic cases. The origin of most sporadic cases is undetermined. In the United States, where people eat outside the home frequently, 58% of cases originate from commercial food facilities (2004 FoodNet data). An outbreak is defined as occurring when two or more people experience similar illness after consuming food from a common source.

Often, a combination of events contributes to an outbreak, for example, food might be left at room temperature for many hours, allowing bacteria to multiply which is compounded by inadequate cooking which results in a failure to kill the dangerously elevated bacterial levels.

Outbreaks are usually identified when those affected know each other. However, more and more, outbreaks are identified by public health staff from unexpected increases in laboratory results for certain strains of bacteria. Outbreak detection and investigation in the United States is primarily handled by local health jurisdictions and is inconsistent from district to district. It is estimated that 1–2% of outbreaks are detected.

Society and Culture

United Kingdom

In postwar Aberdeen (1964) a large-scale (>400 cases) outbreak of typhoid occurred, caused by contaminated corned beef which had been imported from Argentina. The corned beef was placed in cans and because the cooling plant had failed, cold river water from the Plate estuary was used to cool the cans. One of the cans had a defect and the meat inside was contaminated. This meat was then sliced using a meat slicer in a shop in Aberdeen, and a lack of cleaning the machinery led to spreading the contamination to other meats cut in the slicer. These meats were then eaten by the people of Aberdeen who then became ill.

Serious outbreaks of foodborne illness since the 1970s prompted key changes in UK food safety law. These included the death of 19 patients in the Stanley Royd Hospital outbreak and the bovine spongiform encephalopathy (BSE, mad cow disease) outbreak identified in the 1980s. The death of 17 people in the 1996 Wishaw outbreak of *E. coli* O157 was a precursor to the establishment of the Food Standards Agency which, according to Tony Blair in the 1998 white paper *A Force for Change* Cm 3830, "would be powerful, open and dedicated to the interests of consumers".

In May 2015, for the second year running, England's Food Standards Agency devoted its annual Food Safety Week to – "The Chicken Challenge". The focus was on the handling of raw chicken in the home and in catering facilities in a drive to reduce the worryingly high levels of food poisoning from the *campylobacter* bacterium. Anne Hardy argues that widespread public education of food hygiene can be useful, particularly through media (T.V cookery programmes) and advertisement. She points to the examples set by Scandinavian societies.

United States

In 2001, the Center for Science in the Public Interest petitioned the United States Department of Agriculture to require meat packers to remove spinal cords before processing cattle carcasses for human consumption, a measure designed to lessen the risk of infection by variant Creutzfeldt–Jakob disease. The petition was supported by the American Public Health Association, the Consumer

Federation of America, the Government Accountability Project, the National Consumers League, and Safe Tables Our Priority. This was opposed by the National Cattlemen's Beef Association, the National Renderers Association, the National Meat Association, the Pork Producers Council, sheep raisers, milk producers, the Turkey Federation, and eight other organizations from the animal-derived food industry.

None of the US Department of Health and Human Services targets regarding incidence of foodborne infections were reached in 2007.

Organizations

The World Health Organization Department of Food Safety and Zoonoses (FOS) provides scientific advice for organizations and the public on issues concerning the safety of food. Its mission is to lower the burden of foodborne disease, thereby strengthening the health security and sustainable development of Member States. Foodborne and waterborne diarrhoeal diseases kill an estimated 2.2 million people annually, most of whom are children. WHO works closely with the Food and Agriculture Organization of the United Nations (FAO) to address food safety issues along the entire food production chain—from production to consumption—using new methods of risk analysis. These methods provide efficient, science-based tools to improve food safety, thereby benefiting both public health and economic development.

International Food Safety Authorities Network (INFOSAN)

The International Food Safety Authorities Network (INFOSAN) is a joint program of the WHO and FAO. INFOSAN has been connecting national authorities from around the globe since 2004, with the goal of preventing the international spread of contaminated food and foodborne disease and strengthening food safety systems globally. This is done by:

1. Promoting the rapid exchange of information during food safety events;
2. Sharing information on important food safety issues of global interest;
3. Promoting partnership and collaboration between countries; and
4. Helping countries strengthen their capacity to manage food safety risks.

Membership to INFOSAN is voluntary, but is restricted to representatives from national and regional government authorities and requires an official letter of designation. INFOSAN seeks to reflect the multidisciplinary nature of food safety and promote intersectoral collaboration by requesting the designation of Focal Points in each of the respective national authorities with a stake in food safety, and a single Emergency Contact Point in the national authority with the responsibility for coordinating national food safety emergencies; countries choosing to be members of INFOSAN are committed to sharing information between their respective food safety authorities and other INFOSAN members. The operational definition of a food safety authority includes those authorities involved in: food policy; risk assessment; food control and management; food inspection services; foodborne disease surveillance and response; laboratory services for monitoring and surveillance of foods and foodborne diseases; and food safety information, education and communication across the farm-to-table continuum.

Regulatory Steps

Food may be contaminated during all stages of food production and retailing. In order to prevent viral contamination, regulatory authorities in Europe have enacted several measures:

- European Commission Regulation (EC) No 2073/2005 of November 15, 2005
- European Committee for Standardization (CEN): Standard method for the detection of norovirus and hepatitis A virus in food products (shellfish, fruits and vegetables, surfaces and bottled water)
- CODEX Committee on Food Hygiene (CCFH): Guideline for the application of general principles of food hygiene for the control of viruses in food

Pathogenic Bacteria

Pathogenic bacteria are bacteria that can cause infection.

Although most bacteria are harmless or often beneficial, several are pathogenic. One of the bacterial diseases with the highest disease burden is tuberculosis, caused by the bacterium *Mycobacterium tuberculosis*, which kills about 2 million people a year, mostly in sub-Saharan Africa. Pathogenic bacteria contribute to other globally important diseases, such as pneumonia, which can be caused by bacteria such as *Streptococcus* and *Pseudomonas*, and foodborne illnesses, which can be caused by bacteria such as *Shigella*, *Campylobacter*, and *Salmonella*. Pathogenic bacteria also cause infections such as tetanus, typhoid fever, diphtheria, syphilis, and leprosy. Pathogenic bacteria are also the cause of high infant mortality rates in developing countries.

Koch's postulates are the standard to establish a causative relationship between a microbe and a disease.

Diseases

Each species has specific effect and causes symptoms in people who are infected. Some, if not most people who are infected with a pathogenic bacteria do not have symptoms. Immuno-compromised individuals are more susceptible to pathogenic bacteria.

Pathogenic Susceptibility

Some pathogenic bacteria cause disease under certain conditions, such entry through the skin via a cut, through sexual activity or an compromised immune function.

Streptococcus and *Staphylococcus* are part of the normal skin microbiota and typically reside on healthy skin or in the nasopharangeal region. Yet these species can potentially initiate skin infections. They are also able to cause sepsis, pneumonia, meningitis. These infections can become quite serious creating a systemic inflammatory response resulting in massive vasodilation, shock, and death.

Other bacteria are opportunistic pathogens and cause disease mainly in people suffering from immunosuppression or cystic fibrosis Examples of these opportunistic pathogens include *Pseudomonas aeruginosa, Burkholderia cenocepacia,* and *Mycobacterium avium.*

Intracellular

Obligate intracellular parasites (e.g. Chlamydophila, Ehrlichia, Rickettsia) have the ability to only grow and replicate inside other cells. Even these intracellular infections may be asymptomatic, requiring an incubation period. An example of this *Rickettsia* which causes typhus. Another causes Rocky Mountain spotted fever.

Chlamydia is a phylum of intracellular parasites. These pathogens can cause pneumonia or urinary tract infection and may be involved in coronary heart disease.

Other groups of intracellular bacterial pathogens include: *Salmonella, Neisseria, Brucella, Mycobacterium, Nocardia, Listeria, Francisella, Legionella,* and *Yersinia pestis.* These can exist intracellularly, but can exist outside of host cells.

Infections in Specific Tissue

Bacterial pathogens often cause infection in specific areas of the body. Others are generalists.

- Bacterial vaginosis is caused by bacteria that change the vaginal microbiota caused by an overgrowth of bacteria that crowd out the Lactobacilli species that maintain healthy vaginal microbial populations.
- Other non-bacterial vaginal infections include: yeast infection (candidiasis), *Trichomonas vaginalis* (trichomoniasis).
- Bacterial meningitis is a bacterial inflammation of the meninges, that is, the protective membranes covering the brain and spinal cord.
- Bacterial pneumonia is a bacterial infection of the lungs.
- Urinary tract infection is predominantly caused by bacteria. Symptoms include the strong and frequent sensation or urge to urinate, pain during urination, and urine that is cloudy. The main causal agent is *Escherichia coli.* Urine is typically sterile but contains a variety of salts, and waste products. Bacteria can ascend into the bladder or kidney and causing cystitis and nephritis.
- Bacterial gastroenteritis is caused by enteric, pathogenic bacteria. These pathogenic species are usually distinct from the usually harmless bacteria of the normal gut flora. But a different strain of the same species may be pathogenic. The distinction is sometimes difficult as in the case of *Escherichia.*
- Bacterial skin infections include:
    - Impetigo is a highly contagious bacterial skin infection commonly seen in children. It is caused by *Staphylococcus aureus,* and *Streptococcus pyogenes.*
    - Erysipelas is an acute streptococcus bacterial infection of the deeper skin layers that spreads via with lymphatic system.

- Cellulitis is a diffuse inflammation of connective tissue with severe inflammation of dermal and subcutaneous layers of the skin. Cellulitis can be caused by normal skin flora or by contagious contact, and usually occurs through open skin, cuts, blisters, cracks in the skin, insect bites, animal bites, burns, surgical wounds, intravenous drug injection, or sites of intravenous catheter insertion. In most cases it is the skin on the face or lower legs that is affected, though cellulitis can occur in other tissues.

Mechanisms

Nutrients

Iron is required for humans, as well as the growth of most bacteria. To obtain free iron, some pathogens secrete proteins called siderophores, which take the iron away from iron-transport proteins by binding to the iron even more tightly. Once the iron-siderophore complex is formed, it is taken up by siderophore receptors on the bacterial surface and then that iron is brought into the bacterium.

Direct Damage

Once pathogens attach to host cells, they can cause direct damage as the pathogens use the host cell for nutrients and produce waste products. As pathogens multiply and divide inside host cells, the cells usually rupture and the intercellular bacteria are released. Some bacteria such as *E. coli*, *Shigella*, *Salmonella*, and *Neisseria gonorrhoeae*, can induce host epithelial cells to engulf them in a process resembling phagocytosis. The pathogens can then disrupt host cells as they pass through them and be extruded from host cells by a reverse phagocytosis process, enabling them to enter other host cells. Some bacteria can also penetrate host cells by excreting enzymes and by their own motility; such penetration can itself damage the host cell.

Toxin Production

Toxins are poisonous substances that are produced by certain microorganisms and are often the primary factor contributing to the pathogenic properties of the microorganisms. Endotoxins are the lipid portions of lipopolysaccharides that are part of the outer membrane of the cell wall of gram negative bacteria. Endotoxins are released when the bacteria lyses, which is why after antibiotic treatment symptoms can at first worsen as the bacteria are killed and they release their endotoxins. Exotoxins are proteins produced inside pathogenic bacteria as part of their growth and metabolism, most common in gram positive bacteria. The exotoxins are released when the bacteria die and the cell wall breaks apart. Exotoxins are highly specific in the effects on body tissues and work by destroying particular parts of the host cell or by inhibiting certain metabolic functions. Exotoxins are among the most lethal known substances, only 1 mg of the botulinum exotoxin is enough to kill one million guinea pigs. Diseases caused this way are often caused by minute amounts of exotoxins, not by the bacteria themselves.

Identification

Typically identification is done by growing the organism in a wide range of cultures which can take up to 48 hours. The growth is then visually or genomically identified. The cultured organism is then subjected to antibiotics to observe reaction to help further identify species and strain.

Treatment

Bacterial infections may be treated with antibiotics, which are classified as bacteriocidal if they kill bacteria or bacteriostatic if they just prevent bacterial growth. There are many types of antibiotics and each class inhibits a process that is different in the pathogen from that found in the host. For example, the antibiotics chloramphenicol and tetracyclin inhibit the bacterial ribosome but not the structurally different eukaryotic ribosome, so they exhibit selective toxicity. Antibiotics are used both in treating human disease and in intensive farming to promote animal growth. Both uses may be contributing to the rapid development of antibiotic resistance in bacterial populations. Phage therapy can also be used to treat certain bacterial infections. Infections can be prevented by antiseptic measures such as sterilizing the skin prior to piercing it with the needle of a syringe and by proper care of indwelling catheters. Surgical and dental instruments are also sterilized to prevent infection by bacteria. Disinfectants such as bleach are used to kill bacteria or other pathogens on surfaces to prevent contamination and further reduce the risk of infection. Bacteria in food are killed by cooking to temperatures above 73 °C (163 °F).

List of Genera of Pathogenic Bacteria and Microscopy Features

Many genera contain pathogenic bacteria species. They often possess characteristics that help to classify and organize them into groups. The following is a partial listing.

Genus	Species	Gram staining	Shape	Oxygen requirement	Intra/ Extracellular
Bacillus	• *Bacillus anthracis* • *Bacillus cereus*	Positive	Rods	Facultative anaerobic	Extracellular
Bartonella	• *Bartonella henselae* • *Bartonella quintana*	Negative	Rods	Aerobic	Facultative intracellular
Bordetella	• *Bordetella pertussis*	Negative	Small coccobacilli	Aerobic	Extracellular
Borrelia	• *Borrelia burgdorferi* • *Borrelia garinii* • *Borrelia afzelii* • *Borrelia recurrentis*	Negative, stains poorly	spirochete	Anaerobic	Extracellular
Brucella	• *Brucella abortus* • *Brucella canis* • *Brucella melitensis* • *Brucella suis*	Negative	coccobacilli	Aerobic	Intracellular
Campylobacter	• *Campylobacter jejuni*	Negative	Spirochete Bacillus	microaerophilic	extracellular
Chlamydia and *Chlamydophila*	• *Chlamydia pneumoniae* • *Chlamydia trachomatis* • *Chlamydophila psittaci*	(not Gram-stained)	Small, round, ovoid	Facultative or strictly aerobic	Obligate intracellular
Clostridium	• *Clostridium botulinum* • *Clostridium difficile* • *Clostridium perfringens* • *Clostridium tetani*	Positive	Large, blunt-ended rods	Obligate anaerobic	extracellular
Corynebacterium	• *Corynebacterium diphtheriae*	Positive (unevenly)	bacilli	Mostly facultative anaerobic	extracellular
Enterococcus	• *Enterococcus faecalis* • *Enterococcus faecium*	Positive	Cocci	Facultative Anaerobic	extracellular

Escherichia	• *Escherichia coli*	Negative	Bacillus	Facultative anaerobic	extracellular or intracellular
Francisella	• *Francisella tularensis*	Negative	coccobacillus	strictly aerobic	Facultative intracellular
Haemophilus	• *Haemophilus influenzae*	Negative	coccobacilli to long and slender filaments		extracellular
Helicobacter	• *Helicobacter pylori*	Negative	Spirochete	Microaerophile	extracellular
Legionella	• *Legionella pneumophila*	Negative, stains poorly	cocobacilli	aerobic	facultative intracellular
Leptospira	• *Leptospira interrogans* • *Leptospira santarosai* • *Leptospira weilii* • *Leptospira noguchii*	Negative, stains poorly	Spirochete	Strictly aerobic	extracellular
Listeria	• *Listeria monocytogenes*	Positive, darkly	Slender, short rods	Facultative Anaerobic	intracellular
Mycobacterium	• *Mycobacterium leprae* • *Mycobacterium tuberculosis* • *Mycobacterium ulcerans*	(none)	Long, slender rods	aerobic	extracellular
Mycoplasma	• *Mycoplasma pneumoniae*	(none)	'fried egg' appearance, no cell wall	Mostly facultative anaerobic; *M. pneumoniae* strictly aerobic	extracellular
Neisseria	• *Neisseria gonorrhoeae* • *Neisseria meningitidis*	Negative	Kidney bean-shaped	aerobic	*Gonococcus*: facultative intracellular *N. meningitidis*: extracellular
Pseudomonas	• *Pseudomonas aeruginosa*	Negative	rods	Obligate aerobic	extracellular
Rickettsia	• *Rickettsia rickettsii*	Negative, stains poorly	Small, rod-like coccobacillary	Aerobic	Obligate intracellular
Salmonella	• *Salmonella typhi* • *Salmonella typhimurium*	Negative	Bacillus shape	Facultative anaerobica	Facultative intracellular
Shigella	• *Shigella sonnei*	Negative	rods	Facultative anaerobic	extracellular
Staphylococcus	• *Staphylococcus aureus* • *Staphylococcus epidermidis* • *Staphylococcus saprophyticus*	Positive, darkly	Round cocci	Facultative anaerobic	extracellular, facultative intracellular
Streptococcus	• *Streptococcus agalactiae* • *Streptococcus pneumoniae* • *Streptococcus pyogenes*	Positive	ovoid to spherical	Facultative anaerobic	extracellular
Treponema	• *Treponema pallidum*	Negative, stains poorly	Spirochete	Aerobic	extracellular
Ureaplasma	• *Ureaplasma urealyticum*	Stains poorly	indistinct, 'fried egg' appearance, no cell wall	anaerobic	extracellular
Vibrio	• *Vibrio cholerae*	Negative	Spiral with single polar flagellum	Facultative anaerobic	extracellular
Yersinia	• *Yersinia pestis* • *Yersinia enterocolitica* • *Yersinia pseudotuberculosis*	Negative, bipolarly	Small rods	Facultative Anaerobe	Intracellular

List of Species of Pathogenic Bacteria and Clinical Characteristics

This is description of the more common genera and species presented with their clinical characteristics and treatments.

Species of human pathogenic bacteria					
Species		**Transmission**	**Diseases**	**Treatment**	**Prevention**
Actinomyces israelii		Oral flora	Actinomycosis: painful abscesses in the mouth, lungs, or gastrointestinal tract.	Prolonged penicillin G and drainage	
Bacillus anthracis		Contact with cattle, sheep, goats and horses Spores enter through inhalation or through abrasions	Anthrax: pulmonary, gastrointestinal and/or cutaneous symptoms.	In early infection: Penicillin Doxycycline Ciprofloxacin Raxibacumab	Anthrax vaccine Autoclaving of equipment
Bacteroides fragilis		Gut flora	Abscesses in gastrointestinal tract, pelvic cavity and lungs	metronidazole	Wound care Aspiration prevention
Bordetella pertussis		Contact with respiratory droplets expelled by infected human hosts.	Whooping cough Secondary bacterial pneumonia	Macrolides such as erythromycin, before paroxysmal stage	Pertussis vaccine, such as in DPT vaccine
Borrelia	*B. burgdorferi* *B. garinii* *B. afzelii*	Ixodes ticks reservoir in deer and mice	• Lyme disease (B. burgdorferi) • Relapsing fever	Early stages of Lyme disease: • doxycycline • amoxicillin • ceftriaxone in neurological involvement Chronic Lyme disease: • penicillin G Relapsing fever: • doxycycline	Wearing clothing that limits skin exposure to ticks. Insect repellent. Avoid areas where ticks are found.
Brucella	*B. abortus* *B. canis* *B. melitensis* *B. suis*	Direct contact with infected animal Oral, by ingestion of unpasteurized milk or milk products	Brucellosis	doxycycline streptomycin or gentamicin	
Campylobacter jejuni		Fecal-oral from animals (mammals and fowl) Uncooked meat (especially poultry) Contaminated water	• Enteritis, bloody diarrhea • Guillain–Barré syndrome	Treat symptoms Fluoroquinolone such as ciprofloxacin in severe cases	Good hygiene Avoiding contaminated water Pasteurizing milk and milk products Cooking meat (especially poultry)
Chlamydia	*C. pneumoniae*	Respiratory droplets	Atypical pneumonia	Doxycycline Erythromycin	None
	C. trachomatis	vaginal sex oral sex anal sex Vertical from mother to newborn(ICN) Direct or contaminated surfaces and flies (trachoma)	Trachoma Neonatal conjunctivitis Neonatal pneumonia Nongonococcal urethritis (NGU) Urethritis Pelvic inflammatory disease Epididymitis Prostatitis Lymphogranuloma venereum (LGV)	Erythromycin (adults) Doxycycline (infants and pregnant women)	Erythromycin or silver nitrate in newborn's eyes Safe sex Abstinence
Chlamydophila psittaci		Inhalation of dust with secretions or feces from birds (e.g. parrots)	Psittacosis	Tetracycline Doxycycline Erythromycin	-

Clostridium	*C. botulinum*	Spores from soil, persevere in canned food, smoked fish and honey	Botulism: Mainly muscle weakness and paralysis	Antitoxin Penicillin Hyperbaric oxygen Mechanical ventilation	Proper food preservation techniques
	C. difficile	Gut flora, overgrowing when other flora is depleted	Pseudomembranous colitis	Discontinuing responsible antibiotic Vancomycin or metronidazole if severe	Fecal bacteriotherapy
	C. perfringens	Spores in soil Vaginal flora and gut flora	Anaerobic cellulitis Gas gangrene Acute food poisoning	Gas gangrene: Debridement or amputation Hyperbaric medicine High doses of doxycycline or penicillin G and clindamycin Food poisoning: Supportive care is sufficient	Appropriate food handling
	C. tetani	Spores in soil, skin penetration through wounds	Tetanus	Tetanus immune globulin Sedatives Muscle relaxants Mechanical ventilation Penicillin or metronidazole	Tetanus vaccine (such as in the DPT vaccine)
Corynebacterium diptheriae		respiratory droplets part of human flora	Diphtheria	Horse serum antitoxin Erythromycin Penicillin	DPT vaccine
Ehrlichia	*E. canis* *E. chaffeensis*	Dog tick	Ehrlichiosis	• doxycycline • rifampin	
Enterococcus	*E. faecalis* *E. faecium*	Part of gut flora, opportunistic or entering through GI tract or urinary system wounds	bacterial endocarditis biliary tract infections urinary tract infections	Ampicillin (combined with aminoglycoside in endocarditis) Vancomycin	No vaccine Hand washing and other nosocomial prevention
Escherichia	*E. coli* (generally)	• Gut flora, and in urinary tract • Spreading extraintestinally or proliferating in the GI tract	• Diarrhea • Urinary tract infections (UTI) • Meningitis in infants • Hospital-acquired pneumonia • Hospital-acquired sepsis	**UTI:** (resistance-tests are required first) • Co-trimoxazole • Fluoroquinolone, e.g. ciprofloxacin **Meningitis:** • Cephalosporin (e.g. cefotaxime) and gentamicin combination **Diarrhea:** • Antibiotics above shorten duration • Electrolyte and fluid replacement	(no vaccine or preventive drug) • Cooking ground beef and pasteurizing milk against O157:H7 • Hand washing and disinfection
	Enterotoxigenic *E. coli* (ETEC)	• Fecal-oral through food and water • Direct physical contact	• Traveller's diarrhea		
	Enteropathogenic *E. coli*	• Vertical, in utero or at birth	• Diarrhea in infants		
	Enteroinvasive E.coli (EIEC)	• Fecal-oral	• bloody diarrhea and fever		
	Enterohemorrhagic (EHEC), including *E. coli* O157:H7	• Reservoir in cattle	• bloody diarrhea • Hemolytic-uremic syndrome		
Francisella tularensis		• vector-borne by arthropods • Infected wild or domestic animals, birds or house pets	Tularemia: Fever, ulceration at entry site and/or lymphadenopathy. Can cause severe pneumonia.	• Streptomycin • Gentamicin	• Avoiding insect vectors • Precautions when handling wild animals or animal products

Haemophilus influenzae		• Droplet contact • Human flora of e.g. upper respiratory tract	• Bacterial meningitis • Upper respiratory tract infections • Pneumonia, bronchitis • Septic arthritis in infants	**Meningitis:** (resistance-tests are required first) • Third generation cephalosporin, e.g. cefotaxime or ceftriaxone • Ampicillin and sulbactam combination	• Hib vaccine to infants • Rifampin prophylactically
Helicobacter pylori		• Colonizing stomach • Unclear person-to-person transmission	• Peptic ulcer • Chronic gastritis • Risk factor for gastric carcinoma and gastric B-cell lymphoma	• Tetracycline, metronidazole and bismuth salt combination	(No vaccine or preventive drug)
Klebsiella pneumoniae		• Mouth, skin, and gut flora. • Pneumonia upon aspiration	• Klebsiella pneumonia, with significant lung necrosis and hemoptysis • Hospital-acquired Urinary tract infection and sepsis	• 3rd generation cephalosporin • ciprofloxacin	• hand hygiene.
Legionella pneumophila		• Droplet contact, from e.g. cooling towers, humidifiers, air conditioners and water distribution systems	• Legionnaire's Disease • Pontiac fever	• Macrolides, such as erythromycin • Fluoroquinolones • Rifampin	(no vaccine or preventive drug) Heating water
Leptospira species		• Food and water contaminated by urine from infected wild or domestic animals. *Leptospira* survives for weeks in fresh water and moist soil.	• Leptospirosis	• Penicillin G • Tetracycline, e.g. doxycycline	Vaccine not widely used • Doxycycline Prevention of exposure • Rodent control
Listeria monocytogenes		• Raw milk or cheese, ground meats, poultry • Vertically to newborn or fetus	• Listeriosis: • Meningitis • Sepsis	• Ampicillin • Co-trimoxazole	(no vaccine) • Proper food preparation and handling
Mycobacterium	*M. leprae*	• Prolonged human-human contact, e.g. through exudates from skin lesions to abrasion of other person	• Leprosy (Hansen's disease)	Tuberculoid form: • Dapsone and rifampin Lepromatous form: • Clofazimine	• BCG vaccine shows some effects
	M. tuberculosis	• Droplet contact	• Tuberculosis	Standard "short" course: • First 2 months, combination: ○ Isoniazid ○ Rifampicin ○ Pyrazinamide ○ Ethambutol • Further 4 months, combination: ○ Isoniazid ○ Rifampicin	• BCG vaccine • Isoniazid
Mycoplasma pneumoniae		• Human flora • Respiratory droplets	• Mycoplasma pneumonia	• Doxycycline and erythromycin	

Neisseria	*N. gonorrhoeae*	• Sexually transmitted • vertical in birth	• Gonorrhea • Urethritis (men) • Pelvic inflammatory disease (women) • Ophthalmia neonatorum • Septic arthritis	**Uncomplicated gonorrhea:** • Ceftriaxone • Tetracycline, e.g. doxycycline if also chlamydia is suspected • Spectinomycin for resistance or patient allergy to cephalosporin **Ophthalmia neonatorum:** • Erythromycin + ceftriaxone	(No vaccine) • Safe sex • Erythromycin into eyes of newborn at risk
	N. meningitidis	• Droplet transmission	• Meningococcal disease including meningitis • Sepsis, including Waterhouse-Friderichsen syndrome	• Penicillin G • Ceftriaxone	• NmVac4-A/C/Y/W-135 vaccine • Rifampin
Pseudomonas aeruginosa		Opportunistic; Infects damaged tissues or people with immunodeficiency.	Pseudomonas infection: • Pneumonia • Urinary tract infection • Corneal infection • Endocarditis • Osteomyelitis • Burn wound infection • Sepsis • Malignant external otitis	• Anti-pseudomonal penicillins such as ticarcillin • Aminoglycoside	(no vaccine) • Topical silver sulfadiazine for burn wounds
Nocardia asteroides		In soil	Nocardiosis	TMP/SMX	
Rickettsia rickettsii		• Wood or dog tick	• Rocky mountain spotted fever	• Doxycycline • Chloramphenicol	(no preventive drug or approved vaccine) • Vector control, such as clothing • Prompt removal of attached ticks
Salmonella	*S typhi*	• Fecal-oral route, through food or water	• Typhoid fever type salmonellosis (fever, abdominal pain, hepatosplenomegaly, rose spots) • Chronic carrier state	• Ceftriaxone • Fluoroquinolones, e.g. ciprofloxacin	• Ty21a and ViCPS vaccines • Hygiene and food preparation
	Other *Salmonella* species e.g. S. typhimurium	• Fecal-oral • Food contaminated by fowl (e.g. uncooked eggs) or turtles	• Salmonellosis with gastroenteritis • Paratyphoid fever • Osteomyelitis in people with sickle cells • Sepsis	• Fluid and electrolyte replacement for diarrhea • Antibiotics (in neonates and immuno-compromised): • Ciprofloxacin • Ceftriaxone • TMP/SMX • Azithromycin	(No vaccine or preventive drug) • Proper sewage disposal • Food preparation • Good personal hygiene

Shigella	*S. sonnei* *S. dysenteriae*	• Fecal-oral	• Shigellosis (bacillary dysentery)	• Fluid and electrolyte replacement • Fluoroquinolone such as ciprofloxacin if severe	• Protection of water and food supplies • Vaccines are in trial stage
Staphylococcus	*aureus*	• Human flora on mucosae in e.g. anterior nares, skin and vagina, entering through wound	Coagulase-positive staphylococcal infections: • Skin infections, including impetigo • Acute infective endocarditis • Septis • Necrotizing pneumonia • Meningitis • Osteomyelitis • Toxinoses ○ Scalded skin syndrome ○ Toxic shock syndrome ○ Staphylococcal food poisoning	• Incision and drainage of localized lesions • Nafcillin, oxacillin, methicillin • Vancomycin for Methicillin-resistant (MRSA)	(no vaccine or preventive drug) • Barrier precautions, washing hands and fomite disinfection in hospitals
	epidermidis	Human flora in skin, anterior nares and mucous membranes	• Infections of implanted prostheses (e.g. heart valves and joints) and catheters	• Vancomycin	None
	saprophyticus	Part of normal vaginal flora	• Cystitis in women	• TMP/SMX or norfloxacin	None
Streptococcus	*agalactiae*	Human flora in vagina, urethral mucous membranes, rectum • Vertically during childbirth • Sexually	• Neonatal meningitis • Neonatal sepsis • Neonatal pneumonia • Endometritis in postpartum women • Opportunistic infections with septicemia and pneumonia	• Penicillin G • Aminoglycoside in case of lethal infection	None
	pneumoniae	• Respiratory droplets • Human flora in nasopharynx (spreading in immunocompromised)	• Acute bacterial pneumonia & meningitis in adults • Otitis media and sinusitis in children • Sepsis	• Penicillin G	• 23-serotype vaccine for adults (PPV) • Heptavalent conjugated vaccine for children (PCV)
	pyogenes	• Respiratory droplets • Direct physical contact with impetigo lesions	• Streptococcal pharyngitis • Sepsis • Scarlet fever • Rheumatic fever • Impetigo and erysipelas • Puerperal fever • Necrotizing fasciitis • Poststreptococcal glomerulonephritis	• Penicillin G or V • Macrolide, e.g. clarithromycin or erythromycin in penicillin allergy • Drainage and debridement for necrotizing fasciitis	No vaccine • Rapid antibiotic treatment helps prevent rheumatic fever

	viridans	Oral flora, penetration through abrasions	• Subacute bacterial endocarditis • Dental cavities • Abscesses of brain and liver	Penicillin G	
Treponema pallidum		• Sexual	• Syphilis • Congenital syphilis	• Penicillin G • Doxycycline if penicillin allergy	No preventive drug or vaccine • Safe sex • Antibiotics to pregnant women if risk of transmitting to child
Vibrio cholerae		• Fecal-oral route • Contaminated water and raw seafood	• Cholera: Severe "rice water" diarrhea	• Fluid and electrolyte replacement • Doxycycline	• Proper sanitation • Adequate food preparation
Yersinia pestis		• Fleas from animals • Ingestion of animal tissues • Respiratory droplets	Plague: • Bubonic plague • Pneumonic plague	• Streptomycin primarily • Tetracyclin • Supportive therapy for shock	• Plague vaccine • Minimize exposure to rodents and fleas

Bacillus Cereus

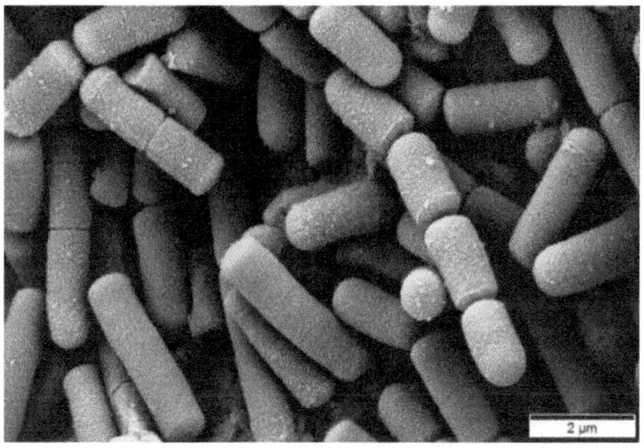

Electron micrograph of *Bacillus cereus*

Bacillus cereus is a Gram-positive, rod-shaped, aerobic, motile, beta hemolytic bacterium commonly found in soil and food. Some strains are harmful to humans and cause foodborne illness, while other strains can be beneficial as probiotics for animals.[not verified in body]. It is the cause of "fried rice syndrome", as the bacteria are classically contracted from fried rice dishes that have been sitting at room temperature for hours (such as at a buffet). *B. cereus* bacteria are facultative anaerobes, and like other members of the genus *Bacillus*, can produce protective endospores. Its virulence factors include cereolysin and phospholipase C.

It was from this species that two new enzymes, named AlkC and AlkD, which are involved in DNA repair, were discovered in 2006.

History

Colonies of *Bacillus cereus* were originally isolated from an agar plate left exposed to the air in a cow shed. In the 2010s, examination of warning letters issued by the US Food and Drug Administration issued to pharmaceutical manufacturing facilities addressing facility microbial contamination revealed that the most common contaminant was *B. cereus*.

Ecology

B. cereus competes with other microorganisms such as *Salmonella* and *Campylobacter* in the gut, so its presence reduces the numbers of those microorganisms. In food animals such as chickens, rabbits and pigs, some harmless strains of *B. cereus* are used as a probiotic feed additive to reduce *Salmonella* in the intestines and cecum. This improves the animals' growth as well as food safety for humans who eat their meat.

Bacillus cereus and other members of *Bacillus* are not easily killed by alcohol; in fact, they have been known to colonize distilled liquors and alcohol-soaked swabs and pads in numbers sufficient to cause infection.

Some strains of *B. cereus* produce cereins, bacteriocins active against different *B. cereus* strains or other Gram-positive bacteria.

Reproduction

At 30 °C (86 °F), a population of *B. cereus* can double in as little as 20 minutes or as long as 3 hours, depending on the food product.

Food	Minutes to double, 30 °C (86 °F)	Hours to multiply by 1,000,000
Milk	20-36	6.6 - 12
Cooked rice	26-31	8.6 - 10.3
Infant formula	56	18.6

Pathogenesis

B. cereus is responsible for a minority of foodborne illnesses (2–5%), causing severe nausea, vomiting, and diarrhea. *Bacillus* foodborne illnesses occur due to survival of the bacterial endospores when food is improperly cooked. Cooking temperatures less than or equal to 100 °C (212 °F) allow some *B. cereus* spores to survive. This problem is compounded when food is then improperly refrigerated, allowing the endospores to germinate. Cooked foods not meant for either immediate consumption or rapid cooling and refrigeration should be kept at temperatures below 10 °C (50 °F) or above 50 °C (122 °F). Germination and growth generally occur between 10 °C and 50 °C, though some strains are psychrotrophic. Bacterial growth results in production of enterotoxins, one of which is highly resistant to heat and acids (pH levels between 2 and 11); ingestion leads to two types of illness, diarrheal and emetic (vomiting) syndrome.

- The diarrheal type is associated with a wide range of foods, has an 8.0- to 16-hour incubation time, and is associated with diarrhea and gastrointestinal pain. Also known as the 'long-incubation' form of *B. cereus* food poisoning, it might be difficult to differentiate from poisoning caused by *Clostridium perfringens*. Enterotoxin can be inactivated after heating at 56 °C (133 °F) for 5 minutes however it is unclear whether its presence in food causes the symptom since it degrades in stomach enzymes; its subsequent production by surviving *B. cereus* spores within the small intestine may be the cause of illness.

- The 'emetic' form is commonly caused by rice cooked for a time and temperature insufficient to kill any spores present, then improperly refrigerated. It can produce a toxin, cereulide, which is not inactivated by later reheating. This form leads to nausea and vomiting one to five hours after consumption. It can be difficult to distinguish from other short-term bacterial foodborne intoxications such as by *Staphylococcus aureus*. Emetic toxin can withstand 121 °C (250 °F) for 90 minutes.

The diarrhetic syndromes observed in patients are thought to stem from the three toxins: hemolysin BL (Hbl), nonhemolytic enterotoxin (Nhe) and cytotoxin K (CytK). The *nhe/hbl/cytK* genes are located on the chromosome of the bacteria. Transcription of these genes is controlled by *PlcR*. These genes occur in the taxonomically related *B. thuringiensis* and *B. anthracis*, as well. These enterotoxins are all produced in the small intestine of the host, thus thwarting digestion by host endogenous enzymes. The Hbl and Nhe toxins are pore-forming toxins closely related to ClyA of *E. coli*. The proteins exhibit a conformation known as "beta-barrel" that can insert into cellular membranes due to a hydrophobic exterior, thus creating pores with hydrophilic interiors. The effect is loss of cellular membrane potential and eventually cell death. CytK is a pore-forming protein more related to other hemolysins.

The timing of the toxin production was previously thought to be possibly responsible for the two different courses of disease, but in fact the emetic syndrome is caused by a toxin, cereulide, found only in emetic strains and is not part of the "standard toolbox" of *B. cereus*. Cereulide is a cyclic polypeptide containing three repeats of four amino acids: D-oxy-Leu—D-Ala—L-oxy-Val—L-Val (similar to valinomycin produced by *Streptomyces griseus*) produced by nonribosomal peptide synthesis. Cereulide is believed to bind to 5-hydroxytryptamine 3 (5-HT3) serotonin receptors, activating them and leading to increased afferent vagus nerve stimulation. It was shown independently by two research groups to be encoded on multiple plasmids: pCERE01 or pBCE4810. Plasmid pBCE4810 shares homology with the *Bacillus anthracis* virulence plasmid pXO1, which encodes the anthrax toxin. Periodontal isolates of *B. cereus* also possess distinct pXO1-like plasmids. Like most of cyclic peptides containing nonproteogenic amino acids, cereulid is resistant to heat, proteolysis, and acid conditions.

B. cereus is also known to cause difficult-to-eradicate chronic skin infections, though less aggressive than necrotizing fasciitis. *B. cereus* can also cause keratitis.

Diagnosis

In case of foodborne illness, the diagnosis of *B. cereus* can be confirmed by the isolation of more than 10^5 *B. cereus* organisms per gram from epidemiologically implicated food, but such testing is often not done because the illness is relatively harmless and usually self-limiting.

Prognosis

Most emetic patients recover within six to 24 hours, but in some cases, the toxin can be fatal. In

2014, 23 neonates receiving total parenteral nutrition contaminated with *B. cereus* developed septicaemia, with three of the infants later dying as a result of infection.

Staphylococcal Enteritis

Staphylococcal enteritis is an inflammation that is usually caused by eating or drinking substances contaminated with staph enterotoxin. The toxin, not the bacterium, settles in the small intestine and cause inflammation and swelling. This in turn can cause abdominal pain, cramping, dehydration, diarrhea and fever.

Staphylococcus aureus is a Gram-positive, facultative anaerobe, coccal (round shaped) bacteria that appears in grape-like clusters that can thrive in high salt and low water activity habitats. *S. aureus* bacteria can live on the skin which is one of the primary modes of transmission. *S. aureus* can cause a range of illnesses from minor skin infections to Staphylococcus aureus food poisoning enteritis. Since humans are the primary source, cross-contamination is the most common way the microorganism is introduced into foods. Foods at high risks are those prepared in large quantities. Staphylococcus aureus is a true food poisoning organism. It produces a heat stable toxin enterotoxin when allowed to grow for several hours in foods such as cream-filled baked goods, poultry meat, gravies, eggs, meat salads, puddings and vegetables. It is important to note that the toxins may be present in dangerous amounts in foods that have no signs of spoilage, such as a bad smell, any off color, odor, or textural or flavor change.

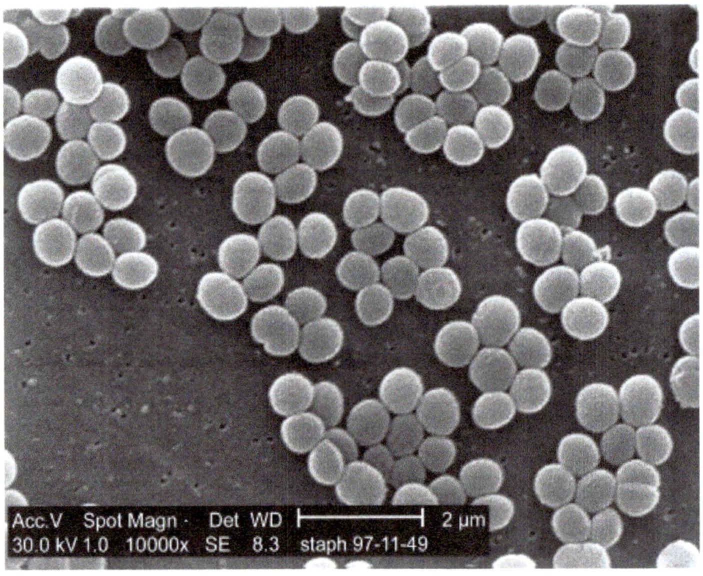

Staphylococcus aureus

Enteritis is the inflammation of the small intestine. It is generally caused by eating or drinking substances that are contaminated with bacteria or viruses. The bacterium and/or toxin settles in the small intestine and cause inflammation and swelling. This in turn can cause abdominal pain, cramping, diarrhea, fever, and dehydration. There are other types of enteritis, the types include: bacterial gastroenteritis, *Campylobacter* enteritis, *E. coli* enteritis, radiation enteritis, *Salmonella* enteritis and *Shigella* enteritis.

Pathogenesis

S. aureus is an enterotoxin producer. Enterotoxins are chromosomally encoded exotoxins that are produced and secreted from several bacterial organisms. It is a heat stable toxin and is resistant to digestive protease. It is the ingestion of the toxin that causes the inflammation and swelling of the intestine.

Symptoms

Common symptoms of *Staphylococcus aureus* food poisoning include: a rapid onset which is usually 1–8 hours, nausea, explosive vomiting for up to 24 hours, abdominal cramps/pain, headache, weakness, diarrhea and usually a subnormal body temperature. Symptoms usually start one to six hours after eating and last less than 12 hours. The duration of some cases may take two or more days to fully resolve.

Tests and Exams

For the detection of *Staphylococcus aureus* food poisoning which can lead to staphylococcal enteritis a stool culture may be required. A stool culture is used to detect the presence of disease-causing bacteria (pathogenic) and help diagnose an infection of the digestive tract. In the case of staphylococcal enteritis, it is conducted to see if the stool is positive for a pathogenic bacterium.

Treatment and Diet

Treatment is supportive and based upon symptoms, with fluid and electrolyte replacement as the primary goal. Dehydration caused by diarrhea and vomiting is the most common complication. To prevent dehydration, it is important to take frequent sips of a rehydration drink (like water) or try to drink a cup of water or rehydration drink for each large, loose stool.

Dietary management of enteritis consists of starting with a clear liquid diet until vomiting and diarrhea end and then slowly introduce the BRATT diet. The BRATT diet consists of bananas, rice, applesauce, tea, and toast. It is also important to avoid foods that are high in fiber or are possibly difficult to digest.

Prevention

Staphylococcal enteritis may be avoided by using proper hygiene and sanitation with food preparation. This includes thoroughly cooking all meats. If food is to be stored longer than two hours, keep hot foods hot (over 140°F) and cold foods cold (40°F or under). Ensure to refrigerate leftovers promptly and store cooked food in a wide, shallow container and refrigerate as soon as possible. Sanitation is very important. Keep kitchens and food-serving areas clean and sanitized. Finally, as most staphylococcal food poisoning are the result of food handling, hand washing is critical. Food handlers should use hand sanitizers with alcohol or thorough hand washing with soap and water.

Tips for hand washing:

1. Wash hands with warm, soapy water before and after handling raw foods.

a. First, wet your hands.

b. Add soap to your hands.

c. Rub both sides for at least 20 seconds.

d. Rinse thoroughly.

e. Air dry, or dry your hands with a clean towel or paper towel.

2. Always wash your hands after using the bathroom, after changing a baby's diaper, after touching pets or other animals, and after sneezing or coughing

3. Properly dress or glove.

Vibrio parahaemolyticus

Vibrio parahaemolyticus is a curved, rod-shaped, Gram-negative bacterium found in brackish saltwater, which, when ingested, causes gastrointestinal illness in humans. *V. parahaemolyticus* is oxidase positive, facultatively aerobic, and does not form spores. Like other members of the genus *Vibrio*, this species is motile, with a single, polar flagellum.

Pathogenesis

While infection can occur by the fecal-oral route, ingestion of bacteria in raw or undercooked seafood, usually oysters, is the predominant cause the acute gastroenteritis caused by *V. parahaemolyticus*. Wound infections also occur, but are less common than seafood-borne disease. The disease mechanism of *V. parahaemolyticus* infections has not been fully elucidated.

Clinical isolates usually possess a pathogenicity island (PAI) on the second chromosome. The PAI can be acquired by horizontal gene transfer and contains genes for several virulence factors. Two fully sequenced variants exist of the *V. parahaemolyticus* PAI with distinctly different lineages. Each PAI variant contains a genetically-distinct Type III Secretion System (T3SS), which is capable of injecting virulence proteins into host cells to disrupt host cell functions or cause cell death by apoptosis. The two known T3SS variants on *V. parahaemolyticus* chromosome 2 are known as T3SS2α and T3SS2β. These variants correspond to the two known PAI variants. Aside from the T3SS, two genes encoding well-characterized virulence proteins are typically found on the PAI, the thermostable direct hemolysin gene (*tdh*) and/or the *tdh*-related hemolysin gene (*trh*). Strains possessing one or both of these hemolysins exhibit beta-hemolysis on blood agar plates. A distinct correlation seems to exist between presence of *tdh*, *trh*, and the two known T3SS variants: observations have shown T3SS2α correlating with *tdh+/trh-* strains, while T3SS2β correlates with *tdh-/trh+* strains.

Signs and Symptoms

The incubation period of about 24 hours is followed by explosive, watery diarrhea accompanied by nausea, vomiting, abdominal cramps, and sometimes fever. Symptoms typically resolve within 72 hours, but can persist for up to 10 days in immunocompromised individuals. As the vast majority of cases of *V. parahaemolyticus* food infection are self-limiting, treatment is not typically necessary. In severe cases, fluid and electrolyte replacement is indicated.

Epidemiology

Outbreaks tend to be concentrated along coastal regions during the summer and early fall when higher water temperatures favor higher levels of bacteria. Seafood most often implicated includes squid, mackerel, tuna, sardines, crab, shrimp, and bivalves, such as oysters and clams. In the Northeast United States, there is an increasing incidence of illness due to oysters contaminated with *V. parahaemolyticus*, which is associated with warmer waters from the Gulf of Mexico moving northward, at least in part due to changes in climate.

Additionally, swimming or working in affected areas can lead to infections of the eyes, ears, or open cuts and wounds. Following Hurricane Katrina, 22 wounds were infected with *Vibrio*, three of which were caused by *V. parahaemolyticus*, and two of these led to death.

Hosts

Hosts of *V. parahaemolyticus* include:

- *Clithon retropictus*
- *Litopenaeus* shrimp (suspected; possibly causes necrotising hepatopancreatitis)
- *Nerita albicilla*

Vibrio Vulnificus

Vibrio vulnificus is a species of Gram-negative, motile, curved, rod-shaped (bacillus), pathogenic bacteria of the genus *Vibrio*. Present in marine environments such as estuaries, brackish ponds, or coastal areas, *V. vulnificus* is related to *V. cholerae*, the causative agent of cholera. Infection with *V. vulnificus* leads to rapidly expanding cellulitis or septicemia. It was first isolated as a source of disease in 1976. The capsule, made of polysaccharides, is thought to protect against phagocytosis. The observed association of the infection with liver disease (associated with increased serum iron) might be due to the capability of more virulent strains to capture iron bound to transferrin. Toxin production plays a relevant role in pathogenicity.

Signs and Symptoms

V. vulnificus is an extremely virulent bacterium that can cause three types of infections:

- Acute gastroenteritis from eating raw or undercooked shellfish: *V. vulnificus* causes an infection often incurred after eating seafood, especially raw or undercooked oysters. It does not alter the appearance, taste, or odor of oysters. Symptoms include vomiting, diarrhea and abdominal pain

- Necrotizing wound infections can occur in injured skin exposed to contaminated marine water. *V. vulnificus* bacteria can enter the body through open wounds when swimming or wading in infected waters, or by puncture wounds from the spines of fish such as tilapia, catfish or stingrays. These patients may develop a blistering dermatitis sometimes mistaken for pemphigus or pemphigoid.

- Invasive septicemia can occur after eating raw or undercooked shellfish, especially oysters. *V. vulnificus* is 80 times more likely to spread into the bloodstream in people with compromised immune systems, especially those with chronic liver disease. When this happens, severe symptoms including blistering skin lesions and septic shock can sometimes lead to death. This severe infection may occur regardless of whether the infection began from contaminated food or an open wound.

Among healthy people, ingestion of *V. vulnificus* can cause vomiting, diarrhea, and abdominal pain. In someone with a compromised immune system, particularly those with chronic liver disease, it can infect the bloodstream, causing a severe and life-threatening illness characterized by fever and chills, decreased blood pressure (septic shock), and blistering skin lesions.

Treatment

V. vulnificus wound infections have a mortality rate around 25%. In patients in whom the infection worsens into septicemia, typically following ingestion, the mortality rate rises to 50%. The majority of these patients die within the first 48 hours of infection. The optimal treatment is not known, but, in one retrospective study of 93 patients in Taiwan, use of a third-generation cephalosporin and a tetracycline (e.g., ceftriaxone and doxycycline, respectively) were associated with an improved outcome. Prospective clinical trials are needed to confirm this finding, but *in vitro* data support the supposition this combination is synergistic against *V. vulnificus*. Likewise, the American Medical Association and the Centers for Disease Control and Prevention (CDC) recommend treating the patient with a quinolone or intravenous doxycycline with ceftazidime. The first successful documented treatment of fulminant *V. vulnificus* sepsis was in 1995. Treatment was Fortaz and intravenous (IV) Cipro and IV doxycycline, which proved successful. Prevention of secondary infections from respiratory failure and acute renal failure are crucial. Key to the diagnosis and treatment was early recognition of bullae in an immunocompromised patient with liver cirrhosis and oyster ingestion within the previous 48 hours, and request by the physician for STAT Gram staining and blood cultures for *V. vulnificus*.

V. vulnificus often causes large, disfiguring ulcers that require extensive debridement or even amputation.

V. vulnificus is commonly found in the Gulf of Mexico, where more than a dozen people have died from the infection since 1990. Most deaths at that time were occurring due to fulminant sepsis either in the area of oyster harvest and ingestion or in tourists returning home. Lack of disease recognition and the risk factors, presentation, and cause were and are major obstacles to good outcome and recovery.

After the successful treatment of the first patient, the Florida Department of Health was able to trace the origin of the outbreak to Apalachicola Bay oysters and their harvesting in water prone to excessive growth of the organism due to warmth of the water and lack of freshwater dilution by reduced flow of the Chattahoochee River into the Apalachicola River into Apalachicola Bay. A similar situation occurred after Hurricane Katrina in New Orleans.

Prognosis

The worst prognosis is in those patients arriving at hospital in a state of shock. Total mortality in treated patients (ingestion and wound) is around 33%.

Patients especially vulnerable are those with liver disease (especially cirrhosis and hepatitis) or immunocompromised states (cancer, bone marrow suppression, HIV, diabetes, etc.). With these cases, *V. vulnificus* usually enters the bloodstream, where it may cause fever and chills, septic shock (with sharply decreased blood pressure), and blistering skin lesions. About half of those who contract blood infections die.

V. vulnificus infections also disproportionately affect males; 85% of those developing endotoxic shock from the bacteria are male. Females having had an oophorectomy experienced increased mortality rates, as estrogen has been shown experimentally to have a protective effect against *V. vulnificus*.

History

The pathogen was first isolated in 1976 from a series of blood culture samples submitted to the CDC in Atlanta. It was described as a "lactose-positive vibrio". It was subsequently given the name *Beneckea vulnifica*, and finally *Vibrio vulnificus* by Farmer in 1979.

Increasing seasonal temperatures and decreasing coastal salinity levels seem to favor a greater concentration of *Vibrio* within filter-feeding shellfish of the US Atlantic seaboard and the Gulf of Mexico, especially oysters (*Crassostrea virginica*). Scientists have frequently demonstrated the presence of *V. vulnificus* in the gut of oysters and other shellfish and in the intestines of fish that inhabit oyster reefs. The vast majority of people who develop sepsis from *V. vulnificus* became ill after they ate raw oysters, most of these cases have been men.

Health officials clearly identified strains of *V. vulnificus* infections among evacuees from New Orleans due to the flooding there caused by Hurricane Katrina.

On Thursday, June 18, 2015, an online news story article, featured on the MSN News webpage, and written by Katy Galimberti, an AccuWeather.com staff writer, with commentary provided by AccuWeather meteorologist Alex Sosnowski, stated that eight cases of *Vibrio vulnificus* infection "have been reported so far in 2015 across six different counties. Two cases resulted in death – one in Brevard County, Florida and one in Marion County, Florida." Mr. Sosnowski then noted that Florida had had warm months previously, and the story said that the pathogen prefers brackish warm water around the Gulf Coastal area. With two deaths out of eight known cases, that localized outbreak would thus far have a fatality (mortality) rate of 25%, higher than many other pathogens, but still lower than many others with even higher fatality rates. Much of the mortality due to *V. vulnificus* occurs in those patients who develop generalized infections, and in turn develop sepsis or septic shock; many, but certainly not all, of those cases are in compromised individuals.

References

- Smith, David F.; Diack, H. Lesley and Pennington, T. Hugh (2005) Food Poisoning, Policy and Politics : Corned Beef and Typhoid in Britain in the 1960s. Boydell Press. ISBN 1-84383-138-4
- Kumar, Vinay; Abbas, Abul K.; Fausto, Nelson; & Mitchell, Richard N. (2007). Robbins Basic Pathology (8th ed.). Saunders Elsevier. pp. 843 ISBN 978-1-4160-2973-1
- Bowden GHW (1996). Baron S; et al., eds. Actinomycosis in: Baron's Medical Microbiology (4th ed.). Univ of Texas Medical Branch. ISBN 0-9631172-1-1. (via NCBI Bookshelf).
- Baron, Samuel (1996). Medical Microbiology (4th ed.). University of Texas Medical Branch at Galveston, Galveston, Texas. ISBN 0-9631172-1-1.
- Ryan, KJ; Ray, CG, eds. (2004). Sherris Medical Microbiology (4th ed.). McGraw Hill. ISBN 0-8385-8529-9.
- Ryan KJ; Ray CG, eds. (2004). Sherris Medical Microbiology (4th ed.). McGraw Hill. ISBN 0-8385-8529-9.
- Turnbull PCB (1996). Baron S; et al., eds. Bacillus. In: Baron's Medical Microbiology (4th ed.). Univ of Texas Medical Branch. ISBN 0-9631172-1-1. (via NCBI Bookshelf).
- Roberts, T. A.; Baird-Parker, A. C.; Tompkin, R. B. (1996). Characteristics of microbial pathogens. London: Blackie Academic & Professional. p. 24. ISBN 0-412-47350-X. Retrieved 25 November 2010.
- Davis, Judi Ratliff; Lawley, Richard; Davis, Judy; Laurie Curtis (2008). The food safety hazard guidebook. Cambridge, UK: RSC Pub. p. 17. ISBN 0-85404-460-4. Retrieved 25 November 2010.
- Ryan KJ, Ray CG, eds. (2004). Sherris Medical Microbiology (4th ed.). McGraw Hill. ISBN 0-8385-8529-9.
- Oliver JD, Kaper J (2001). Vibrio species. pp. 263-300 In: Food Microbiology: Fundamentals and Frontiers. (Doyle MP et al., editors) (2nd ed.). ASM Press. ISBN 1-55581-117-5.
- James, William D.; Berger, Timothy G. (2006). Andrews' Diseases of the Skin: Clinical Dermatology. Saunders Elsevier. ISBN 0-7216-2921-0.
- Oliver JD, Kaper J (2005). Vibrio vulnificus. In: Oceans and Health: Pathogens in the Marine Environment. (Belken SS, Colwell RR, editors) (2nd ed.). Springer Science. ISBN 0-387-23708-9.
- "The Food Standards Agency: A Force for Change". gov.uk. Food Standards Agency, United Kingdom. January 14, 1998. Retrieved 14 August 2016.
- Hardy, Anne (13 January 2016). "Food Poisoning: An On-going Saga". History and Policy. History and Policy. Retrieved 4 July 2016.
- "Meat Produced by Advanced Meat/Bone Separation Machinery and Meat Recovery (AMR) Systems". Federal Register. U.S. National Archive and Records Administration. Retrieved 3 July 2016.
- "Livestock Industry Opposed to Stricter Laws on Mad Cow Prevention". January 2003. Retrieved 3 July 2016.
- Casey, Michael. "New Hampshire Looks for Answers Behind Oyster Outbreaks". R&D Magazine. Associated Press. Retrieved 5 December 2016.
- Flynn, Dan (November 22, 2011). "Still Too Many Raw Oyster Deaths in Gulf States". Food Safety News. Retrieved August 1, 2016.
- Katy Galimberti (June 18, 2015). "Flesh-Eating Bacteria Kills Two in Florida as Water Temperatures Rise". msn.com. Retrieved August 1, 2016.
- "Thayer Martin Agar (Modified) Procedure" (PDF). University of Nebraska-Medical Center, Clinical Laboratory Science Program. Retrieved 2015-05-03.
- Mabeza, GF; Macfarlane J (March 2003). "Pulmonary actinomycosis". European Respiratory Journal. ERS Journals Ltd. 21 (3): 545–551. doi:10.1183/09031936.03.00089103. PMID 12662015. Retrieved 2008-07-21.
- Itzhak Brook (Jan 28, 2014). "Bacteroides Infection Follow-up". Medscape. Retrieved 2015-09-25.

- "Signs & Symptoms". Centers for Disease Control and Prevention. Page last reviewed: October 26, 2015
- Mikkola, Raimo. Food and Indoor Air Isolated Bacillus Non-Protein Toxins: Structures, Physico-Chemical Properties and Mechanisms of Effects on Eukaryotic Cells (PDF). p. 12. Retrieved 2015-10-24.

4

Various Foodborne Diseases

Diseases that are related to food contamination are cholera, gastroenteritis, shigellosis, botulism, sal-monellosis, Gerstmann-Straussler-Scheinker syndrome and kuru. Cholera is an infection caused by the bacterium vibrio cholera; the symptoms are vomiting and diarrhea. The section serves as a source to understand the diseases related to food contamination.

Cholera

Cholera is an infection of the small intestine by some strains of the bacterium *Vibrio cholerae*. Symptoms may range from none, to mild, to severe. The classic symptom is large amounts of watery diarrhea that lasts a few days. Vomiting and muscle cramps may also occur. Diarrhea can be so severe that it leads within hours to severe dehydration and electrolyte imbalance. This may result in sunken eyes, cold skin, decreased skin elasticity, and wrinkling of the hands and feet. The dehydration may result in the skin turning bluish. Symptoms start two hours to five days after exposure.

Cholera is caused by a number of types of *Vibrio cholerae*, with some types producing more severe disease than others. It is spread mostly by unsafe water and unsafe food that has been contaminated with human feces containing the bacteria. Undercooked seafood is a common source. Humans are the only animal affected. Risk factors for the disease include poor sanitation, not enough clean drinking water, and poverty. There are concerns that rising sea levels will increase rates of disease. Cholera can be diagnosed by a stool test. A rapid dipstick test is available but is not as accurate.

Prevention involves improved sanitation and access to clean water. Cholera vaccines that are given by mouth provide reasonable protection for about six months. They have the added benefit of protecting against another type of diarrhea caused by *E. coli*. The primary treatment is oral rehydration therapy—the replacement of fluids with slightly sweet and salty solutions. Rice-based solutions are preferred. Zinc supplementation is useful in children. In severe cases, intravenous fluids, such as Ringer's lactate, may be required, and antibiotics may be beneficial. Testing to see which antibiotic the cholera is susceptible to can help guide the choice.

Cholera affects an estimated 3–5 million people worldwide and causes 58,000–130,000 deaths a year as of 2010. While it is currently classified as a pandemic, it is rare in the developed world. Children are mostly affected. Cholera occurs as both outbreaks and chronically in certain areas. Areas with an ongoing risk of disease include Africa and south-east Asia. While the risk of death among those affected is usually less than 5%, it may be as high as 50% among some groups who do not have access to treatment. Historical descriptions of cholera are found as early as the 5th century BC in Sanskrit. The study of cholera by John Snow between 1849 and 1854 led to significant advances in the field of epidemiology.

Signs and Symptoms

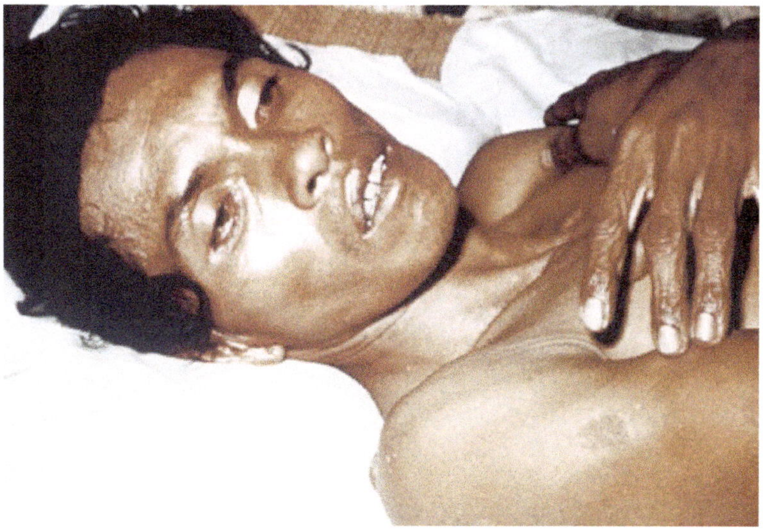

A person with severe dehydration due to cholera. Note the sunken eyes and decreased skin turgor which produces wrinkled hands and skin

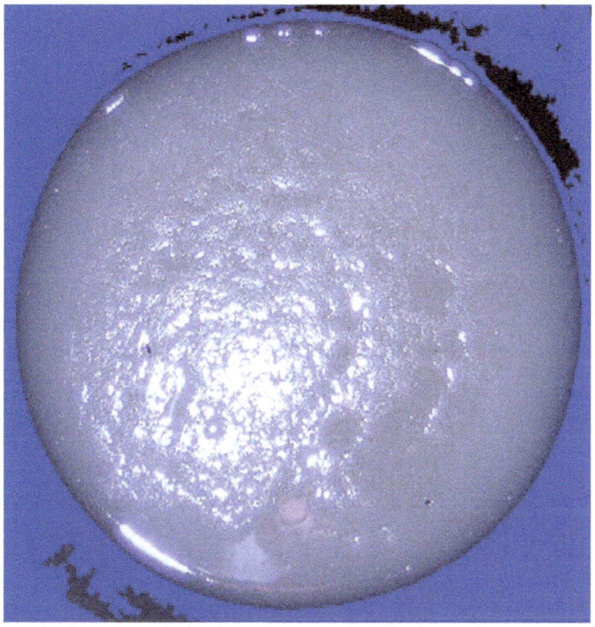

Typical "rice water" diarrhea

The primary symptoms of cholera are profuse diarrhea and vomiting of clear fluid. These symptoms usually start suddenly, half a day to five days after ingestion of the bacteria. The diarrhea is frequently described as "rice water" in nature and may have a fishy odor. An untreated person with cholera may produce 10 to 20 litres (3 to 5 US gal) of diarrhea a day. Severe cholera, without treatment, kills about half of affected individuals. If the severe diarrhea is not treated, it can result in life-threatening dehydration and electrolyte imbalances. Estimates of the ratio of asymptomatic to symptomatic infections have ranged from 3 to 100. Cholera has been nicknamed the "blue death" because a person's skin may turn bluish-gray from extreme loss of fluids.

Fever is rare and should raise suspicion for secondary infection. Patients can be lethargic, and might have sunken eyes, dry mouth, cold clammy skin, decreased skin turgor, or wrinkled hands and feet. Kussmaul breathing, a deep and labored breathing pattern, can occur because of acidosis from stool bicarbonate losses and lactic acidosis associated with poor perfusion. Blood pressure drops due to dehydration, peripheral pulse is rapid and thready, and urine output decreases with time. Muscle cramping and weakness, altered consciousness, seizures, or even coma due to electrolyte losses and ion shifts are common, especially in children.

Cause

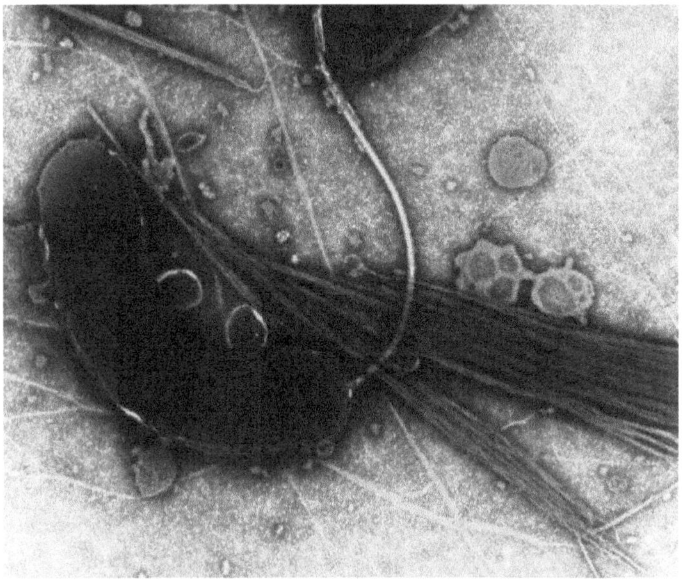

Vibrio cholerae, the bacterium that causes cholera

Transmission

Cholera has been found in two animal populations: shellfish and plankton.

Transmission is usually through the fecal-oral route of contaminated food or water caused by poor sanitation. Most cholera cases in developed countries are a result of transmission by food, while in the developing world it is more often water. Food transmission can occur when people harvest seafood such as oysters in waters infected with sewage, as *Vibrio cholerae* accumulates in planktonic crustaceans and the oysters eat the zooplankton.

People infected with cholera often have diarrhea, and disease transmission may occur if this highly liquid stool, colloquially referred to as "rice-water", contaminates water used by others. The source of the contamination is typically other cholera sufferers when their untreated diarrheal discharge is allowed to get into waterways, groundwater or drinking water supplies. Drinking any infected water and eating any foods washed in the water, as well as shellfish living in the affected waterway, can cause a person to contract an infection. Cholera is rarely spread directly from person to person.

Both toxic and non-toxic strains exist. Non-toxic strains can acquire toxicity through a temperate bacteriophage.

Susceptibility

About 100 million bacteria must typically be ingested to cause cholera in a normal healthy adult. This dose, however, is less in those with lowered gastric acidity (for instance those using proton pump inhibitors). Children are also more susceptible, with two- to four-year-olds having the highest rates of infection. Individuals' susceptibility to cholera is also affected by their blood type, with those with type O blood being the most susceptible. Persons with lowered immunity, such as persons with AIDS or children who are malnourished, are more likely to experience a severe case if they become infected. Any individual, even a healthy adult in middle age, can experience a severe case, and each person's case should be measured by the loss of fluids, preferably in consultation with a professional health care provider.

The cystic fibrosis genetic mutation known as delta-F508 in humans has been said to maintain a selective heterozygous advantage: heterozygous carriers of the mutation (who are thus not affected by cystic fibrosis) are more resistant to *V. cholerae* infections. In this model, the genetic deficiency in the cystic fibrosis transmembrane conductance regulator channel proteins interferes with bacteria binding to the gastrointestinal epithelium, thus reducing the effects of an infection.

Mechanism

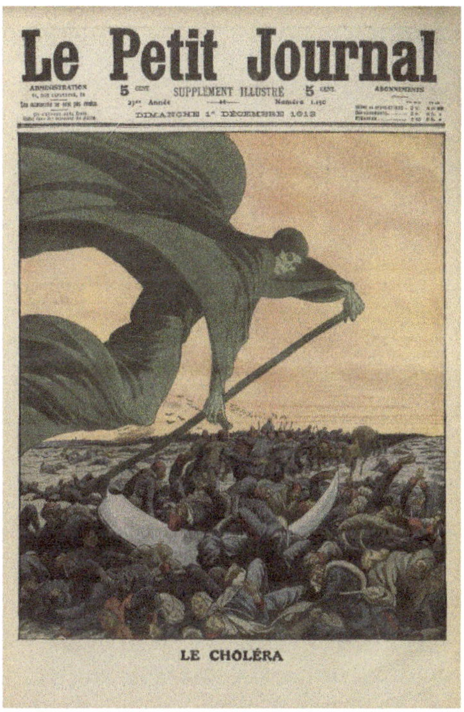

Drawing of Death bringing cholera, in *Le Petit Journal* (1912)

When consumed, most bacteria do not survive the acidic conditions of the human stomach. The few surviving bacteria conserve their energy and stored nutrients during the passage through the stomach by shutting down much protein production. When the surviving bacteria exit the stomach and reach the small intestine, they must propel themselves through the thick mucus that lines the small intestine to reach the intestinal walls where they can attach and thrive.

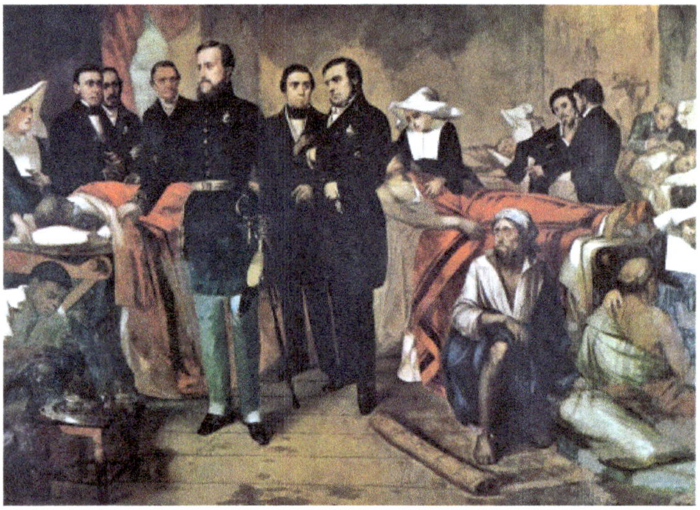

Emperor Pedro II of Brazil visiting people with cholera in 1855.

Once the cholera bacteria reach the intestinal wall they no longer need the flagella to move. The bacteria stop producing the protein flagellin to conserve energy and nutrients by changing the mix of proteins which they express in response to the changed chemical surroundings. On reaching the intestinal wall, *V. cholerae* start producing the toxic proteins that give the infected person a watery diarrhea. This carries the multiplying new generations of *V. cholerae* bacteria out into the drinking water of the next host if proper sanitation measures are not in place.

The cholera toxin (CTX or CT) is an oligomeric complex made up of six protein subunits: a single copy of the A subunit (part A), and five copies of the B subunit (part B), connected by a disulfide bond. The five B subunits form a five-membered ring that binds to GM1 gangliosides on the surface of the intestinal epithelium cells. The A1 portion of the A subunit is an enzyme that ADP-ribosylates G proteins, while the A2 chain fits into the central pore of the B subunit ring. Upon binding, the complex is taken into the cell via receptor-mediated endocytosis. Once inside the cell, the disulfide bond is reduced, and the A1 subunit is freed to bind with a human partner protein called ADP-ribosylation factor 6 (Arf6). Binding exposes its active site, allowing it to permanently ribosylate the Gs alpha subunit of the heterotrimeric G protein. This results in constitutive cAMP production, which in turn leads to secretion of H_2O, Na^+, K^+, Cl^-, and HCO_3^- into the lumen of the small intestine and rapid dehydration. The gene encoding the cholera toxin was introduced into *V. cholerae* by horizontal gene transfer. Virulent strains of *V. cholerae* carry a variant of a temperate bacteriophage called CTXφ.

Microbiologists have studied the genetic mechanisms by which the *V. cholerae* bacteria turn off the production of some proteins and turn on the production of other proteins as they respond to the series of chemical environments they encounter, passing through the stomach, through the mucous layer of the small intestine, and on to the intestinal wall. Of particular interest have been the genetic mechanisms by which cholera bacteria turn on the protein production of the toxins that interact with host cell mechanisms to pump chloride ions into the small intestine, creating an ionic pressure which prevents sodium ions from entering the cell. The chloride and sodium ions create a salt-water environment in the small intestines, which through osmosis can pull up to six litres of water per day through the intestinal cells, creating the massive amounts of diarrhea. The host can become rapidly dehydrated unless an appropriate mixture of dilute salt water and sugar is taken to replace the blood's water and salts lost in the diarrhea.

By inserting separate, successive sections of *V. cholerae* DNA into the DNA of other bacteria, such as *E. coli* that would not naturally produce the protein toxins, researchers have investigated the mechanisms by which *V. cholerae* responds to the changing chemical environments of the stomach, mucous layers, and intestinal wall. Researchers have discovered a complex cascade of regulatory proteins controls expression of *V. cholerae* virulence determinants. In responding to the chemical environment at the intestinal wall, the *V. cholerae* bacteria produce the TcpP/TcpH proteins, which, together with the ToxR/ToxS proteins, activate the expression of the ToxT regulatory protein. ToxT then directly activates expression of virulence genes that produce the toxins, causing diarrhea in the infected person and allowing the bacteria to colonize the intestine. Current research aims at discovering "the signal that makes the cholera bacteria stop swimming and start to colonize (that is, adhere to the cells of) the small intestine."

Genetic Structure

Amplified fragment length polymorphism fingerprinting of the pandemic isolates of *V. cholerae* has revealed variation in the genetic structure. Two clusters have been identified: Cluster I and Cluster II. For the most part, Cluster I consists of strains from the 1960s and 1970s, while Cluster II largely contains strains from the 1980s and 1990s, based on the change in the clone structure. This grouping of strains is best seen in the strains from the African continent.

Antibiotic Resistance

In many areas of the world, antibiotic resistance is increasing. In Bangladesh, for example, most cases are resistant to tetracycline, trimethoprim-sulfamethoxazole, and erythromycin. Rapid diagnostic assay methods are available for the identification of multiple drug-resistant cases. New generation antimicrobials have been discovered which are effective against in *in vitro* studies.

Diagnosis

A rapid dipstick test is available to determine the presence of *V. cholerae*. In those samples that test positive, further testing should be done to determine antibiotic resistance. In epidemic situations, a clinical diagnosis may be made by taking a patient history and doing a brief examination. Treatment is usually started without or before confirmation by laboratory analysis.

Stool and swab samples collected in the acute stage of the disease, before antibiotics have been administered, are the most useful specimens for laboratory diagnosis. If an epidemic of cholera is suspected, the most common causative agent is *V. cholerae* O1. If *V. cholerae* serogroup O1 is not isolated, the laboratory should test for *V. cholerae* O139. However, if neither of these organisms is isolated, it is necessary to send stool specimens to a reference laboratory.

Infection with *V. cholerae* O139 should be reported and handled in the same manner as that caused by *V. cholerae* O1. The associated diarrheal illness should be referred to as cholera and must be reported in the United States.

Prevention

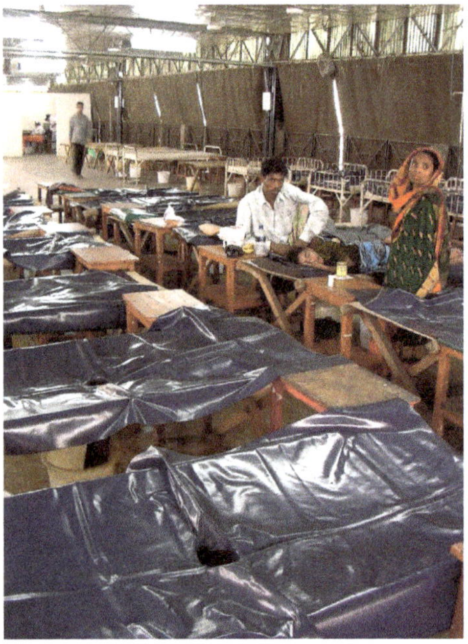

Cholera hospital in Dhaka, showing typical "cholera beds"

The World Health Organization (WHO) recommends focusing on prevention, preparedness, and response to combat the spread of cholera. They also stress the importance of an effective surveillance system. Governments can play a role in all of these areas, and in preventing cholera or indirectly facilitating its spread.

Although cholera may be life-threatening, prevention of the disease is normally straightforward if proper sanitation practices are followed. In developed countries, due to nearly universal advanced water treatment and sanitation practices, cholera is no longer a major health threat. The last major outbreak of cholera in the United States occurred in 1910–1911. Effective sanitation practices, if instituted and adhered to in time, are usually sufficient to stop an epidemic. There are several points along the cholera transmission path at which its spread may be halted:

- Sterilization: Proper disposal and treatment of infected fecal waste water produced by cholera victims and all contaminated materials (e.g. clothing, bedding, etc.) are essential. All materials that come in contact with cholera patients should be sanitized by washing in hot water, using chlorine bleach if possible. Hands that touch cholera patients or their clothing, bedding, etc., should be thoroughly cleaned and disinfected with chlorinated water or other effective antimicrobial agents.

- Sewage: antibacterial treatment of general sewage by chlorine, ozone, ultraviolet light or other effective treatment before it enters the waterways or underground water supplies helps prevent undiagnosed patients from inadvertently spreading the disease.

- Sources: Warnings about possible cholera contamination should be posted around contaminated water sources with directions on how to decontaminate the water (boiling, chlorination etc.) for possible use.

- Water purification: All water used for drinking, washing, or cooking should be sterilized by either boiling, chlorination, ozone water treatment, ultraviolet light sterilization (e.g. by solar water disinfection), or antimicrobial filtration in any area where cholera may be present. Chlorination and boiling are often the least expensive and most effective means of halting transmission. Cloth filters or sari filtration, though very basic, have significantly reduced the occurrence of cholera when used in poor villages in Bangladesh that rely on untreated surface water. Better antimicrobial filters, like those present in advanced individual water treatment hiking kits, are most effective. Public health education and adherence to appropriate sanitation practices are of primary importance to help prevent and control transmission of cholera and other diseases.

Handwashing with soap and/or ash after visiting toilets and before handling food or eating is also recommended for cholera prevention by WHO Africa.

Surveillance

Surveillance and prompt reporting allow for containing cholera epidemics rapidly. Cholera exists as a seasonal disease in many endemic countries, occurring annually mostly during rainy seasons. Surveillance systems can provide early alerts to outbreaks, therefore leading to coordinated response and assist in preparation of preparedness plans. Efficient surveillance systems can also improve the risk assessment for potential cholera outbreaks. Understanding the seasonality and location of outbreaks provides guidance for improving cholera control activities for the most vulnerable. For prevention to be effective, it is important that cases be reported to national health authorities.

Vaccine

A number of safe and effective oral vaccines for cholera are available. Dukoral, an orally administered, inactivated whole cell vaccine, has an overall efficacy of about 52% during the first year after being given and 62% in the second year, with minimal side effects. It is available in over 60 countries. However, it is not currently recommended by the Centers for Disease Control and Prevention (CDC) for most people traveling from the United States to endemic countries. One injectable vaccine was found to be effective for two to three years. The protective efficacy was 28% lower in children less than 5 years old. However, as of 2010, it has limited availability. Work is under way to investigate the role of mass vaccination. The World Health Organization (WHO) recommends immunization of high-risk groups, such as children and people with HIV, in countries where this disease is endemic. If people are immunized broadly, herd immunity results, with a decrease in the amount of contamination in the environment.

Sari Filtration

An effective and relatively cheap method to prevent the transmission of cholera is the use of a folded *sari* (a long cloth garment) to filter drinking water. In Bangladesh this practice was found to decrease rates of cholera by nearly half. It involves folding a *sari* four to eight times. Between uses the cloth should be rinsed in clean water and dried in the sun to kill any bacteria on it. A nylon cloth appears to work as well.

Treatment

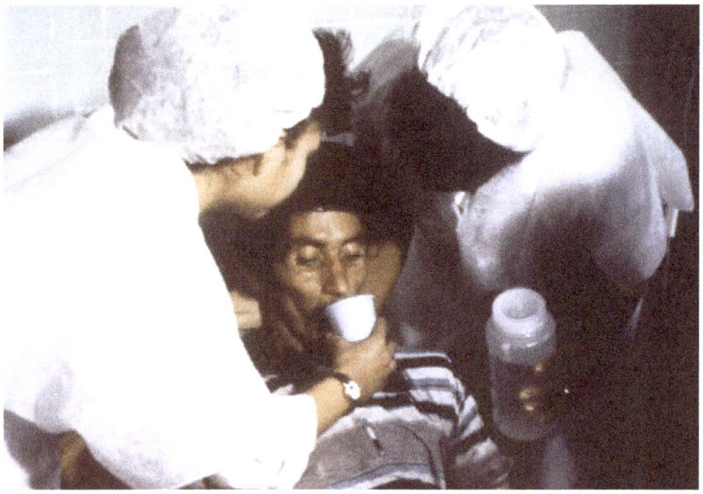

Cholera patient being treated by medical staff in 1992

Continued eating speeds the recovery of normal intestinal function. The World Health Organization recommends this generally for cases of diarrhea no matter what the underlying cause. A CDC training manual specifically for cholera states: "Continue to breastfeed your baby if the baby has watery diarrhea, even when traveling to get treatment. Adults and older children should continue to eat frequently."

Fluids

The most common error in caring for patients with cholera is to underestimate the speed and volume of fluids required. In most cases, cholera can be successfully treated with oral rehydration therapy, which is highly effective, safe, and simple to administer. Rice-based solutions are preferred to glucose-based ones due to greater efficiency. In severe cases with significant dehydration, intravenous rehydration may be necessary. Ringer's lactate is the preferred solution, often with added potassium. Large volumes and continued replacement until diarrhea has subsided may be needed. Ten percent of a person's body weight in fluid may need to be given in the first two to four hours. This method was first tried on a mass scale during the Bangladesh Liberation War, and was found to have much success. Despite widespread beliefs, fruit juices and commercial fizzy drinks like cola, are not ideal for rehydration of people with serious infections of the intestines, and the too high sugar content may even harm water uptake.

If commercially produced oral rehydration solutions are too expensive or difficult to obtain, solutions can be made. One such recipe calls for 1 liter of boiled water, 1/2 teaspoon of salt, 6 teaspoons of sugar, and added mashed banana for potassium and to improve taste.

Electrolytes

As there frequently is initially acidosis, the potassium level may be normal, even though large losses have occurred. As the dehydration is corrected, potassium levels may decrease rapidly, and thus need to be replaced. This may be done by eating foods high in potassium like bananas or green coconut water.

Antibiotics

Antibiotic treatments for one to three days shorten the course of the disease and reduce the severity of the symptoms. Use of antibiotics also reduces fluid requirements. People will recover without them, however, if sufficient hydration is maintained. The World Health Organization only recommends antibiotics in those with severe dehydration.

Doxycycline is typically used first line, although some strains of *V. cholerae* have shown resistance. Testing for resistance during an outbreak can help determine appropriate future choices. Other antibiotics proven to be effective include cotrimoxazole, erythromycin, tetracycline, chloramphenicol, and furazolidone. Fluoroquinolones, such as ciprofloxacin, also may be used, but resistance has been reported.

Antibiotics improve outcomes in those who are both severely and not severely dehydrated. Azithromycin and tetracycline may work better than doxycycline or ciprofloxacin.

Zinc Supplementation

In Bangladesh zinc supplementation reduced the duration and severity of diarrhea in children with cholera when given with antibiotics and rehydration therapy as needed. It reduced the length of disease by eight hours and the amount of diarrhea stool by 10%. Supplementation appears to be also effective in both treating and preventing infectious diarrhea due to other causes among children in the developing world.

Prognosis

If people with cholera are treated quickly and properly, the mortality rate is less than 1%; however, with untreated cholera, the mortality rate rises to 50–60%. For certain genetic strains of cholera, such as the one present during the 2010 epidemic in Haiti and the 2004 outbreak in India, death can occur within two hours of becoming ill.

Epidemiology

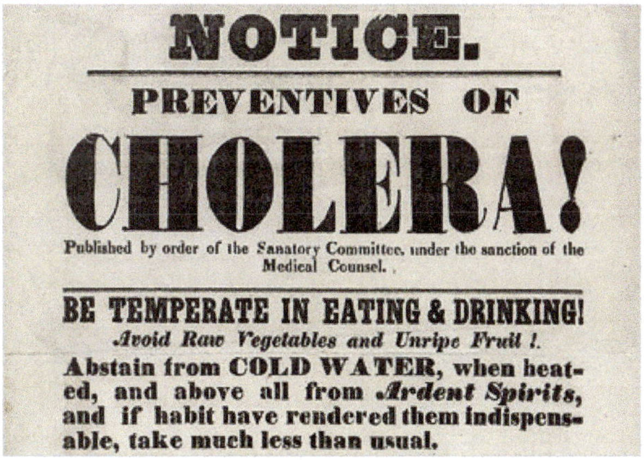

Hand bill from the New York City Board of Health, 1832—the outdated public health advice demonstrates the lack of understanding of the disease and its actual causative factors.

Cholera affects an estimated 3–5 million people worldwide, and causes 58,000–130,000 deaths a year as of 2010. This occurs mainly in the developing world. In the early 1980s, death rates are believed to have been greater than 3 million a year. It is difficult to calculate exact numbers of cases, as many go unreported due to concerns that an outbreak may have a negative impact on the tourism of a country. Cholera remains both epidemic and endemic in many areas of the world.

Although much is known about the mechanisms behind the spread of cholera, this has not led to a full understanding of what makes cholera outbreaks happen in some places and not others. Lack of treatment of human feces and lack of treatment of drinking water greatly facilitate its spread, but bodies of water can serve as a reservoir, and seafood shipped long distances can spread the disease. Cholera was not known in the Americas for most of the 20th century, but it reappeared towards the end of that century.

History

Cholera likely has its origins in the Indian subcontinent as evidenced by its prevalence in the region for centuries. Early outbreaks in the Indian subcontinent are believed to have been the result of poor living conditions as well as the presence of pools of still water, both of which provide ideal conditions for cholera to thrive. The disease first spread by trade routes (land and sea) to Russia in 1817, later to the rest of Europe, and from Europe to North America and the rest of the world. Seven cholera pandemics have occurred in the past 200 years, with the seventh pandemic originating in Indonesia in 1961.

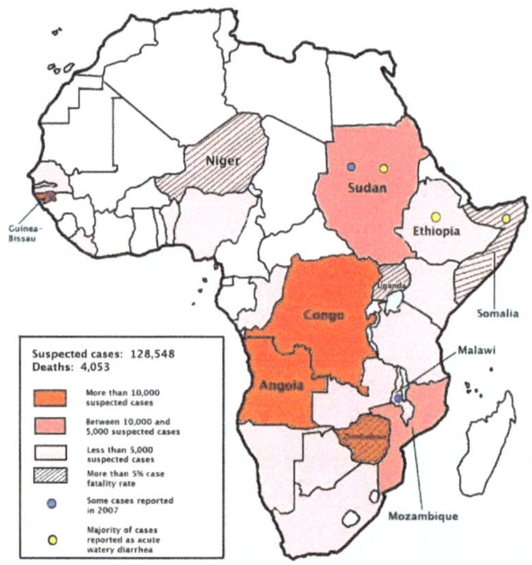

Map of the 2008–2009 cholera outbreak in sub-Saharan Africa showing the statistics as of 12 February 2009.

The first cholera pandemic occurred in the Bengal region of India, near Calcutta starting in 1817 through 1824. The disease dispersed from India to Southeast Asia, the Middle East, Europe, and Eastern Africa through trade routes. The second pandemic lasted from 1827 to 1835 and particularly affected North American and Europe due to the result of advancements in transportation and global trade, and increased human migration, including soldiers. The third pandemic erupted in 1839, persisted until 1856, extended to North Africa, and reached South America, for the first time specifically affecting Brazil. The fourth pandemic lasted from 1863 to 1875 spread from India to Naples and Spain. The fifth pandemic was from 1881-1896 and started in India and spread to

Europe, Asia, and South America. The sixth pandemic started 1899–1923. These epidemics were less fatal due to a greater understanding of the cholera bacteria. Egypt, the Arabian peninsula, Persia, India, and the Philippines were hit hardest during these epidemics, while other areas, like Germany in 1892 and Naples from 1910–1911, also experienced severe outbreaks. The final pandemic originated in 1961 in Indonesia and is marked by the emergence of a new strain, nicknamed *El Tor*, which still persists today in developing countries.

Since it became widespread in the 19th century, cholera has killed tens of millions of people. In Russia alone, between 1847 and 1851, more than one million people perished of the disease. It killed 150,000 Americans during the second pandemic. Between 1900 and 1920, perhaps eight million people died of cholera in India. Cholera became the first reportable disease in the United States due to the significant effects it had on health. John Snow, in England, was the first to identify the importance of contaminated water as its cause in 1854. Cholera is now no longer considered a pressing health threat in Europe and North America due to filtering and chlorination of water supplies, but still heavily affects populations in developing countries.

In the past, vessels flew a yellow quarantine flag if any crew members or passengers were suffering from cholera. No one aboard a vessel flying a yellow flag would be allowed ashore for an extended period, typically 30 to 40 days. In modern sets of international maritime signal flags, the quarantine flag is yellow and black.

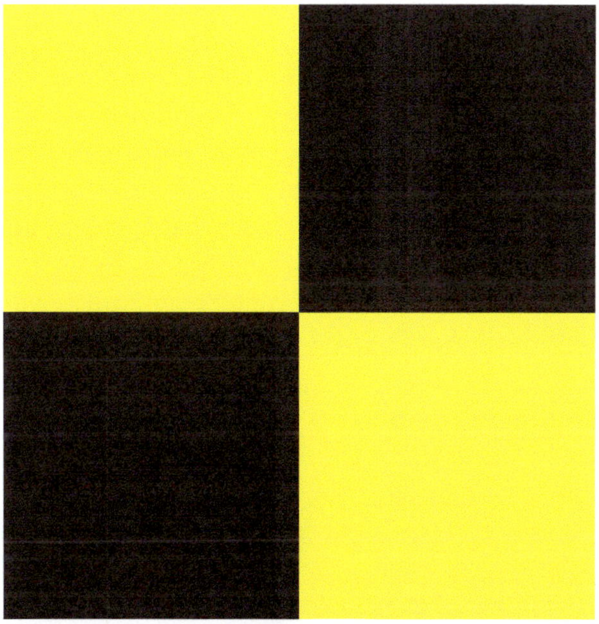

Signal flag "Lima" called the "Yellow Jack" which when flown in harbor means ship is under quarantine. A simple yellow flag (also called the "Yellow Jack") had historically been used to signal quarantine (it stands for **Q** among signal flags), but now indicates the opposite, as a signal of a ship free of disease that requests boarding and inspection.

Historically many different claimed remedies have existed in folklore. Many of the older remedies were based on the miasma theory. Some believed that abdominal chilling made one more susceptible and flannel and cholera belts were routine in army kits. In the 1854–1855 outbreak in Naples homeopathic Camphor was used according to Hahnemann. T. J. Ritter's "Mother's Remedies" book lists tomato syrup as a home remedy from northern America. Elecampane was recommended in the United Kingdom according to William Thomas Fernie

Cholera cases are much less frequent in developed countries where governments have helped to establish water sanitation practices and effective medical treatments. The United States, for example, used to have a severe cholera problem similar to those in some developing countries. There were three large cholera outbreaks in the 1800s, which can be attributed to *Vibrio cholerae's* spread through interior waterways like the Erie Canal and routes along the Eastern Seaboard. The island of Manhattan in New York City touched the Atlantic Ocean, where cholera collected just off the coast. At this time, New York City did not have as effective a sanitation system as it does today, so cholera was able to spread.

Cholera morbus is a historical term that was used to refer to gastroenteritis rather than specifically cholera.

Research

The bacterium was isolated in 1854 by Italian anatomist Filippo Pacini, but its exact nature and his results were not widely known.

Spanish physician Jaume Ferran i Clua developed a cholera inoculation in 1885, the first to immunize humans against a bacterial disease.

Russian-Jewish bacteriologist Waldemar Haffkine developed the first cholera vaccine in July 1892.

One of the major contributions to fighting cholera was made by the physician and pioneer medical scientist John Snow (1813–1858), who in 1854 found a link between cholera and contaminated drinking water. Dr. Snow proposed a microbial origin for epidemic cholera in 1849. In his major "state of the art" review of 1855, he proposed a substantially complete and correct model for the etiology of the disease. In two pioneering epidemiological field studies, he was able to demonstrate human sewage contamination was the most probable disease vector in two major epidemics in London in 1854. His model was not immediately accepted, but it was seen to be the more plausible, as medical microbiology developed over the next 30 years or so.

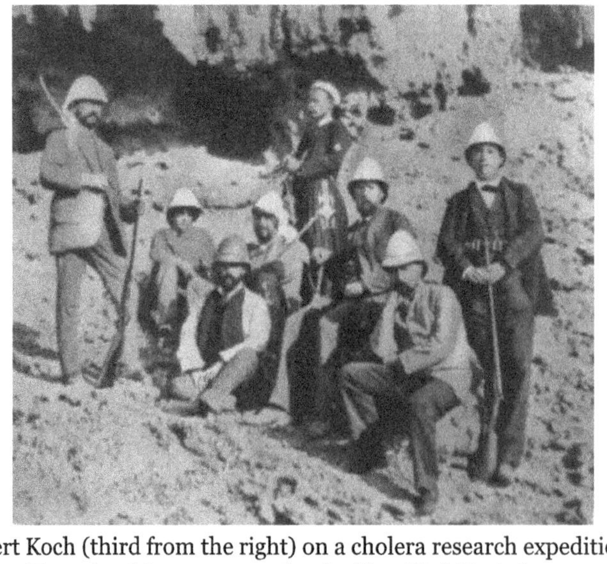

Robert Koch (third from the right) on a cholera research expedition in Egypt in 1884, one year after he identified *V. cholerae*.

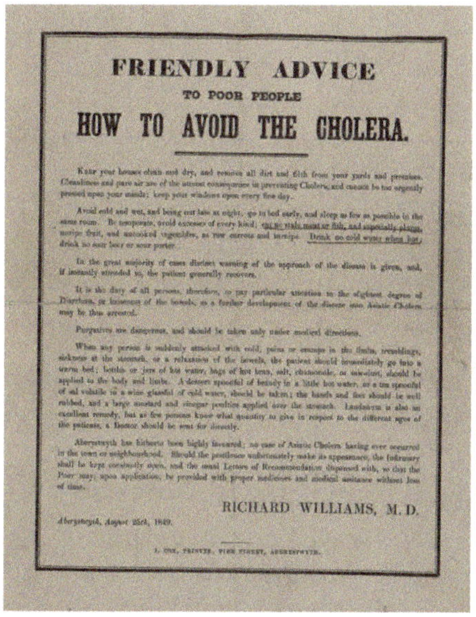

FRIENDLY ADVICE

TO POOR PEOPLE

HOW TO AVOID THE CHOLERA.

Keep your houses clean and dry, and remove all dirt and filth from your yards and premises. Cleanliness and pure air are of the utmost consequence in preventing Cholera, and cannot be too urgently pressed upon your minds; keep your windows open every fine day.

Avoid cold and wet, and being out late at night; go to bed early, and sleep as few as possible in the same room. Be temperate, avoid excesses of every kind; eat no stale meat or fish, and especially plums, unripe fruit, and uncooked vegetables, as raw carrots and turnips. Drink no cold water when hot; drink no sour beer or sour porter.

In the great majority of cases distinct warning of the approach of the disease is given, and, if instantly attended to, the patient generally recovers.

It is the duty of all persons, therefore, to pay particular attention to the slightest degree of Diarrhoea, or looseness of the bowels, as a further development of the disease into Asiatic Cholera may be thus arrested.

Purgatives are dangerous, and should be taken only under medical directions.

When any person is suddenly attacked with cold, pains or cramps in the limbs, tremblings, sickness at the stomach, or a relaxation of the bowels, the patient should immediately go into a warm bed; bottles or jars of hot water, bags of hot bran, salt, chamomile, or saw-dust, should be applied to the body and limbs. A dessert spoonful of brandy in a little hot water, or a tea spoonful of sal volatile in a wine glassful of cold water, should be taken; the hands and feet should be well rubbed, and a large mustard and vinegar poultice applied over the stomach. Laudanum is also an excellent remedy, but as few persons know what quantity to give in respect to the different ages of the patients, a Doctor should be sent for directly.

Aberystwyth has hitherto been highly favoured; no case of Asiatic Cholera having ever occurred in the town or neighbourhood. Should the pestilence unfortunately make its appearance, the Infirmary shall be kept constantly open, and the usual Letters of Recommendation dispensed with, so that the Poor may, upon application, be provided with proper medicines and medical assistance without loss of time.

RICHARD WILLIAMS, M. D.

Aberystwyth, August 25th, 1849.

J. COX, PRINTER, PIER STREET, ABERYSTWYTH.

How to avoid the cholera leaflet; Aberystwyth; August 1849

Cities in developed nations made massive investment in clean water supply and well-separated sewage treatment infrastructures between the mid-1850s and the 1900s. This eliminated the threat of cholera epidemics from the major developed cities in the world. In 1883, Robert Koch identified *V. cholerae* with a microscope as the bacillus causing the disease.

Robert Allan Phillips, working at the US Naval Medical Research Unit Two in Southeast Asia, evaluated the pathophysiology of the disease using modern laboratory chemistry techniques and developed a protocol for rehydration. His research led the Lasker Foundation to award him its prize in 1967.

More recently, in 2002, Alam, *et al.*, studied stool samples from patients at the International Centre for Diarrhoeal Disease in Dhaka, Bangladesh. From the various experiments they conducted, the researchers found a correlation between the passage of *V. cholerae* through the human digestive system and an increased infectivity state. Furthermore, the researchers found the bacterium creates a hyperinfected state where genes that control biosynthesis of amino acids, iron uptake systems, and formation of periplasmic nitrate reductase complexes were induced just before defecation. These induced characteristics allow the cholera vibrios to survive in the "rice water" stools, an environment of limited oxygen and iron, of patients with a cholera infection.

Society and Culture

Health Policy

In many developing countries, cholera still reaches its victims through contaminated water sources, and countries without proper sanitation techniques have greater incidence of the disease. Governments can play a role in this. In 2008, for example, the Zimbabwean cholera outbreak was due partly to the government's role, according to a report from the James Baker Institute. The Haitian government's inability to provide safe drinking water after the 2010 earthquake led to an increase in cholera cases as well.

Similarly, South Africa's cholera outbreak was exacerbated by the government's policy of privatizing water programs. The wealthy elite of the country were able to afford safe water while others had to use water from cholera-infected rivers.

According to Rita R. Colwell of the James Baker Institute, if cholera does begin to spread, government preparedness is crucial. A government's ability to contain the disease before it extends to other areas can prevent a high death toll and the development of an epidemic or even pandemic. Effective disease surveillance can ensure that cholera outbreaks are recognized as soon as possible and dealt with appropriately. Oftentimes, this will allow public health programs to determine and control the cause of the cases, whether it is unsanitary water or seafood that have accumulated a lot of *Vibrio cholerae* specimens. Having an effective surveillance program contributes to a government's ability to prevent cholera from spreading. In the year 2000 in the state of Kerala in India, the Kottayam district was determined to be "Cholera-affected"; this pronouncement led to task forces that concentrated on educating citizens with 13,670 information sessions about human health. These task forces promoted the boiling of water to obtain safe water, and provided chlorine and oral rehydration salts. Ultimately, this helped to control the spread of the disease to other areas and minimize deaths. On the other hand, researchers have shown that most of the citizens infected during the 1991 cholera outbreak in Bangladesh lived in rural areas, and were not recognized by the government's surveillance program. This inhibited physicians' abilities to detect cholera cases early.

According to Colwell, the quality and inclusiveness of a country's health care system affects the control of cholera, as it did in the Zimbabwean cholera outbreak. While sanitation practices are important, when governments respond quickly and have readily available vaccines, the country will have a lower cholera death toll. Affordability of vaccines can be a problem; if the governments do not provide vaccinations, only the wealthy may be able to afford them and there will be a greater toll on the country's poor. The speed with which government leaders respond to cholera outbreaks is important.

Besides contributing to an effective or declining public health care system and water sanitation treatments, government can have indirect effects on cholera control and the effectiveness of a response to cholera. A country's government can impact its ability to prevent disease and control its spread. A speedy government response backed by a fully functioning health care system and financial resources can prevent cholera's spread. This limits cholera's ability to cause death, or at the very least a decline in education, as children are kept out of school to minimize the risk of infection.

Notable Cases

- Tchaikovsky's death has traditionally been attributed to cholera, most probably contracted through drinking contaminated water several days earlier. "Since the water was not boiled and cholera was affecting Saint Petersburg, such a connection is quite plausible ...." Tchaikovsky's mother died of cholera, and his father became sick with cholera at this time but made a full recovery. Some scholars, however, including English musicologist and Tchaikovsky authority David Brown and biographer Anthony Holden, have theorized that his death was a suicide.
- 2010 Haiti cholera outbreak. Ten months after the 2010 earthquake, an outbreak swept over Haiti, traced to a United Nations base of peacekeepers from Nepal. This marks the

worst cholera outbreak in recent history, as well as the best documented cholera outbreak in modern public health.

- Sadi Carnot, Physicist, a founder of thermodynamics (d. 1832)
- Charles X, King of France (d. 1836)
- James K. Polk, eleventh president of the United States (d. 1849)
- Carl von Clausewitz, Prussian soldier and German military theorist (d. 1831)
- Elliot Bovill, Chief Justice of the Straits Settlements (1893)

Gastroenteritis

Gastroenteritis, also known as infectious diarrhea, is inflammation of the gastrointestinal tract that involves the stomach and small intestine. Signs and symptoms include some combination of diarrhea, vomiting, and abdominal pain. Fever, lack of energy, and dehydration may also occur. This typically lasts less than two weeks. It is unrelated to influenza though it has been called the stomach flu.

Gastroenteritis can be due to infections by viruses, bacteria, parasites, and fungus. The most common cause is viruses. In children rotavirus is the most common cause of severe disease. In adults, norovirus and *Campylobacter* are common. Transmission may occur due to eating improperly prepared foods, drinking contaminated water, or through close contact with an individual who is infected. Testing to confirm the diagnosis is typically not needed.

Prevention includes hand washing with soap, drinking clean water, proper disposal of human waste, and breastfeeding babies instead of using formula. The rotavirus vaccine is recommended in children. Treatment involves getting enough fluids. For mild or moderate cases, this can typically be achieved by drinking oral rehydration solution (a combination of water, salts, and sugar). In those who are breast fed, continued breastfeeding is recommended. For more severe cases, intravenous fluids may be needed. Fluids may also be given by a nasogastric tube. Zinc supplementation is recommended in children. Antibiotics are generally not needed.

It is estimated that three to five billion cases of gastroenteritis resulting in 1.4 million deaths occur globally each year. Children and those in the developing world are most commonly affected. As of 2011, in those below age five, there were about 1.7 billion cases resulting in 0.7 million deaths. In the developing world children less than two years of age frequently get six or more infections a year. It is less common in adults, partly due to the development of immunity.

Signs and Symptoms

Gastroenteritis typically involves both diarrhea and vomiting, or less commonly, presents with only one or the other. Abdominal cramping may also be present. Signs and symptoms usually begin 12–72 hours after contracting the infectious agent. If due to a viral agent, the condition usually resolves within one week. Some viral causes may also be associated with fever, fatigue, headache, and muscle pain. If the stool is bloody, the cause is less likely to be viral and more likely to be bacterial. Some bacterial infections may be associated with severe abdominal pain and may persist for several weeks.

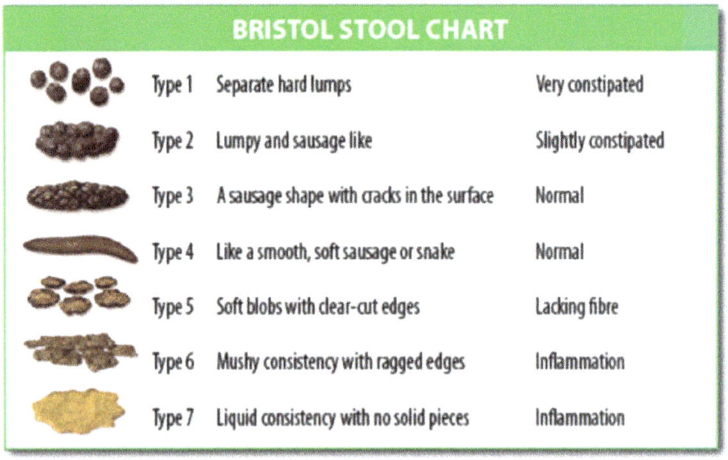

Bristol stool chart

Children infected with rotavirus usually make a full recovery within three to eight days. However, in poor countries treatment for severe infections is often out of reach and persistent diarrhea is common. Dehydration is a common complication of diarrhea, and a child with a significant degree of dehydration may have a prolonged capillary refill, poor skin turgor, and abnormal breathing. Repeat infections are typically seen in areas with poor sanitation, and malnutrition, stunted growth, and long-term cognitive delays can result.

Reactive arthritis occurs in 1% of people following infections with *Campylobacter* species, and Guillain–Barré syndrome occurs in 0.1%. Hemolytic uremic syndrome (HUS) may occur due to infection with Shiga toxin-producing *Escherichia coli* or *Shigella* species, causing low platelet counts, poor kidney function, and low red blood cell count (due to their breakdown). Children are more predisposed to getting HUS than adults. Some viral infections may produce benign infantile seizures.

Cause

Viruses (particularly rotavirus) and the bacteria *Escherichia coli* and *Campylobacter* species are the primary causes of gastroenteritis. There are, however, many other infectious agents that can cause this syndrome. Non-infectious causes are seen on occasion, but they are less likely than a viral or bacterial cause. Risk of infection is higher in children due to their lack of immunity and relatively poor hygiene.

Viral

Rotavirus, norovirus, adenovirus, and astrovirus are known to cause viral gastroenteritis. Rotavirus is the most common cause of gastroenteritis in children, and produces similar rates in both the developed and developing world. Viruses cause about 70% of episodes of infectious diarrhea in the pediatric age group. Rotavirus is a less common cause in adults due to acquired immunity. Norovirus is the cause in about 18% of all cases.

Norovirus is the leading cause of gastroenteritis among adults in America, causing greater than 90% of outbreaks. These localized epidemics typically occur when groups of people spend time in close physical proximity to each other, such as on cruise ships, in hospitals, or in restaurants. People may remain infectious even after their diarrhea has ended. Norovirus is the cause of about 10% of cases in children.

Bacterial

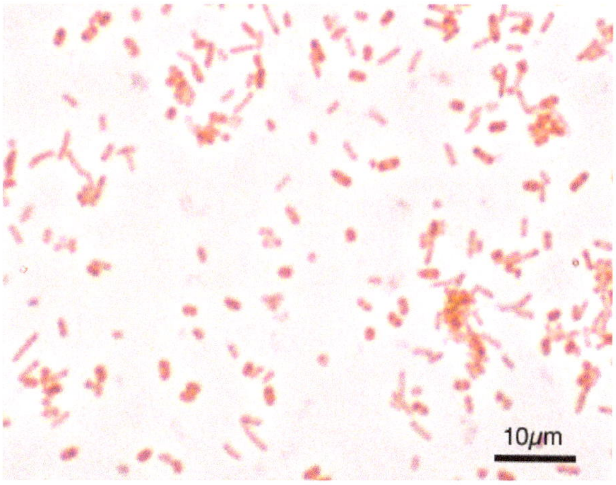

Salmonella enterica serovar Typhimurium (ATCC 14028) as seen with a microscope at 1000 fold magnification and following Gram staining.

In the developed world *Campylobacter jejuni* is the primary cause of bacterial gastroenteritis, with half of these cases associated with exposure to poultry. In children, bacteria are the cause in about 15% of cases, with the most common types being *Escherichia coli*, *Salmonella*, *Shigella*, and *Campylobacter* species. If food becomes contaminated with bacteria and remains at room temperature for a period of several hours, the bacteria multiply and increase the risk of infection in those who consume the food. Some foods commonly associated with illness include raw or undercooked meat, poultry, seafood, and eggs; raw sprouts; unpasteurized milk and soft cheeses; and fruit and vegetable juices. In the developing world, especially sub-Saharan Africa and Asia, cholera is a common cause of gastroenteritis. This infection is usually transmitted by contaminated water or food.

Toxigenic *Clostridium difficile* is an important cause of diarrhea that occurs more often in the elderly. Infants can carry these bacteria without developing symptoms. It is a common cause of diarrhea in those who are hospitalized and is frequently associated with antibiotic use. *Staphylococcus aureus* infectious diarrhea may also occur in those who have used antibiotics. Acute "traveler's diarrhea" is usually a type of bacterial gastroenteritis, while the persistent form is usually parasitic. Acid-suppressing medication appears to increase the risk of significant infection after exposure to a number of organisms, including *Clostridium difficile*, *Salmonella*, and *Campylobacter* species. The risk is greater in those taking proton pump inhibitors than with H2 antagonists.

Parasitic

A number of protozoa can cause gastroenteritis – most commonly *Giardia lamblia* – but *Entamoeba histolytica*, *Cryptosporidium* spp., and other species have also been implicated. As a group, these agents comprise about 10% of cases in children. *Giardia* occurs more commonly in the developing world, but this etiologic agent causes this type of illness to some degree nearly everywhere. It occurs more commonly in persons who have traveled to areas with high prevalence, children who attend day care, men who have sex with men, and following disasters.

Transmission

Transmission may occur via consumption of contaminated water, or when people share personal objects. In places with wet and dry seasons, water quality typically worsens during the wet season, and this correlates with the time of outbreaks. In areas of the world with four seasons, infections are more common in the winter. Bottle-feeding of babies with improperly sanitized bottles is a significant cause on a global scale. Transmission rates are also related to poor hygiene, especially among children, in crowded households, and in those with pre-existing poor nutritional status. After developing tolerance, adults may carry certain organisms without exhibiting signs or symptoms, and thus act as natural reservoirs of contagion. While some agents (such as *Shigella*) only occur in primates, others may occur in a wide variety of animals (such as *Giardia*).

Non-infectious

There are a number of non-infectious causes of inflammation of the gastrointestinal tract. Some of the more common include medications (like NSAIDs), certain foods such as lactose (in those who are intolerant), and gluten (in those with celiac disease). Crohn's disease is also a non-infectious source of (often severe) gastroenteritis. Disease secondary to toxins may also occur. Some food-related conditions associated with nausea, vomiting, and diarrhea include: ciguatera poisoning due to consumption of contaminated predatory fish, scombroid associated with the consumption of certain types of spoiled fish, tetrodotoxin poisoning from the consumption of puffer fish among others, and botulism typically due to improperly preserved food.

In the United States, rates of emergency department use for noninfectious gastroenteritis dropped 30% from 2006 until 2011. Of the twenty most common conditions seen in the emergency department, rates of noninfectious gastroenteritis had the largest decrease in visits in that time period.

Pathophysiology

Gastroenteritis is defined as vomiting or diarrhea due to infection of the small or large bowel. The changes in the small bowel are typically noninflammatory, while the ones in the large bowel are inflammatory. The number of pathogens required to cause an infection varies from as few as one (for *Cryptosporidium*) to as many as 10^8 (for *Vibrio cholerae*).

Diagnosis

Gastroenteritis is typically diagnosed clinically, based on a person's signs and symptoms. Determining the exact cause is usually not needed as it does not alter management of the condition. However, stool cultures should be performed in those with blood in the stool, those who might have been exposed to food poisoning, and those who have recently traveled to the developing world. Diagnostic testing may also be done for surveillance. As hypoglycemia occurs in approximately 10% of infants and young children, measuring serum glucose in this population is recommended. Electrolytes and kidney function should also be checked when there is a concern about severe dehydration.

Dehydration

A determination of whether or not the person has dehydration is an important part of the assessment, with dehydration typically divided into mild (3–5%), moderate (6–9%), and severe (≥10%) cases. In children, the most accurate signs of moderate or severe dehydration are a prolonged capillary refill, poor skin turgor, and abnormal breathing. Other useful findings (when used in combination) include sunken eyes, decreased activity, a lack of tears, and a dry mouth. A normal urinary output and oral fluid intake is reassuring. Laboratory testing is of little clinical benefit in determining the degree of dehydration. Thus the use of urine testing or ultrasounds is generally not needed.

Differential Diagnosis

Other potential causes of signs and symptoms that mimic those seen in gastroenteritis that need to be ruled out include appendicitis, volvulus, inflammatory bowel disease, urinary tract infections, and diabetes mellitus. Pancreatic insufficiency, short bowel syndrome, Whipple's disease, coeliac disease, and laxative abuse should also be considered. The differential diagnosis can be complicated somewhat if the person exhibits *only* vomiting or diarrhea (rather than both).

Appendicitis may present with vomiting, abdominal pain, and a small amount of diarrhea in up to 33% of cases. This is in contrast to the large amount of diarrhea that is typical of gastroenteritis. Infections of the lungs or urinary tract in children may also cause vomiting or diarrhea. Classical diabetic ketoacidosis (DKA) presents with abdominal pain, nausea, and vomiting, but without diarrhea. One study found that 17% of children with DKA were initially diagnosed as having gastroenteritis.

Prevention

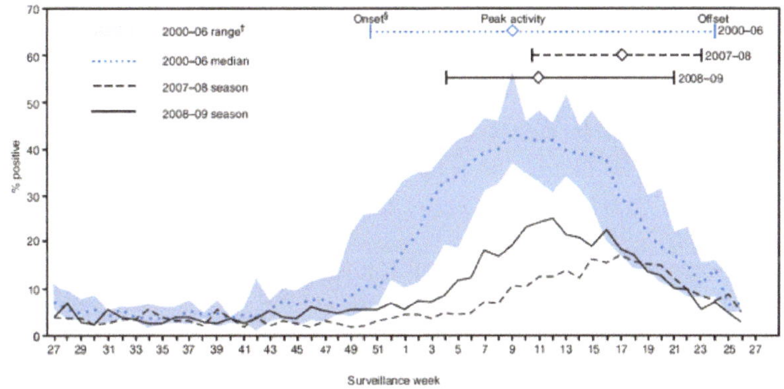

Percentage of rotavirus tests with positive results, by surveillance week, United States, July 2000 – June 2009.

Lifestyle

A supply of easily accessible uncontaminated water and good sanitation practices are important for reducing rates of infection and clinically significant gastroenteritis. Personal measures (such as hand washing with soap) have been found to decrease rates of gastroenteritis in both the developing and developed world by as much as 30%. Alcohol-based gels may also be effective. Breastfeeding is important, especially in places with poor hygiene, as is improvement of hygiene generally. Breast milk reduces both the frequency of infections and their duration. Avoiding contaminated food or drink should also be effective.

Vaccination

Due to both its effectiveness and safety, in 2009 the World Health Organization recommended that the rotavirus vaccine be offered to all children globally. Two commercial rotavirus vaccines exist and several more are in development. In Africa and Asia these vaccines reduced severe disease among infants and countries that have put in place national immunization programs have seen a decline in the rates and severity of disease. This vaccine may also prevent illness in non-vaccinated children by reducing the number of circulating infections. Since 2000, the implementation of a rotavirus vaccination program in the United States has substantially decreased the number of cases of diarrhea by as much as 80 percent. The first dose of vaccine should be given to infants between 6 and 15 weeks of age. The oral cholera vaccine has been found to be 50–60% effective over 2 years.

Management

Gastroenteritis is usually an acute and self-limiting disease that does not require medication. The preferred treatment in those with mild to moderate dehydration is oral rehydration therapy (ORT). For children at risk of dehydration from vomiting, taking a single dose of the anti vomiting medication metoclopramide or ondansetron, may be helpful, and butylscopolamine is useful in treating abdominal pain.

Rehydration

The primary treatment of gastroenteritis in both children and adults is rehydration. This is preferably achieved by drinking rehydration solution, although intravenous delivery may be required if there is a decreased level of consciousness or if dehydration is severe. Drinking replacement therapy products made with complex carbohydrates (i.e. those made from wheat or rice) may be superior to those based on simple sugars. Drinks especially high in simple sugars, such as soft drinks and fruit juices, are not recommended in children under 5 years of age as they may *increase* diarrhea. Plain water may be used if more specific ORT preparations are unavailable or the person is not willing to drink them. A nasogastric tube can be used in young children to administer fluids if warranted. In those who require intravenous fluids, one to four hours' worth is often sufficient.

Dietary

It is recommended that breast-fed infants continue to be nursed in the usual fashion, and that formula-fed infants continue their formula immediately after rehydration with ORT. Lactose-free or lactose-reduced formulas usually are not necessary. Children should continue their usual diet during episodes of diarrhea with the exception that foods high in simple sugars should be avoided. The BRAT diet (bananas, rice, applesauce, toast and tea) is no longer recommended, as it contains insufficient nutrients and has no benefit over normal feeding.

Some probiotics have been shown to be beneficial in reducing both the duration of illness and the frequency of stools. They may also be useful in preventing and treating antibiotic associated diarrhea. Fermented milk products (such as yogurt) are similarly beneficial. Zinc supplementation appears to be effective in both treating and preventing diarrhea among children in the developing world.

Antiemetics

Antiemetic medications may be helpful for treating vomiting in children. Ondansetron has some utility, with a single dose being associated with less need for intravenous fluids, fewer hospitalizations, and decreased vomiting. Metoclopramide might also be helpful. However, the use of ondansetron might possibly be linked to an increased rate of return to hospital in children. The intravenous preparation of ondansetron may be given orally if clinical judgment warrants. Dimenhydrinate, while reducing vomiting, does not appear to have a significant clinical benefit.

Antibiotics

Antibiotics are not usually used for gastroenteritis, although they are sometimes recommended if symptoms are particularly severe or if a susceptible bacterial cause is isolated or suspected. If antibiotics are to be employed, a macrolide (such as azithromycin) is preferred over a fluoroquinolone due to higher rates of resistance to the latter. Pseudomembranous colitis, usually caused by antibiotic use, is managed by discontinuing the causative agent and treating it with either metronidazole or vancomycin. Bacteria and protozoans that are amenable to treatment include *Shigella Salmonella typhi*, and *Giardia* species. In those with *Giardia* species or *Entamoeba histolytica*, tinidazole treatment is recommended and superior to metronidazole. The World Health Organization (WHO) recommends the use of antibiotics in young children who have both bloody diarrhea and fever.

Antimotility Agents

Antimotility medication has a theoretical risk of causing complications, and although clinical experience has shown this to be unlikely, these drugs are discouraged in people with bloody diarrhea or diarrhea that is complicated by fever. Loperamide, an opioid analogue, is commonly used for the symptomatic treatment of diarrhea. Loperamide is not recommended in children, however, as it may cross the immature blood–brain barrier and cause toxicity. Bismuth subsalicylate, an insoluble complex of trivalent bismuth and salicylate, can be used in mild to moderate cases, but salicylate toxicity is theoretically possible.

Epidemiology

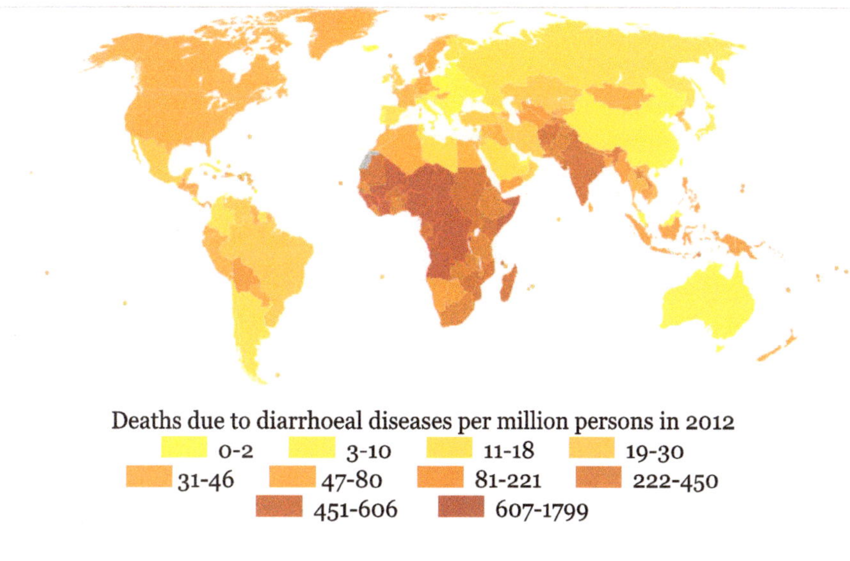

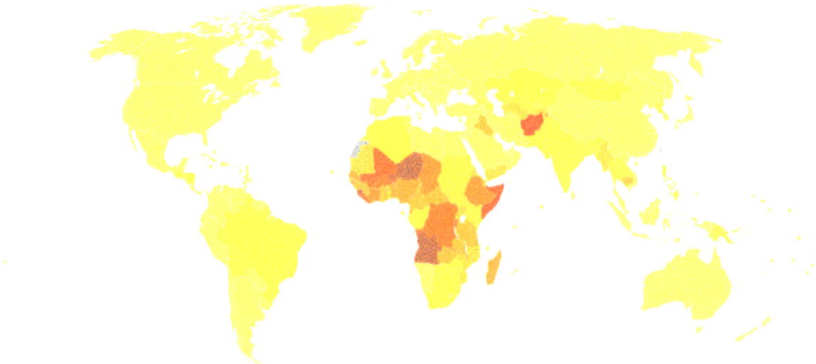

Disability-adjusted life year for diarrhea per 100,000 inhabitants in 2004.

- no data
- ≤less 500
- 500–1000
- 1000–1500
- 1500–2000
- 2000–2500
- 2500–3000
- 3000–3500
- 3500–4000
- 4000–4500
- 4500–5000
- 5000–6000
- ≥6000

It is estimated that three to five billion cases of gastroenteritis resulting in 1.4 million deaths occur globally on an annual basis. Children and those in the developing world are most commonly affected. As of 2011, in those less than five, there were about 1.7 billion cases resulting in 0.7 million deaths, with most of these occurring in the world's poorest nations. More than 450,000 of these fatalities are due to rotavirus in children under 5 years of age. Cholera causes about three to five million cases of disease and kills approximately 100,000 people yearly. In the developing world, children less than two years of age frequently get six or more infections a year that result in significant gastroenteritis. It is less common in adults, partly due to the development of acquired immunity.

In 1980, gastroenteritis from all causes caused 4.6 million deaths in children, with the majority occurring in the developing world. Death rates were reduced significantly (to approximately 1.5 million deaths annually) by the year 2000, largely due to the introduction and widespread use of oral rehydration therapy. In the US, infections causing gastroenteritis are the second most common infection (after the common cold), and they result in between 200 and 375 million cases of acute diarrhea and approximately ten thousand deaths annually, with 150 to 300 of these deaths in children less than five years of age.

History

The first usage of "gastroenteritis" was in 1825. Before this time it was commonly known as typhoid fever or "cholera morbus", among others, or less specifically as "griping of the guts", "surfeit", "flux", "colic", "bowel complaint", or any one of a number of other archaic names for acute diarrhea. Cholera morbus is a historical term that was used to refer to gastroenteritis rather than specifically cholera.

Society and Culture

Gastroenteritis is associated with many colloquial names, including “Montezuma’s revenge”, “Delhi belly”, “la turista”, and “back door sprint”, among others. It has played a role in many military campaigns and is believed to be the origin of the term “no guts no glory”.

Gastroenteritis is the main reason for 3.7 million visits to physicians a year in the United States and 3 million visits in France. In the United States gastroenteritis as a whole is believed to result in costs of 23 billion USD per year with that due to rotavirus alone resulting in estimated costs of 1 billion USD a year.

Research

There are a number of vaccines against gastroenteritis in development. For example, vaccines against *Shigella* and enterotoxigenic *Escherichia coli* (ETEC), two of the leading bacterial causes of gastroenteritis worldwide.

Other Animals

Many of the same agents cause gastroenteritis in cats and dogs as in humans. The most common organisms are *Campylobacter*, *Clostridium difficile*, *Clostridium perfringens*, and *Salmonella*. A large number of toxic plants may also cause symptoms.

Some agents are more specific to a certain species. Transmissible gastroenteritis coronavirus (TGEV) occurs in pigs resulting in vomiting, diarrhea, and dehydration. It is believed to be introduced to pigs by wild birds and there is no specific treatment available. It is not transmissible to humans.

Shigellosis

Shigellosis, also known as bacillary dysentery or Marlow syndrome, in its most severe manifestation, is a foodborne illness caused by infection by bacteria of the genus *Shigella*. Shigellosis rarely occurs in animals other than humans.

The causative organism is frequently found in water polluted with human feces, and is transmitted via the fecal-oral route. The usual mode of transmission is directly person-to-person hand-to-mouth, in the setting of poor hygiene among children.

Shigella is one of the leading bacterial causes of diarrhea worldwide and is a top pathogen causing moderate-to-severe diarrhea in African and South Asian children. It is also a major cause of illness in military personnel and travelers.

Signs and Symptoms

Signs and symptoms may range from mild abdominal discomfort to full-blown dysentery characterized by cramps, diarrhea, with slimy-consistent stools, fever, blood, pus, or mucus in stools or tenesmus. Onset time is 12 to 96 hours, and recovery takes 5 to 7 days.

Infections are associated with mucosal ulceration, rectal bleeding, and drastic dehydration. Reactive arthritis and hemolytic uremic syndrome are possible sequelae that have been reported in the aftermath of shigellosis.

Shigella can be transmitted through food, including salads (potato, tuna, shrimp, macaroni, and chicken), raw vegetables, milk and dairy products, and meat. Contamination of these foods is usually through the fecal-oral route. Fecally contaminated water and unsanitary handling by food handlers are the most common causes of contamination. Apart from hand-to-mouth infection, shigellosis is transmitted through fomites, water and mechanical vectors like houseflies.

The most common neurological symptom includes seizures.

Prevention

Simple precautions can be taken to prevent getting shigellosis: wash hands before handling food and thoroughly cook all food before eating. The primary prevention methods are improved sanitation and personal and food hygiene, but a low-cost and efficacious vaccine would complement these methods.

Since shigellosis is spread very quickly among children, keeping infected children out of daycare for 24 hours after their symptoms have disappeared, will decrease the occurrence of shigellosis in daycares.

Currently, no licensed vaccine targeting *Shigella* exists. Several vaccine candidates for *Shigella* are in various stages of development including live attenuated, conjugate, ribosomal, and proteosome vaccines. *Shigella* has been a longstanding World Health Organization target for vaccine development, and sharp declines in age-specific diarrhea/dysentery attack rates for this pathogen indicate that natural immunity does develop following exposure; thus, vaccination to prevent the disease should be feasible. Shigellosis is resistant to many antibiotics used to treat the disease, so vaccination is an important part of the strategy to reduce morbidity and mortality.

Treatment

Treatment consists mainly of replacing fluids and salts lost because of diarrhea. Oral replacement is satisfactory for most people, but some may need to receive fluids intravenously. In most cases, the disease resolves within four to eight days without antibiotics. Severe infections may last three to six weeks. Antibiotics, such as trimethoprim-sulfamethoxazole (Co-Trimoxazole), ciprofloxacin may be given when the person is very young or very old, when the disease is severe, or when the risk of the infection spreading to other people is high. Additionally, ampicillin (but not amoxicillin) was effective in treating this disease previously, but now the first choice of drug is pivmecillinam.

The severity of the symptoms and the length of time the stool contains *Shigella* are reduced with antibiotics. However, many strains of *Shigella* are becoming resistant to common antibiotics, and effective medications are often in short supply in developing countries. Antidiarrheal drugs (such as diphenoxylate or loperamide) may prolong the infection and should not be used.

Epidemiology

Insufficient data exist, but it is estimated to have caused the death of 34,000 children under the age of five in 2013, and 40,000 deaths in people over five years of age. *Shigella* also causes about 580,000 cases annually among travelers and military personnel from industrialized countries.

An estimated 500,000 cases of shigellosis occur annually in the United States. Infants, the elderly, and the critically ill are susceptible to the most severe symptoms of disease, but all humans are susceptible to some degree. Individuals with acquired immune deficiency syndrome (AIDS) are more frequently infected with *Shigella*. Shigellosis is a more common and serious condition in the developing world; fatality rates of shigellosis epidemics in developing countries can be 5–15%.

Orthodox Jewish communities (OJCs) are a known risk group for shigellosis; *Shigella sonnei* is cyclically epidemic in these communities in Israel, with sporadic outbreaks occurring elsewhere in among these communities. "Through phylogenetic and genomic analysis, we showed that strains from outbreaks in OJCs outside of Israel are distinct from strains in the general population and relate to a single multidrug-resistant sublineage of *S. sonnei* that prevails in Israel. Further Bayesian phylogenetic analysis showed that this strain emerged approximately 30 years ago, demonstrating the speed at which antimicrobial drug–resistant pathogens can spread widely through geographically dispersed, but internationally connected, communities."

Listeriosis

Listeriosis is a bacterial infection most commonly caused by *Listeria monocytogenes*, although *L. ivanovii* and *L. grayi* have been reported in certain cases. *Listeria* primarily causes infections of the central nervous system (meningitis, meningoencephalitis, brain abscess, cerebritis) and bacteremia in those who are immunocompromised, pregnant women, and those at the extremes of age (newborns and the elderly), as well as gastroenteritis in healthy persons who have been severely infected. *Listeria* is ubiquitous and is primarily transmitted via the oral route after ingestion of contaminated food products, after which the organism penetrates the intestinal tract to cause systemic infections. The diagnosis of listeriosis requires the isolation of the organism from the blood and/or the cerebrospinal fluid. Treatment includes prolonged administration of antibiotics, primarily ampicillin and gentamicin, to which the organism is usually susceptible.

Signs and Symptoms

The disease primarily affects older adults, persons with weakened immune systems, pregnant women, and newborns. Rarely, people without these risk factors can also be affected. A person with listeriosis usually has fever and muscle aches, often preceded by diarrhea or other gastrointestinal symptoms. Almost everyone who is diagnosed with listeriosis has invasive infection (meaning that the bacteria spread from their intestines to their blood stream or other body sites). Disease may occur as much as two months after eating contaminated food.

The symptoms vary with the infected person:

- High-risk persons other than pregnant women: Symptoms can include fever, muscle aches, headache, stiff neck, confusion, loss of balance, and convulsions.
- Pregnant women: Pregnant women typically experience only a mild, flu-like illness. However, infections during pregnancy can lead to miscarriage, stillbirth, premature delivery, or life-threatening infection of the newborn.
- Previously healthy persons: People who were previously healthy but were exposed to a very large dose of Listeria can develop a non-invasive illness (meaning that the bacteria have not spread into their blood stream or other body sites). Symptoms can include diarrhea and fever.

If an animal has eaten food contaminated with Listeria and does not have any symptoms, most experts believe that no tests or treatment are needed, even for people at high risk for listeriosis.

Cause

Listeria monocytogenes is ubiquitous in the environment. The main route of acquisition of *Listeria* is through the ingestion of contaminated food products. *Listeria* has been isolated from raw meat, dairy products, vegetables, fruit and seafood. Soft cheeses, unpasteurized milk and unpasteurised pâté are potential dangers; however, some outbreaks involving post-pasteurized milk have been reported.

Rarely listeriosis may present as cutaneous listeriosis. This infection occurs after direct exposure to *L. monocytogenes* by intact skin and is largely confined to veterinarians who are handling diseased animals, most often after a listerial abortion.

Diagnosis

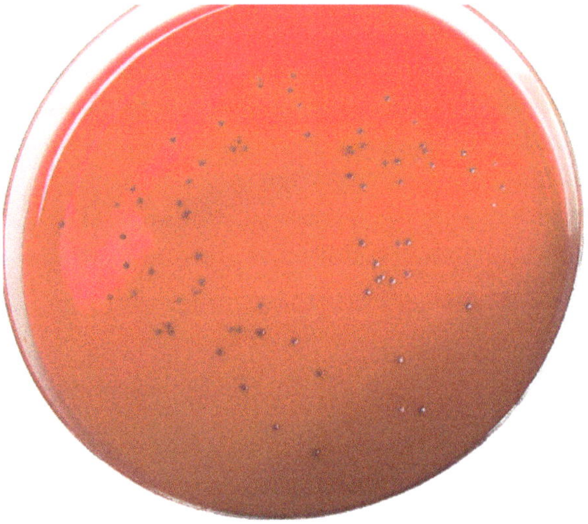

Listeria monocytogenes grown on Biorad RAPID'L.Mono Agar

In CNS infection cases, *L. monocytogenes* can often be cultured from the blood or from the CSF (Cerebrospinal fluid).

Prevention

The main means of prevention is through the promotion of safe handling, cooking and consumption of food. This includes washing raw vegetables and cooking raw food thoroughly, as well as reheating leftover or ready-to-eat foods like hot dogs until steaming hot.

Another aspect of prevention is advising high-risk groups such as pregnant women and immunocompromised patients to avoid unpasteurized pâtés and foods such as soft cheeses like feta, Brie, Camembert cheese, and bleu. Cream cheeses, yogurt, and cottage cheese are considered safe. In the United Kingdom, advice along these lines from the Chief Medical Officer posted in maternity clinics led to a sharp decline in cases of listeriosis in pregnancy in the late 1980s.

Treatment

Bacteremia should be treated for 2 weeks, meningitis for 3 weeks, and brain abscess for at least 6 weeks. Ampicillin generally is considered antibiotic of choice; gentamicin is added frequently for its synergistic effects. Overall mortality rate is 20–30%; of all pregnancy-related cases, 22% resulted in fetal loss or neonatal death, but mothers usually survive.

Epidemiology

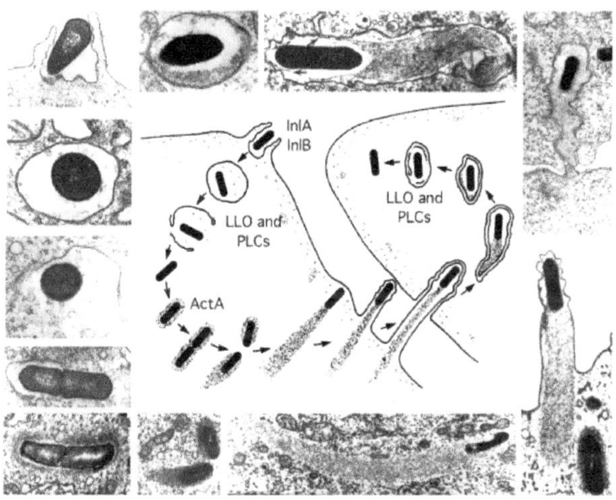

Stages in the intracellular life-cycle of *Listeria monocytogenes*. (Center) Cartoon depicting entry, escape from a vacuole, actin nucleation, actin-based motility, and cell-to-cell spread. (Outside) Representative electron micrographs from which the cartoon was derived. LLO, PLCs, and ActA are all described in the text. The cartoon and micrographs were adapted from Tilney and Portnoy (1989).

Incidence in 2004–2005 was 2.5–3 cases per million population a year in the United States, where pregnant women accounted for 30% of all cases. Of all nonperinatal infections, 70% occur in immunocompromised patients. Incidence in the U.S. has been falling since the 1990s, in contrast to Europe where changes in eating habits have led to an increase during the same time. In Sweden, it has stabilized at around 5 cases per annum per million population, with pregnant women typically accounting for 1–2 of some 40 total yearly cases.

There are four distinct clinical syndromes:

- Infection in pregnancy: *Listeria* can proliferate asymptomatically in the vagina and uterus.

If the mother becomes symptomatic, it is usually in the third trimester. Symptoms include fever, myalgias, arthralgias and headache. Miscarriage, stillbirth and preterm labor are complications of this infection. Symptoms last 7–10 days.

- Neonatal infection (granulomatosis infantiseptica): There are two forms. One, an early-onset sepsis, with *Listeria* acquired in utero, results in premature birth. *Listeria* can be isolated in the placenta, blood, meconium, nose, ears, and throat. Another, late-onset meningitis is acquired through vaginal transmission, although it also has been reported with caesarean deliveries.

- Central nervous system (CNS) infection: *Listeria* has a predilection for the brain parenchyma, especially the brain stem, and the meninges. It can cause cranial nerve palsies, encephalitis, meningitis, meningoencephalitis and abscesses. Mental status changes are common. Seizures occur in at least 25% of patients.

- Gastroenteritis: *L. monocytogenes* can produce food-borne diarrheal disease, which typically is noninvasive. The median incubation period is 21 days, with diarrhea lasting anywhere from 1–3 days. Patients present with fever, muscle aches, gastrointestinal nausea or diarrhea, headache, stiff neck, confusion, loss of balance, or convulsions.

Listeria has also been reported to colonize the hearts of some patients. The overall incidence of cardiac infections caused by *Listeria* is relatively low, with 7-10% of case reports indicating some form of heart involvement. There is some evidence that small subpopulations of clinical isolates are more capable of colonizing the heart throughout the course of infection, but cardiac manifestations are usually sporadic and may rely on a combination of bacterial factors and host predispositions, as they do with other strains of cardiotropic bacteria.

Recent Outbreaks

According to the Centers for Disease Control and Prevention (CDC) there are about 1,600 cases of listeriosis annually in the United States. Compared to 1996-1998, the incidence of listeriosis had declined by about 38% by 2003. However, illnesses and deaths continue to occur. On average from 1998-2008, 2.4 outbreaks per year were reported to the CDC. A large outbreak occurred in 2002, when 54 illnesses, 8 deaths, and 3 fetal deaths in 9 states were found to be associated with consumption of contaminated turkey deli meat.

The 2008 Canadian listeriosis outbreak, an outbreak of listeriosis in Canada linked to a Maple Leaf Foods plant in Toronto, Ontario killed 22 people.

On March 13, 2015, the Centers for Disease Control and Prevention that State and local health officials, CDC, and FDA are collaborating to investigate an outbreak of Listeria. The joint investigation found that certain Blue Bell brand ice cream products are the likely source for some or all of these illnesses. Upon further investigation the CDC claimed Blue Bell ice cream had evidence of listeria bacteria in its Oklahoma manufacturing plant as far back as March 2013, which led to 3 deaths in Kansas.

On March 14, 2015, an outbreak of listeriosis in Kansas was linked to certain Blue Bell Ice Cream products (Blue Bell Chocolate Chip Country Cookies, Great Divide Bars, Sour Pop Green Apple

Bars, Cotton Candy Bars, Scoops, Vanilla Stick Slices, Almond Bars, and No Sugar Added Moo Bars). Blue Bell, the nation's third most popular ice cream brand, says its regular Moo Bars were untainted, as were its ice cream varieties in three-gallon, half-gallon, quart, pint and single-serving containers and its take-home frozen snack novelties. It was the first outbreak of a foodborne illness in the company's history. The items came from the company's production facility located in Broken Arrow, Oklahoma, according to the U.S. Food and Drug Administration (FDA), in Washington, D.C. The Atlanta-based U.S. Centers for Disease Control and Prevention (CDC), also a branch of the U.S. Department of Health and Human Services (DHHS), stated that all five of the sickened individuals, including the three who have died (60% mortality rate) were receiving treatment at the same Kansas hospital before developing the listeriosis, suggesting their infections with the *Listeria* bacteria were nosocomial (acquired, while eating the products, in the hospital). That might also help to explain the higher mortality rate in these cases (60%, versus the more normal 20%-30%): the people, who were all older (three of the five were women) were already hospitalized.

On April 20, 2015, Blue Bell issued a voluntary recall of all its products, citing further internal testing that found *Listeria monocytogenes* in an additional half gallon of ice cream from the Brenham facility.

2011 United States Listeriosis Outbreak

On September 14, 2011, the U.S. Food and Drug Administration warned consumers not to eat cantaloupes shipped by Jensen Farms from Granada, Colorado due to a potential link to a multistate outbreak of listeriosis. At that time Jensen Farms voluntarily recalled cantaloupes shipped from July 29 through September 10, and distributed to at least 17 states with possible further distribution. The CDC reported that at least 22 people in seven states had been infected as of September 14.

On September 26, the Centers for Disease Control and Prevention reported that a total of 72 persons had been infected with the four outbreak-associated strains of Listeria monocytogenes which had been reported to the CDC from 18 states. All illnesses started on or after July 31, 2011 and by September 26, thirteen deaths had been reported: 2 in Colorado, 1 in Kansas, 1 in Maryland, 1 in Missouri, 1 in Nebraska, 4 in New Mexico, 1 in Oklahoma, and 2 in Texas. On September 30, 2011, a random sample of romaine lettuce taken by the U.S. Food and Drug Administration tested positive for listeria on lettuce shipped on September 12 and 13 by an Oregon distributor to at least two other states—Washington and Idaho.

By October 18, the CDC reported that 12 states are now linked to listeria in cantaloupe and that 123 people have been sickened and a total of 25 have died. While the tainted cantaloupes should be off store shelves by now, the number of illnesses may still continue to grow. The CDC confirmed a sixth death in Colorado and a second in New York; Indiana, Kansas, Louisiana, Maryland, Missouri, Nebraska, New Mexico, Oklahoma, Texas and Wyoming have also reported deaths.

A final count on December 8 put the death toll at 30: Colorado (8), Indiana (1), Kansas (3), Louisiana (2), Maryland (1), Missouri (3), Nebraska (1), New Mexico (5), New York (2), Oklahoma (1), Texas (2), and Wyoming (1). Among persons who died, ages ranged from 48 to 96 years, with a median age of 82.5 years. In addition, one woman pregnant at the time of illness had a miscarriage.

Botulism

Botulism is a rare and potentially fatal illness caused by a toxin, produced by the bacterium *Clostridium botulinum*. The disease begins with weakness, trouble seeing, feeling tired, and trouble speaking. This may then be followed by weakness of the arms, chest muscles, and legs. The disease does not usually affect consciousness or cause a fever.

Botulism can be spread several different ways. The bacterial spores which cause it are common in both soil and water. They produce the botulinum toxin when exposed to low oxygen levels and certain temperatures. Foodborne botulism happens when food containing the toxin is eaten. Infant botulism happens when the bacteria develops in the intestines and releases the toxin. This typically only occurs in children less than six months old, as protective mechanisms develop after that time. Wound botulism is found most often among those who inject street drugs. In this situation, spores enter a wound, and in the absence of oxygen, release the toxin. It is not passed directly between people. The diagnosis is confirmed by finding the toxin or bacteria in the person in question.

Prevention is primarily by proper food preparation. The toxin, though not the organism, is destroyed by heating it to more than 85 °C (185 °F) for longer than 5 minutes. Honey can contain the organism, and for this reason, honey should not be fed to children under 12 months. Treatment is with an antitoxin. In those who lose their ability to breathe on their own, mechanical ventilation may be necessary for months. Antibiotics may be used for wound botulism. Death occurs in 5 to 10% of people. Botulism can affect many other animals.

Signs and Symptoms

The muscle weakness of botulism characteristically starts in the muscles supplied by the cranial nerves—a group of twelve nerves that control eye movements, the facial muscles and the muscles controlling chewing and swallowing. Double vision, drooping of both eyelids, loss of facial expression and swallowing problems may therefore occur. In addition to affecting the voluntary muscles, it can also cause disruptions in the autonomic nervous system. This is experienced as a dry mouth and throat (due to decreased production of saliva), postural hypotension (decreased blood pressure on standing, with resultant lightheadedness and risk of blackouts), and eventually constipation (due to decreased peristalsis). Some of the toxins (B and E) also precipitate nausea, vomiting, and difficulty with talking. The weakness then spreads to the arms (starting in the shoulders and proceeding to the forearms) and legs (again from the thighs down to the feet).

Severe botulism leads to reduced movement of the muscles of respiration, and hence problems with gas exchange. This may be experienced as dyspnea (difficulty breathing), but when severe can lead to respiratory failure, due to the buildup of unexhaled carbon dioxide and its resultant depressant effect on the brain. This may lead to coma and eventually death if untreated.

Clinicians frequently think of the symptoms of botulism in terms of a classic triad: bulbar palsy and descending paralysis, lack of fever, and clear senses and mental status ("clear sensorium").

Infant Botulism

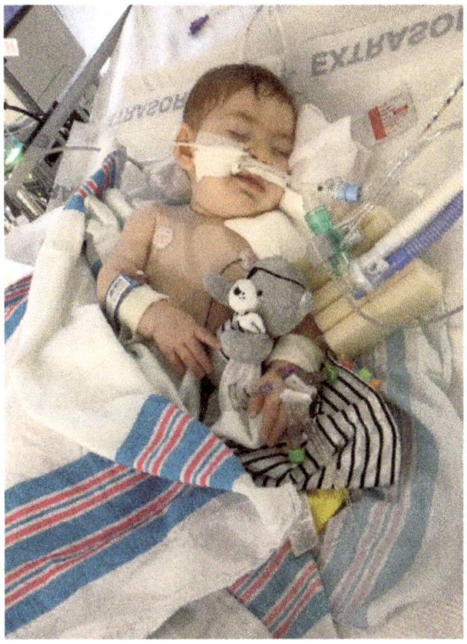

Infant with botulism. He is unable to move or open his eyes. His cry was weak. He is not asleep or sedated.

Infant botulism (also referred to as floppy baby syndrome) was first recognized in 1976, and is the most common form of botulism in the United States. There were 17 diagnosed cases of infant botulism in the United States in 2013. Infants are susceptible to infant botulism in the first year of life, with more than 90% of cases occurring in infants younger than six months. Infant botulism results from the ingestion of the *C. botulinum* spores, and subsequent colonization of the small intestine. The infant gut may be colonized when the composition of the intestinal microflora (normal flora) is insufficient to competitively inhibit the growth of *C. botulinum* and levels of bile acids (which normally inhibit clostridial growth) are lower than later in life.

The growth of the spores releases botulinum toxin, which is then absorbed into the bloodstream and taken throughout the body, causing paralysis by blocking the release of acetylcholine at the neuromuscular junction. Typical symptoms of infant botulism include constipation, lethargy, weakness, difficulty feeding and an altered cry, often progressing to a complete descending flaccid paralysis. Although constipation is usually the first symptom of infant botulism, it is commonly overlooked.

Honey is a known dietary reservoir of *C. botulinum* spores and has been linked to infant botulism. For this reason honey is not recommended for infants less than one year of age. Most cases of infant botulism, however, are thought to be caused by acquiring the spores from the natural environment. *Clostridium botulinum* is a ubiquitous soil-dwelling bacterium. Many infant botulism patients have been demonstrated to live near a construction site or an area of soil disturbance.

Infant botulism has been reported in 49 of 50 US states, and cases have been recognized in 26 countries on five continents.

Complications

Infant botulism has no long-term side effects, but can be complicated by hospital-acquired infections. The case fatality rate is less than 1% for hospitalized infants with botulism.

Botulism can result in death due to respiratory failure. However, in the past 50 years, the proportion of patients with botulism who die has fallen from about 50% to 7% due to improved supportive care. A patient with severe botulism may require mechanical ventilation (breathing support through a ventilator) as well as intensive medical and nursing care, sometimes for several months. The respiratory failure and paralysis that occur with severe botulism may require a person to be on a breathing machine (ventilator) for weeks or months. The person may require rehabilitation therapy after leaving the hospital.

Cause

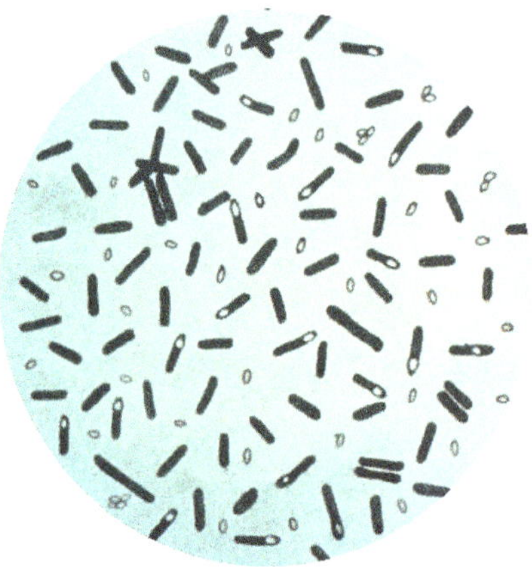

A photomicrograph of Clostridium botulinum bacteria.

Clostridium botulinum is an anaerobic, Gram positive, spore-forming rod. Botulinum toxin is one of the most powerful known toxins: about one microgram is lethal to humans when inhaled. It acts by blocking nerve function (neuromuscular blockade) through inhibition of the excitatory neurotransmitter acetylcholine's release from the presynaptic membrane of neuromuscular junctions in the somatic nervous system. This causes paralysis. Advanced botulism can cause respiratory failure by paralysing the muscles of the chest; this can progress to respiratory arrest.

In all cases, illness is caused by the botulinum toxin produced by the bacterium *C. botulinum* in anaerobic conditions and not by the bacterium itself. The pattern of damage occurs because the toxin affects nerves that fire (depolarise) at a higher frequency first.

Mechanisms of entry into the human body for botulinum toxin are described below.

Colonization of the Gut

The most common form in Western countries is infant botulism. This occurs in infants who are colonized with the bacterium in the small intestine during the early stages of their lives. The bacterium then produces the toxin, which is absorbed into the bloodstream. The consumption of honey during the first year of life has been identified as a risk factor for infant botulism; it is a factor in a fifth of all cases. The adult form of infant botulism is termed *adult intestinal toxemia*, and is exceedingly rare.

Food

Toxin that is produced by the bacterium within containers of food that have been improperly preserved is the most common cause of food-borne botulism. Fish that has been pickled without the salinity or acidity of brine that contains acetic acid and high sodium levels, as well as smoked fish stored at too high a temperature, presents a risk, as does improperly canned food.

Food borne botulism results from contaminated food in which *C. botulinum* spores have been allowed to germinate in low-oxygen conditions. This typically occurs in home-canned food substances and fermented uncooked dishes. Given that multiple people often consume food from the same source, it is common for more than a single person to be affected simultaneously. Symptoms usually appear 12–36 hours after eating, but can also appear within 2 hours to 10 days.

Wound

Wound botulism results from the contamination of a wound with the bacteria, which then secrete the toxin into the bloodstream. This has become more common in intravenous drug users since the 1990s, especially people using black tar heroin and those injecting heroin into the skin rather than the veins. Wound botulism accounts for 29% of cases.

Inhalation

Isolated cases of botulism have been described after inhalation by laboratory workers.

Injection

Botulism has occurred after cosmetic use of inappropriate strengths of Botox.

Mechanism

The toxin is the protein botulinum toxin produced under anaerobic conditions (where there is no oxygen) by the bacterium *Clostridium botulinum.*

Clostridium botulinum is a large anaerobic Gram-positive bacillus that forms subterminal endospores.

There are eight serological varieties of the bacterium denoted by the letters A to H. The toxin from all of these acts in the same way and produces similar symptoms: the motor nerve endings are prevented from releasing acetylcholine, causing flaccid paralysis and symptoms of blurred vision, ptosis, nausea, vomiting, diarrhea and/or constipation, cramps, and respiratory difficulty.

Botulinum toxin is broken into 8 neurotoxins (labeled as types A, B, C [C1, C2], D, E, F, and G), which are antigenically and serologically distinct but structurally similar. Human botulism is caused mainly by types A, B, E, and (rarely) F. Types C and D cause toxicity only in other animals.

In October 2013, scientists released news of the discovery of type H, the first new botulism neurotoxin found in forty years. However, further information about type H has not been disclosed because of its potential for abuse as a lethal bioweapon and lack of a known antitoxin.

Some types produce a characteristic putrefactive smell and digest meat (types A and some of B and F); these are said to be proteolytic; type E and some types of B, C, D and F are nonproteolytic and can go undetected because there is no strong odor associated with them.

When the bacteria are under stress, they develop spores, which are inert. Their natural habitats are in the soil, in the silt that comprises the bottom sediment of streams, lakes and coastal waters and ocean, while some types are natural inhabitants of the intestinal tracts of mammals (e.g., horses, cattle, humans), and are present in their excreta. The spores can survive in their inert form for many years.

Toxin is produced by the bacteria when environmental conditions are favourable for the spores to replicate and grow, but the gene that encodes for the toxin protein is actually carried by a virus or phage that infects the bacteria. Unfortunately, little is known about the natural factors that control phage infection and replication within the bacteria.

The spores require warm temperatures, a protein source, an anaerobic environment, and moisture in order to become active and produce toxin. In the wild, decomposing vegetation and invertebrates combined with warm temperatures can provide ideal conditions for the botulism bacteria to activate and produce toxin that may affect feeding birds and other animals. Spores are not killed by boiling, but botulism is uncommon because special, rarely obtained conditions are necessary for botulinum toxin production from C. botulinum spores, including an anaerobic, low-salt, low-acid, low-sugar environment at ambient temperatures.

Botulinum inhibits the release within the nervous system of acetylcholine, a neurotransmitter, responsible for communication between motor neurons and muscle cells. All forms of botulism lead to paralysis that typically starts with the muscles of the face and then spreads towards the limbs. In severe forms, botulism leads to paralysis of the breathing muscles and causes respiratory failure. In light of this life-threatening complication, all suspected cases of botulism are treated as medical emergencies, and public health officials are usually involved to identify the source and take steps to prevent further cases from occurring.

Botulinum toxin A, C, and E cleave the SNAP-25, ultimately leading to paralysis.

Diagnosis

For botulism in babies, diagnosis should be made on signs and symptoms. Confirmation of the diagnosis is made by testing of a stool or enema specimen with the mouse bioassay.

Physicians may consider diagnosing botulism if the patient's history and physical examination suggest botulism. However, these clues are often not enough to allow a diagnosis. Other diseases such as Guillain–Barré syndrome, stroke, and myasthenia gravis can appear similar to botulism, and special tests may be needed to exclude these other conditions. These tests may include a brain scan, cerebrospinal fluid examination, nerve conduction test (electromyography, or EMG), and an edrophonium chloride (Tensilon) test for myasthenia gravis. A definite diagnosis can be made if botulinum toxin is identified in the food, stomach or intestinal contents, vomit or feces. The toxin is occasionally found in the blood in peracute cases. Botulinum toxin can be detected by a variety of techniques, including enzyme-linked immunosorbent assays (ELISAs), electrochemiluminescent (ECL) tests and mouse inoculation or feeding trials. The toxins can be typed with neutralization tests in mice. In toxicoinfectious botulism, the organism can be cultured from tissues. On egg yolk medium, toxin-producing colonies usually display surface iridescence that extends beyond the colony.

Prevention

Although the botulinum toxin is destroyed by thorough cooking over the course of a few minutes, the spore itself is not killed by the temperatures reached with normal sea-level-pressure boiling, leaving it free to grow and again produce the toxin when conditions are right.

A recommended prevention measure for infant botulism is to avoid giving honey to infants less than 12 months of age, as botulinum spores are often present. In older children and adults the normal intestinal bacteria suppress development of *C. botulinum.*

While commercially canned goods are required to undergo a "botulinum cook" in a pressure cooker at 121 °C (250 °F) for 3 minutes, and so rarely cause botulism, there have been notable exceptions such as the 1978 Alaskan salmon outbreak and the 2007 Castleberry's Food Company outbreak. Foodborne botulism is the rarest form though, accounting for only around 15% of cases (US) and has more frequently been from home-canned foods with low acid content, such as carrot juice, asparagus, green beans, beets, and corn. However, outbreaks of botulism have resulted from more unusual sources. In July 2002, fourteen Alaskans ate *muktuk* (whale meat) from a beached whale, and eight of them developed symptoms of botulism, two of them requiring mechanical ventilation.

Other, but much rarer sources of infection (about every decade in the US) include garlic or herbs stored covered in oil without acidification, chili peppers, improperly handled baked potatoes wrapped in aluminum foil, tomatoes, and home-canned or fermented fish.

When canning or preserving food at home, attention should be paid to hygiene, pressure, temperature, refrigeration and storage. When making home preserves, only acidic fruit such as apples, pears, stone fruits and berries should be bottled. Tropical fruit and tomatoes are low in acidity and must have some acidity added before they are bottled.

Oils infused with fresh garlic or herbs should be acidified and refrigerated. Potatoes which have been baked while wrapped in aluminum foil should be kept hot until served or refrigerated. Because the botulism toxin is destroyed by high temperatures, home-canned foods are best boiled for 10 minutes before eating. Metal cans containing food in which bacteria, possibly botulinum, are growing may bulge outwards due to gas production from bacterial growth; such cans should be discarded.

Any container of food which has been heat-treated and then assumed to be airtight which shows signs of not being so, e.g., metal cans with pinprick holes from rust or mechanical damage, should also be discarded. Contamination of a canned food solely with *C. botulinum* may not cause any visual defects (e.g. bulging). Only sufficient thermal processing during production should be used as a food safety control.

Vaccine

There is a vaccine but its usefulness is unclear as it is associated with significant adverse effects. As of 2013 there are efforts ongoing to develop a better vaccine.

Treatment

Botulism is generally treated with botulism antitoxin and supportive care.

Supportive care for botulism includes monitoring of respiratory function. Respiratory failure due to paralysis may require mechanical ventilation for 2 to 8 weeks, plus intensive medical and nursing care. After this time, paralysis generally improves as new neuromuscular connections are formed.

In some abnormal cases, physicians may try to remove contaminated food still in the digestive tract by inducing vomiting and/or using enemas. Wounds should be treated, usually surgically, to remove the source of the toxin-producing bacteria.

Antitoxin

In adults, botulism can be treated by passive immunization with a horse-derived antitoxin, which blocks the action of the toxin circulating in the blood. A trivalent antitoxin containing antibodies raised against botulinum toxin types A, B, and E is used most commonly, however a heptavalent botulism antitoxin has also been developed and was approved by the U.S. FDA in 2013. In infants, horse-derived antitoxin is sometimes avoided for fear of infants developing serum sickness or lasting hypersensitivity to horse-derived proteins. To avoid this, a human-derived antitoxin has been developed and approved by the U.S. FDA in 2003 for the treatment of infant botulism. This human-derived antitoxin has been shown to be both safe and effective for the treatment of infant botulism. However, the danger of equine-derived antitoxin to infants has not been clearly established, and one study showed the equine-derived antitoxin to be both safe and effective for the treatment of infant botulism.

Trivalent (A,B,E) botulinum antitoxin is derived from equine sources utilizing whole antibodies (Fab and Fc portions). In the United States, this antitoxin is available from the local health department via the CDC. The second antitoxin, heptavalent (A,B,C,D,E,F,G) botulinum antitoxin, is derived from "despeciated" equine IgG antibodies which have had the Fc portion cleaved off leaving the F(ab')2 portions. This less immunogenic antitoxin is effective against all known strains of botulism where not contraindicated.

Prognosis

The paralysis caused by botulism can persist for 2 to 8 weeks, during which supportive care and ventilation may be necessary to keep the patient alive. Botulism is fatal in 5 to 10% of people who are affected. However, if left untreated, botulism is fatal in 40 to 50% of cases.

The mortality rate for wound botulism is about 10%.

Infant botulism has no long-term side effects but can be complicated by nosocomial adverse events. The case fatality rate is less than 1% for hospitalized infants with botulism. In part because the vast majority of infants with botulism are hospitalized, the overall infant botulism mortality rate is about 1.3%.

Epidemiology

Globally, botulism is fairly rare. In the United States, for example, an average of 145 cases are reported each year. Of these, roughly 65% are infant botulism, 20% are wound botulism, and 15% are foodborne. Infant botulism is predominantly sporadic and not associated with epidemics, but great geographic variability exists. From 1974 to 1996, for example, 47.2% of all infant botulism cases reported in the U.S. occurred in California.

Between 1990 and 2000, the Centers for Disease Control and Prevention reported 263 individual foodborne cases from 160 botulism events in the United States with a case-fatality rate of 4%. Thirty-nine percent (103 cases and 58 events) occurred in Alaska, all of which were attributable to traditional Alaska aboriginal foods. In the lower 49 states, home-canned food was implicated in 70 (91%) events with canned asparagus being the most numerous cause. Two restaurant-associated outbreaks affected 25 persons. The median number of cases per year was 23 (range 17–43), the median number of events per year was 14 (range 9–24). The highest incidence rates occurred in Alaska, Idaho, Washington, and Oregon. All other states had an incidence rate of 1 case per ten million people or less.

The number of cases of food borne and infant botulism has changed little in recent years, but wound botulism has increased because of the use of black tar heroin, especially in California.

United States

All data regarding botulism antitoxin releases and laboratory confirmation of cases in the US are recorded annually by the Centers for Disease Control and Prevention and published on their website.

- 1971 Bon Vivant botulism case On July 2, 1971, the U.S. Food and Drug Administration (FDA) released a public warning after learning that a New York man had died and his wife had become seriously ill due to botulism after eating a can of Bon Vivant vichyssoise soup.
- Between March 31 and April 6, 1977, 59 individuals developed type B botulism. All ill persons had eaten at the same Mexican restaurant in Pontiac, Michigan and all had consumed a hot sauce made with improperly home-canned jalapeño peppers, either by adding it to their food, or by eating a nacho that had had hot sauce used in its preparation. The full clinical spectrum (mild symptomatology with neurologic findings through life-threatening ventilatory paralysis) of type B botulism was documented.
- In April 1994, the largest outbreak of botulism in the United States since 1978 occurred in El Paso, Texas. Thirty persons were affected; 4 required mechanical ventilation. All ate food from a Greek restaurant. The attack rate among persons who ate a potato-based dip was 86% (19/22) compared with 6% (11/176) among persons who did not eat the dip (relative risk [RR] Å 13.8; 95% confidence interval [CI], 7.6–25.1). The attack rate among persons who ate an eggplant-based dip was 67% (6/9) compared with 13% (24/189) among persons who did not (RR Å 5.2; 95% CI, 2.9–9.5). Botulism toxin type A was detected from patients and in both dips. Toxin formation resulted from holding aluminum foil-wrapped baked potatoes at room temperature, apparently for several days, before they were used in the dips. Food handlers should be informed of the potential hazards caused by holding foil-wrapped potatoes at ambient temperatures after cooking.
- Beginning in late June 2007, 8 people contracted botulism poisoning by eating canned food products produced by Castleberry's Food Company in its Augusta, Georgia plant. It was later identified that the Castleberry's plant had serious production problems on a specific line of retorts that had under-processed the cans of food. These issues included broken

cooking alarms, leaking water valves and inaccurate temperature devices, all the result of poor management of the company. All of the victims were hospitalized and placed on mechanical ventilation. The Castleberry's Food Company outbreak was the first instance of botulism in commercial canned foods in the United States in over 30 years.

- One person died, 21 cases were confirmed, and 10 more were suspected in Lancaster, Ohio when a botulism outbreak occurred after a church potluck in April 2015. The suspected source was a salad made from home-canned potatoes.

United Kingdom

The largest recorded outbreak of foodborne botulism in the United Kingdom occurred in June 1989. A total of 27 patients were affected; one patient died. Twenty-five of the patients had eaten one brand of hazelnut yogurt in the week before the onset of symptoms. This yogurt contained hazelnut conserve sweetened with aspartame rather than sugar. Control measures included the cessation of all yogurt production by the implicated producer, the withdrawal of the firm's yogurts from sale, the recall of cans of the hazelnut conserve, and advice to the general public to avoid the consumption of all hazelnut yogurts.

Other Species

Botulism can occur in many vertebrates and invertebrates. Botulism has been reported in rats, mice, chicken, frogs, toads, goldfish, aplysia, squid, crayfish, drosophila, leeches, etc.

Death from botulism is common in waterfowl; an estimated 10,000 to 100,000 birds die of botulism annually. In some large outbreaks, a million or more birds may die. Ducks appear to be affected most often. Botulism also affects commercially raised poultry. In chickens, the mortality rate varies from a few birds to 40% of the flock.

Botulism seems to be relatively uncommon in domestic mammals; however, in some parts of the world, epidemics with up to 65% mortality are seen in cattle. The prognosis is poor in large animals that are recumbent.

In cattle, the symptoms may include drooling, restlessness, uncoordination, urine retention, dysphagia, and sternal recumbency. Laterally recumbent animals are usually very close to death. In sheep, the symptoms may include drooling, a serous nasal discharge, stiffness, and incoordination. Abdominal respiration may be observed and the tail may switch on the side. As the disease progresses, the limbs may become paralyzed and death may occur. Phosphorus-deficient cattle, especially in southern Africa, are inclined to ingest bones and carrion containing clostridial toxins and consequently suffer *lame sickness* or *lamsiekte.*

A recent study has demonstrated an effective vaccine against cattle botulism associated with Clostridium botulinum serotypes C and D.

The clinical signs in horses are similar to cattle. The muscle paralysis is progressive; it usually begins at the hindquarters and gradually moves to the front limbs, neck, and head. Death generally occurs 24 to 72 hours after initial symptoms and results from respiratory paralysis. Some foals are found dead without other clinical signs.

Domestic dogs may develop systemic toxemia after consuming C. botulinum type C exotoxin or spores within bird carcasses or other infected meat but are generally resistant to the more severe effects of Clostridium botulinum type C. Symptoms include flaccid muscle paralysis; dogs with breathing difficulties will require more intensive care monitoring. Muscle paralysis can lead to death due to cardiac and respiratory arrest.

Pigs are relatively resistant to botulism. Reported symptoms include anorexia, refusal to drink, vomiting, pupillary dilation, and muscle paralysis.

In poultry and wild birds, flaccid paralysis is usually seen in the legs, wings, neck and eyelids. Broiler chickens with the toxicoinfectious form may also have diarrhea with excess urates.

Salmonellosis

Salmonellosis is an infection caused by *Salmonella* bacteria. Most people infected with *Salmonella* develop diarrhea, fever, vomiting, and abdominal cramps 12 to 72 hours after infection. In most cases, the illness lasts four to seven days, and most people recover without treatment. In some cases, the diarrhea may be so severe that the patient becomes dangerously dehydrated and must be hospitalized.

Intravenous fluids may be used to treat dehydration. Medications may be used to provide symptomatic relief, such as fever reduction. In severe cases, the *Salmonella* infection may spread from the intestines to the blood stream, and then to other body sites; this is known as typhoid fever and is treated with antibiotics.

The elderly, infants, and those with impaired immune systems are more likely to develop severe illness. Some people afflicted with salmonellosis later experience reactive arthritis, which can have long-lasting, disabling effects. The only two species of *Salmonella* are *Salmonella bongori* and *Salmonella enterica*. The latter is divided in six subspecies: *S. e. enterica, S. e. salamae, S. e. arizonae, S. e. diazonae, S. e. houtenase*, and *S. e. indica*. These subspecies are further divided into numerous serovars. Because the serovars only differ in serotypes, and therefore in infection potential, the serovars are not italicised and are written with a capital letter as they still belong to the same subspecies.

The species *Salmonella enterica* subsp. *enterica* contains over 60% of the total number of serovars and 99% of the serovars that are capable of infecting cold- and warm-blooded animals, as well as humans. Infections are usually contracted from sources such as:

- Poultry, pork, beef, and fish (seafood), if the meat is prepared incorrectly or is infected with the bacteria after preparation
- Infected eggs, egg products, and milk when not prepared, handled, or refrigerated properly
- Tainted fruits and vegetables

Reptiles such as red-eared slider turtles and green iguanas may carry *Salmonella bongori* (which inhabits cold-blooded animals) in their intestines which can cause intestinal infections. The most severe human *Salmonella* infection is caused by *S. enterica* subsp. *enterica* ser. typhi which leads to typhoid fever, an infection that often proves fatal if not treated with the appropriate antibiotics.

This serovar is restricted to humans and is usually contracted through direct contact with the fecal matter of an infected person. Typhoid fever is endemic in the developing world, where unsanitary conditions are more likely to prevail, and which can affect as many as 21.5 million people each year. Recorded cases of typhoid fever in the developed world are mostly related to recent travel in areas where *Salmonella* typhi is endemic.

Signs and Symptoms

Enteritis

After a short incubation period of a few hours to one day, the bacteria multiply in the intestinal lumen, causing an intestinal inflammation. Most people with salmonellosis develop diarrhea, fever, vomiting, and abdominal cramps 12 to 72 hours after infection. Diarrhea is often mucopurulent (containing mucus or pus) and bloody. In most cases, the illness lasts four to seven days, and most people recover without treatment. In some cases, though, the diarrhea may be so severe that the patient becomes dangerously dehydrated and must be taken to a hospital. At the hospital, the patient may receive intravenous fluids to treat the dehydration, and may be given medications to provide symptomatic relief, such as fever reduction. In severe cases, the *Salmonella* infection may spread from the intestines to the blood stream, and then to other body sites, and can cause death, unless the person is treated promptly with antibiotics.

In otherwise healthy adults, the symptoms can be mild. Normally, no sepsis occurs, but it can occur exceptionally as a complication in the immunocompromised. However, in people at risk such as infants, small children, and the elderly, *Salmonella* infections can become very serious, leading to complications. In infants, dehydration can cause a state of severe toxicity. Extraintestinal localizations are possible, especially *Salmonella* meningitis in children, osteitis, etc. Children with sickle-cell anemia who are infected with *Salmonella* may develop osteomyelitis. Treatment of osteomyelitis, in this case, will be to use fluoroquinolones (ciprofloxacin, levofloxacin, etc., and nalidixic acid).

Those whose only symptom is diarrhea usually completely recover, but their bowel habits may not return to normal for several months.

Typhoid Fever

Typhoid fever occurs when *Salmonella* bacteria enter the lymphatic system and cause a systemic form of salmonellosis. Endotoxins first act on the vascular and nervous apparatus, resulting in increased permeability and decreased tone of the vessels, upset thermal regulation, vomiting, and diarrhea. In severe forms of the disease, enough liquid and electrolytes are lost to upset the water-salt metabolism, decrease the circulating blood volume and arterial pressure, and cause hypovolemic shock. Septic shock may also develop. Shock of mixed character (with signs of both hypovolemic and septic shock) are more common in severe salmonellosis. Oliguria and azotemia develop in severe cases as a result of renal involvement due to hypoxia and toxemia.

Long-term

Salmonellosis is associated with later irritable bowel syndrome and inflammatory bowel disease. Evidence however does not support it being a direct cause of the latter.

A small number of people afflicted with salmonellosis experience reactive arthritis, which can last months or years and can lead to chronic arthritis. In sickle-cell anemia, osteomyelitis due to *Salmonella* infection is much more common than in the general population. Though *Salmonella* infection is frequently the cause of osteomyelitis in sickle-cell anemia patients, it is not the most common cause, which remains to be *Staphylococcus* infection.

Those infected may become asymptomatic carriers, but it is relatively uncommon, with shedding observed in only 0.2 to 0.6% of cases after a year.

Causes

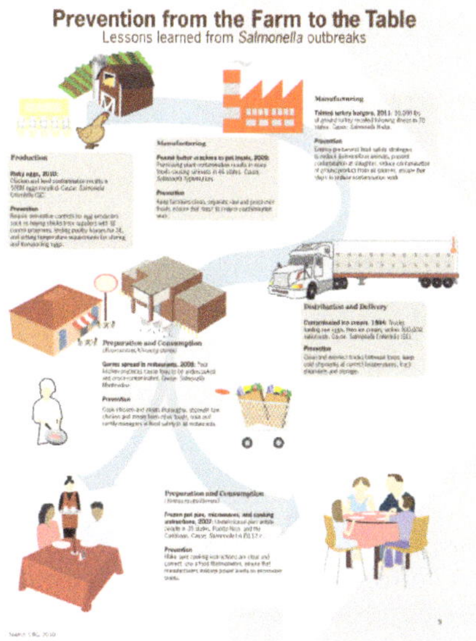

An infographic illustrating how *Salmonella* bacteria spread from the farm

- Contaminated food, often having no unusual look or smell
- Poor kitchen hygiene, especially problematic in institutional kitchens and restaurants because this can lead to a significant outbreak
- Excretions from either sick or infected but apparently clinically healthy people and animals (especially dangerous are caregivers and animals)
- Polluted surface water and standing water
- Unhygienically thawed poultry (the meltwater contains many bacteria)
- An association with reptiles (pet tortoises, snakes, iguanas, and aquatic turtles) is well described.
- Amphibians such as frogs

Salmonella bacteria can survive for some time without a host; thus, they are frequently found in polluted water, with contamination from the excrement of carrier animals being particularly important.

The European Food Safety Authority highly recommends that when handling raw turkey meat, consumers and people involved in the food supply chain should pay attention to personal and food hygiene.

An estimated 142,000 Americans are infected each year with *Salmonella* Enteritidis from chicken eggs, and about 30 die. The shell of the egg may be contaminated with *Salmonella* by feces or environment, or its interior (yolk) may be contaminated by penetration of the bacteria through the porous shell or from a hen whose infected ovaries contaminate the egg during egg formation.

Nevertheless, such interior egg yolk contamination is theoretically unlikely. Even under natural conditions, the rate of infection was very small (0.6% in a study of naturally contaminated eggs and 3.0% among artificially and heavily infected hens).

Prevention

The FDA has published guidelines to help reduce the chance of food-borne salmonellosis. Food must be cooked to 68–72°C (145–160°F), and liquids such as soups or gravies must be boiled. Freezing kills some *Salmonella*, but it is not sufficient to reliably reduce them below infectious levels. While *Salmonella* is usually heat-sensitive, it does acquire heat resistance in high-fat environments such as peanut butter.

Vaccine

Antibodies against nontyphoidal *Salmonella* were first found in Malawi children in research published in 2008. The Malawian researchers have identified an antibody that protects children against bacterial infections of the blood caused by nontyphoidal *Salmonella*. A study at Queen Elizabeth Hospital in Blantyre found that children up to two years old develop antibodies that aid in killing the bacteria. This could lead to a possible *Salmonella* vaccine for humans.

A recent study has tested a vaccine on chickens which offered efficient protection against salmonellosis.

Vaccination of chickens against *Salmonella* essentially wiped out the disease in the United Kingdom. A similar approach has been considered in the United States, but the Food and Drug Administration decided not to mandate vaccination of hens.

Industrial Hygiene

Since 2011, Denmark has had zero cases of human salmonella poisoning. The country eradicated salmonella without vaccines and antibiotics by focusing on eliminating the infection from "breeder stocks", implementing various measures to prevent infection, and taking a zero-tolerance policy towards salmonella in chickens.

Treatment

Electrolytes may be replenished with oral rehydration supplements (typically containing salts sodium chloride and potassium chloride).

Appropriate antibiotics, such as ceftriaxone, may be given to kill the bacteria but are not necessary in most cases. Azithromycin has been suggested to be better at treating typhoid in resistant populations than both fluoroquinolone drugs and ceftriaxone. Antibiotic resistance rates are increasing throughout the world, so health care providers should check current recommendations before choosing an antibiotic.

Epidemiology

In the mid- to late 20th century, *Salmonella enterica* serovar Enteritidis was a common contaminant of eggs. Depending on the region, this is less common now with the advent of hygiene measures in egg production, and the vaccination of laying hens to prevent *Salmonella* colonization. Various *Salmonella* serovars (strains) also cause severe diseases in animals.

United States

About 142,000 people in the United States are infected each year with *Salmonella* Enteritidis from chicken eggs, and about 30 die.

In 2010, an analysis of death certificates in the United States identified a total of 1,316 *Salmonella*-related deaths from 1990 to 2006. These were predominantly among older adults and those who were immunocompromised. The U.S. government reported as many as 20% of all chickens were contaminated with *Salmonella* in the late 1990s, and 16.3% were contaminated in 2005.

The United States has struggled to control salmonella infections, with the rate of infection rising from 2001 to 2011. In 1998, the USDA moved to close plants if salmonella was found in excess of 20 percent, which was the industry's average at the time, for three consecutive tests. Texas-based Supreme Beef Processors, Inc. sued on the argument that Salmonella is naturally occurring and ultimately prevailed when a federal appeals court affirmed a lower court. These issues were highlighted in a proposed Kevin's Law (formally proposed as the Meat and Poultry Pathogen Reduction and Enforcement Act of 2003), of which components were included the Food Safety Modernization Act passed in 2011, but that law applies only to the FDA and not the USDA. The USDA proposed a regulatory initiative in 2011 to Office of Management and Budget.

Europe

Since July 2012, an outbreak of salmonellosis occurred in Northern Europe caused by *Salmonella thompson*. The infections were linked to smoked salmon from the manufacturer Foppen, where the contamination had occurred. Most infections were reported in the Netherlands, over 1060 infections with this subspecies have been confirmed, as well as four mortalities.

A case of widespread infection was detected mid-2012 in seven EU countries. Over 400 people had been infected with *Salmonella enterica* serovar Stanley (*S.* Stanley) that usually appears in the regions of Southeast Asia. After several DNA analyses seemed to point to a specific Belgian strain, the "Joint ECDC/E FSA Rapid Risk Assessment" report detected turkey production as the source of infection.

In Germany, food poisoning infections must be reported. Between 1990 and 2005, the number of officially recorded cases decreased from about 200,000 to about 50,000 cases.

Elsewhere

In March 2007, around 150 people were diagnosed with salmonellosis after eating tainted food at a governor's reception in Krasnoyarsk, Russia. Over 1,500 people attended the ball on March 1, and fell ill as a consequence of ingesting *Salmonella*-tainted sandwiches.

About 150 people were sickened by *Salmonella*-tainted chocolate cake produced by a major bakery chain in Singapore, in December 2007.

History

Both salmonellosis and the *Salmonella* genus of microorganisms derive their names from a modern Latin coining after Daniel E. Salmon (1850–1914), an American veterinary surgeon. He had help from Theobald Smith, and together they found the bacterium in pigs.

Four-inch Regulation

The "Four-inch regulation" or "Four-inch law" is a colloquial name for a regulation issued by the U.S. FDA in 1975, restricting the sale of turtles with a carapace length less than four inches (10 cm).

The regulation was introduced, according to the FDA, "because of the public health impact of turtle-associated salmonellosis." Cases had been reported of young children placing small turtles in their mouths, which led to the size-based restriction.

Creutzfeldt–Jakob Disease

Creutzfeldt–Jakob disease (CJD) is an incurable and universally fatal neurodegenerative disease. CJD is at times called a human form of mad cow disease (bovine spongiform encephalopathy or BSE). However, given that BSE is believed to be the cause of Variant Creutzfeldt–Jakob disease (vCJD) in humans, the two are often confused.

CJD is caused by an infectious agent called a prion. Prions are misfolded proteins that replicate by converting their properly folded counterparts, in their host, to the same misfolded structure they possess. CJD causes the brain tissue to degenerate rapidly, and as the disease destroys the brain, the brain develops holes and the texture changes to resemble that of a kitchen sponge.

Classification

Types of CJD include:

- variant (vCJD):

  This is thought to be caused by the consumption of food contaminated with prions, which also cause BSE.

- sporadic (sCJD):

This accounts for 85% of cases of CJD.

- familial (fCJD):

  This accounts for the majority of the other 15% cases of CJD.

- iatrogenic:

  This form of CJD arises from contamination with tissue from an infected person, usually as the result of a medical procedure. Medical procedures that are associated with the spread of this form of CJD include blood transfusion from the infected person, use of human-derived pituitary growth hormones, gonadotropin hormone therapy, and corneal and meningeal transplants.

Signs and Symptoms

The first symptom of CJD is rapidly progressive dementia, leading to memory loss, personality changes, and hallucinations. Other frequently occurring features include anxiety, depression, paranoia, obsessive-compulsive symptoms, and psychosis. This is accompanied by physical problems such as speech impairment, jerky movements (myoclonus), balance and coordination dysfunction (ataxia), changes in gait, rigid posture, and seizures. In most patients, these symptoms are followed by involuntary movements and the appearance of an atypical diagnostic electroencephalogram tracing. The duration of the disease varies greatly, but sporadic (non-inherited) CJD can be fatal within months or even weeks. Most victims die six months after initial symptoms appear, often of pneumonia due to impaired coughing reflexes. About 15% of patients survive for two or more years. Some patients have been known to live four to five years with mostly psychological symptoms while the disease progresses. It then causes more physical symptoms that lead to diagnosis, after which death usually occurs within a year.

The symptoms of CJD are caused by the progressive death of the brain's nerve cells, which is associated with the build-up of abnormal prion proteins forming amyloids. When brain tissue from a CJD patient is examined under a microscope, many tiny holes can be seen where whole areas of nerve cells have died. The word "spongiform" in "transmissible spongiform encephalopathies" refers to the sponge-like appearance of the brain tissue.

Cause

Transmissible spongiform encephalopathy diseases are caused by prions. Prions are proteins that occur normally in neurons of the central nervous system (CNS). As of 2007, these proteins are thought to affect signaling processes, damaging neurons and resulting in degeneration that causes the spongiform appearance in the affected brain.

The CJD prion is dangerous because it promotes refolding of native proteins into the diseased state. The number of misfolded protein molecules will increase exponentially and the process leads to a large quantity of insoluble protein in affected cells. This mass of misfolded proteins disrupts neuronal cell function and causes cell death. Mutations in the gene for the prion protein can cause a misfolding of the dominantly alpha helical regions into beta pleated sheets. This change in conformation disables the ability of the protein to undergo digestion. Once the prion is transmitted, the defective proteins invade the brain and are produced in a self-sustaining feedback loop.

These neurodegenerative diseases are commonly called *prion diseases.*

People can also acquire CJD genetically through a mutation of the gene that codes for the prion protein (PRNP). This occurs in only 5-10% of all CJD cases. An EU study determined that "87% of cases were sporadic, 8% genetic, and 5% iatrogenic."

Transmission

The defective protein can be transmitted by contaminated harvested human brain products, corneal grafts (in at least one reported case), dural grafts or electrode implants (acquired or iatrogenic form (iCJD)); it can be familial (fCJD); or it may appear for the first time in the patient (sporadic form: sCJD). In the familial form, a mutation occurs in the gene for PrP, PRNP. Ten to fifteen percent of CJD cases are familial.

The disease has also been shown to result from use of human growth hormone obtained from the pituitary glands of people who died from Creutzfeldt–Jakob disease, though the known incidence of this cause is (as of April 2004) quite small. The risk of infection via cadaveric HGH in the US ceased when the medication was withdrawn in 1985.

It is thought that humans can contract the disease by consuming material from animals infected with the bovine form of the disease. The only suspected cases to arise thus far have been vCJD with cases in the UK and Canada. But there are also fears—based on animal studies—that consuming beef or beef products containing prion particles can also cause the development of classic CJD. When BSE material infects humans, the resulting disease is known as (new) variant CJD (nvCJD).

Cannibalism has also been implicated as a transmission mechanism for abnormal prions, causing the disease known as kuru, once found primarily among women and children of the Fore people in Papua New Guinea. While the men of the tribe ate the body of the deceased and rarely contracted the disease, the women and children, who ate the less desirable body parts, including the brain, were eight times more likely than men to contract kuru from infected tissue.

Prions, the infectious agent of CJD, may not be inactivated by means of routine surgical instrument sterilization procedures. The World Health Organization and the US Centers for Disease Control and Prevention recommend that instrumentation used in such cases be immediately destroyed after use; short of destruction, it is recommended that heat and chemical decontamination be used in combination to process instruments that come in contact with high-infectivity tissues. No cases of iatrogenic transmission of CJD have been reported subsequent to the adoption of current sterilization procedures, or since 1976. Copper-hydrogen peroxide has been suggested as an alternative to the current recommendation of sodium hydroxide or sodium hypochlorite. Thermal depolymerization also destroys prions in infected organic and inorganic matter, since the process chemically attacks protein at the molecular level, although more effective and practical methods involve destruction by combinations of detergents and enzymes similar to biological washing powders.

Blood Donor Restrictions

In 2004, a report published in the *Lancet* medical journal showed that vCJD can be transmitted by blood transfusions. The finding alarmed healthcare officials because a large epidemic of the disease could result in the near-future. A blood test for vCJD infection is possible but is not yet available for screening blood donations. Significant restrictions exist to protect the blood supply. The UK government banned anyone who had received a blood transfusion since January 1980 from donating blood. From 1999 there has been a ban in the UK for using UK blood to manufacture fractional products such as albumin. Whilst these restrictions may go some way to preventing a self-sustaining epidemic of secondary infections the number of infected blood donations is unknown and could be considerable as a study by the Health Protection Agency show around 1 in 2000 people in the UK shows signs of abnormal prion accumulation. In June 2013 the government was warned that deaths—then at 176—could rise five-fold through blood transfusions.

On May 28, 2002, the United States Food and Drug Administration instituted a policy that excludes from donation anyone having spent at least six months in certain European countries (or three months in the United Kingdom) from 1980 to 1996. Given the large number of U.S. military personnel and their dependents residing in Europe, it was expected that over 7% of donors would be deferred due to the policy. Later changes to this policy have relaxed the restriction to a cumulative total of five years or more of civilian travel in European countries (six months or more if military). The three-month restriction on travel to the UK, however, has not been changed.

The American Red Cross' policy is as follows: During the period January 1, 1980, to December 31, 1996, spending a total time of three months or more in the United Kingdom, Channel Islands, the Falkland Islands and Gibraltar precludes individuals from donating. Moreover, spending a total time of five years or more after January 1, 1980 (to present), in the above-mentioned countries and/or any country in Europe (except the former USSR), also precludes donation. People with a biologic relative having been diagnosed with CJD or vCJD are unable to donate. Biologic relative in this setting means mother, father, sibling, grandparent, aunt, uncle, or child.

A similar policy applies to potential donors to the Australian Red Cross Blood Service, precluding people who have spent a cumulative time of six months or more in the United Kingdom between 1980 and 1996.

The Singapore Red Cross precludes potential donors having spent a cumulative time of three months or more in the United Kingdom between 1980 and 1996.

In New Zealand, the New Zealand Blood Service (NZBS) in 2000 introduced measures to preclude permanently donors having resided in the United Kingdom (including the Isle of Man and the Channel Islands) for a total of six months or more between January 1980 and December 1996. The measure resulted in ten percent of New Zealand's active blood donors at the time becoming ineligible to donate blood. In 2003, the NZBS further extended restrictions to preclude permanently donors having had received a blood transfusion in the United Kingdom since January 1980, and in April 2006, restrictions were further extended to include the Republic of Ireland and France.

Similar regulations are in place in France and in Germany, where anyone having spent six months or more living in the UK between January 1980 and December 1996 is permanently banned from donating blood.

In Canada, individuals are not eligible to donate blood or plasma if they have spent a cumulative total of three months or more in the United Kingdom (UK) or France from January 1, 1980, to December 31, 1996. They are also ineligible if they have spent a cumulative total of five years or more in Western Europe outside the U.K. or France since January 1, 1980 through December 31, 2007 or Spent a cumulative total of six months or more in Saudi Arabia from January 1, 1980 through December 31, 1996 or if they have had a blood transfusion in the U.K., France or Western Europe since 1980.

The Association of Blood Donors of Denmark precludes potential donors having spent a cumulative time of at least 12 months in the United Kingdom between 1 January 1980 and 31 December 1996.

The Swiss Blutspendedienst SRK precludes potential donors having spent a cumulative time of at least six months in the United Kingdom between 1 January 1980 and 31 December 1996.

In Poland, anyone having spent cumulatively six months or longer between 1 January 1980 and 31 December 1996 in the UK, Ireland, or France is permanently barred from donating.

In the Czech Republic, anyone having spent more than six months in the UK or France between the years 1980 and 1996 or received transfusion in the UK after the year 1980 is not allowed to donate blood. In South Korea, anyone having spent more than three months in the UK after 1997, or more than a month between 1980 and 1996 is banned from donating blood.

Sperm Donor Restrictions

In the U.S., the FDA has banned import of any donor sperm, motivated by a risk of Creutzfeldt–Jakob disease, inhibiting the once popular import of Scandinavian sperm. The risk, however, is not known, since artificial insemination has not been studied as a route of transmission.

Diagnosis

The diagnosis of CJD is suspected when there are typical clinical symptoms and signs such as rapidly progressing dementia with startle myoclonus. Further investigation can then be performed to support the diagnosis including

- Electroencephalography—often has characteristic generalized periodic sharp wave pattern (~80% of pts by 6 months)
- Cerebrospinal fluid analysis for 14-3-3 protein
- MRI of the brain—often shows high signal intensity in the caudate nucleus and putamen bilaterally on T2-weighted images.
- Research in 2010 and 2011 identified a possible blood test for CJD. The test attempts to identify the prion responsible for the disease. However, it has not yet been demonstrated if it is able to detect the prions in early stages of the disease.

Diffusion Weighted Imaging (DWI) images are the most sensitive. In about 24% of cases DWI shows only cortical hyperintensity; in 68%, cortical and subcortical abnormalities; and in 5%, only subcortical anomalies. The involvement of the thalamus can be found in sCJD, is even stronger and constant in vCJD.

Clinical testing for CJD has always been an issue. Diagnosis has been based mostly on clinical and physical examination of symptoms. In recent years, studies have shown that the tumour marker Neuron-specific enolase (NSE) is often elevated in CJD cases, however its diagnostic utility is seen primarily when combined with a test for the 14-3-3 protein. As of 2010 , screening tests to identify infected asymptomatic individuals, such as blood donors, are not yet available, though methods have been proposed and evaluated.

In 2010, a team from New York described detection of PrP^{Sc} even when initially present at only one part in one hundred billion (10^{-11}) in brain tissue. The method combines amplification with a novel technology called surround optical fiber immunoassay (SOFIA) and some specific antibodies against PrP^{Sc}. After amplifying and then concentrating any PrP^{Sc}, the samples are labelled with a fluorescent dye using an antibody for specificity and then finally loaded into a micro-capillary tube. This tube is placed in a specially constructed apparatus so that it is totally surrounded by optical fibres to capture all light emitted once the dye is excited using a laser. The technique allowed detection of PrP^{Sc} after many fewer cycles of conversion than others have achieved, substantially reducing the possibility of artefacts, as well as speeding up the assay. The researchers also tested their method on blood samples from apparently healthy sheep that went on to develop scrapie. The animals' brains were analysed once any symptoms became apparent. The researchers could therefore compare results from brain tissue and blood taken once the animals exhibited symptoms of the diseases, with blood obtained earlier in the animals' lives, and from uninfected animals. The results showed very clearly that PrP^{Sc} could be detected in the blood of animals long before the symptoms appeared. After further development and testing, this method could be of great value in surveillance as a blood or urine-based screening test for CJD. In 2014 a human study showed a nasal brushing method that can accurately detect PrP in the olfactory epithelial of CJD patients. . This finding creates new opportunities for minimally invasive detection of CJD.

In one-third of patients with sporadic CJD, deposits of "prion protein (scrapie)," PrP^{Sc}, can be found in the skeletal muscle and/or the spleen. Diagnosis of vCJD can be supported by biopsy of the tonsils, which harbour significant amounts of PrPSc; however, biopsy of brain tissue is the definitive diagnostic test for all other forms of prion disease. Due to its invasiveness, biopsy will not be done if clinical suspicion is sufficiently high or low. A negative biopsy does not rule out CJD, since it may predominate in a specific part of the brain.

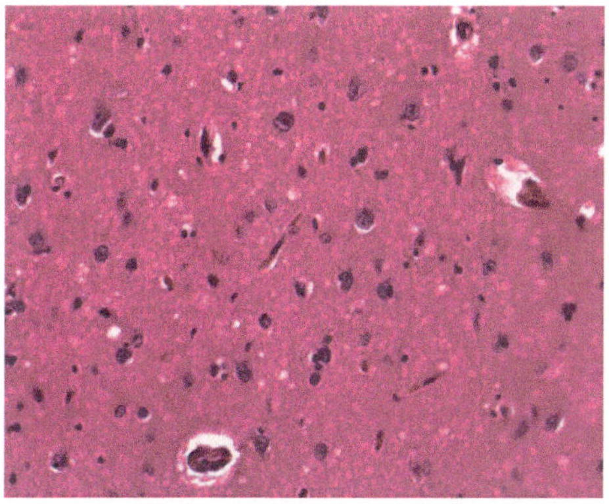

Spongiform change in CJD

The classic histologic appearance is spongiform change in the gray matter: the presence of many round vacuoles from one to 50 micrometres in the neuropil, in all six cortical layers in the cerebral cortex or with diffuse involvement of the cerebellar molecular layer. These vacuoles appear glassy or eosinophilic and may coalesce. Neuronal loss and gliosis are also seen. Plaques of amyloid-like material can be seen in the neocortex in new-variant CJD.

However, vacuolization can be seen in other disease states. Diffuse cortical vacuolization occurs in Alzheimer's disease, and superficial cortical vacuolization occurs in ischemia and frontotemporal dementia. These vacuoles appear clear and punched-out. Larger vacuoles encircling neurons, vessels, and glia are a possible processing artifact.

- Clinical and Pathologic Characteristics:

Characteristic	Classic CJD	Variant CJD
Median age at death	68 years	28 years
Median duration of illness	4–5 months	13–14 months
Clinical signs and symptoms	Dementia; early neurologic signs	Prominent psychiatric/behavioral symptoms; painful dysesthesias; delayed neurologic signs
Periodic sharp waves on electroencephalogram	Often present	Often absent
Signal hyperintensity in the caudate nucleus and putamen on diffusion-weighted and FLAIR MRI	Often present	Often absent
Pulvinar sign-bilateral high signal intensities on axial fluid attenuated inversion recovery (FLAIR) MRI. Also posterior thalami involvement on sagittal T2 sequences	Not reported	Present in >75% of cases
Immunohistochemical analysis of brain tissue	Variable accumulation.	Marked accumulation of protease-resistant prion protein
Presence of agent in lymphoid tissue	Not readily detected	Readily detected
Increased glycoform ratio on immunoblot analysis of protease-resistant prion protein	Not reported	Marked accumulation of protease-resistant prion protein
Presence of amyloid plaques in brain tissue	May be present	May be present

- An abnormal signal in the posterior thalamus on T2- and diffusion-weighted images and fluid-attenuated inversion recovery sequences on brain magnetic resonance imaging (MRI); in the appropriate clinical context, this signal is highly specific for vCJD. (Source: CDC)

Treatment

As of 2016, no generally accepted treatment for CJD exists; though research continues, the disease is invariably fatal. An experimental treatment was given to a Northern Irish teenager, Jonathan Simms, beginning in January 2003. The medication, called pentosan polysulphate (PPS) and used to treat interstitial cystitis, is infused into the patient's lateral ventricle within the brain. PPS does not seem to stop the disease from progressing, and both brain function and tissue continue to be lost. However, the treatment is alleged to slow the progression of the otherwise untreatable disease, and may have contributed to the longer than expected survival of the seven patients studied. Simms died in 2011. The CJD Therapy Advisory Group to the UK Health Departments advises that data are not sufficient to support claims that pentosan polysulphate is an effective treatment and suggests that further research in animal models is appropriate. A 2007 review of the treatment of 26 patients with PPS finds no proof of efficacy because of the lack of accepted objective criteria.

Scientists have investigated using RNA interference to slow the progression of scrapie in mice. The RNA blocks production of the protein that the CJD process transforms into prions. This research is unlikely to lead to a human therapy for many years.

Both amphotericin B and doxorubicin have been investigated as potentially effective against CJD, but as yet there is no strong evidence that either drug is effective in stopping the disease. Further study has been taken with other medical drugs, but none are effective. However, anticonvulsants and anxiolytic agents, such as valproate or a benzodiazepine, may be administered to relieve associated symptoms.

Scientists from the University of California, San Francisco are currently running a treatment trial for sporadic CJD using quinacrine, a medicine originally created for malaria. Pilot studies showed quinacrine permanently cleared abnormal prion proteins from cell cultures, but results have not yet been published on their clinical study. The efficacy of quinacrine was also assessed in a rigorous clinical trial in the UK and the results were published in Lancet Neurology, and concluded that quinacrine had no measurable effect on the clinical course of CJD.

In a 2013 paper published in the Proceedings of the National Academy of Sciences, scientists from The Scripps Research Institute reported that Astemizole, a medication approved for human use, has been found to have anti-prion activity and may lead to a treatment for Creutzfeldt–Jakob disease.

Epidemiology

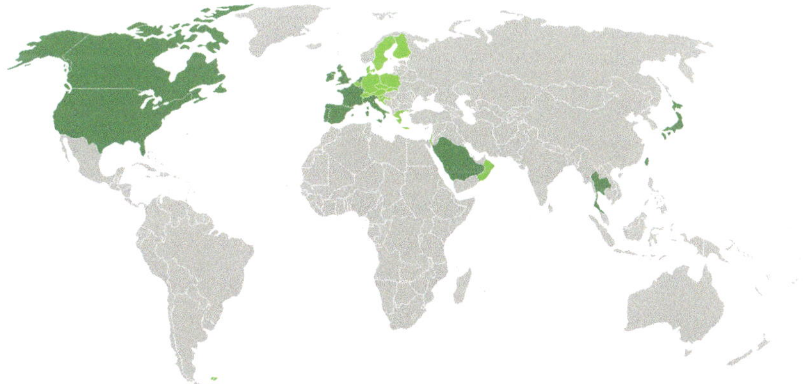

Dark green areas are countries that have confirmed human cases of variant Creutzfeldt–Jakob disease and light green are countries that have bovine spongiform encephalopathy cases.

Although CJD is the most common human prion disease, it is still believed to be rare, estimated to occur in about one out of every one million people every year, however, an autopsy study published in 1989 and others suggest that between 3-13% of people diagnosed with alzheimers were actually misdiagnosed, and instead had CJD, not alzheimers. Presumably the people became infected through prion contaminated beef from cattle with subclinical atypical BSE, which has a very long incubation period. CJD usually affects people aged 45–75, most commonly appearing in people between the ages of 60–65. The exception to this is the more recently recognised 'variant' CJD (vCJD), which occurs in younger people.

CDC monitors the occurrence of CJD in the United States through periodic reviews of national mortality data. According to the CDC:

- CJD occurs worldwide at a rate of about 1 case per million population per year.
- On the basis of mortality surveillance from 1979 to 1994, the annual incidence of CJD remained stable at approximately 1 case per million people in the United States.
- In the United States, CJD deaths among people younger than 30 years of age are extremely rare (fewer than five deaths per billion per year).
- The disease is found most frequently in patients 55–65 years of age, but cases can occur in people older than 90 years and younger than 55 years of age.
- In more than 85% of cases, the duration of CJD is less than 1 year (median: four months) after onset of symptoms.

Additional Concerns

In *The Lancet* (June 2006), a University College London team suggested that it may take more than 50 years for vCJD to develop, from their studies of kuru, a similar disease in Papua New Guinea. The reasoning behind the claim is that kuru was possibly transmitted through cannibalism in Papua New Guinea when family members would eat the body of a dead relative as a sign of mourning. In the 1950s, cannibalism was banned in Papua New Guinea. In the late 20th century, however, kuru reached epidemic proportions in certain Papua New Guinean communities, therefore suggesting that vCJD may also have a similar incubation period of 20 to 50 years. A critique to this theory is that while mortuary cannibalism was banned in Papua New Guinea in the 1950s, that does not necessarily mean that the practice ended. 15 years later Jared Diamond was informed by Papuans that the practice continued. Kuru may have passed to the Fore people through the preparation of the dead body for burial.

These researchers noticed a genetic variation in some kuru patients that has been known to promote long incubation periods. They have also proposed that individuals having contracted CJD in the early 1990s represent a distinct genetic subpopulation, with unusually short incubation periods for bovine spongiform encephalopathy (BSE). This means that there may be many more vCJD patients with longer incubation periods, which may surface many years later.

In 1997, a number of people from Kentucky, US, developed CJD. It was discovered that all the victims had consumed squirrel brains, although a coincidental relationship between the disease and this dietary practice may have been involved. In 2008, UK scientists expressed concern over the possibility of a second wave of human cases due to the wide exposure and long incubation of some cases of vCJD.

History

The disease was first described by German neurologist Hans Gerhard Creutzfeldt in 1920 and shortly afterward by Alfons Maria Jakob, giving it the name Creutzfeldt–Jakob. Some of the clinical findings described in their first papers do not match current criteria for Creutzfeldt–Jakob disease, and it has been speculated that at least two of the patients in initial studies were suffering from a different ailment. An early description of familial CJD stems from the German psychiatrist and neurologist Friedrich Meggendorfer (1880–1953). A study published in 1997 counted more than 100 cases worldwide of transmissible CJD and new cases continued to appear at the time.

The first report of suspected iatrogenic CJD was published in 1974. Animal experiments showed that corneas of infected animals could transmit CJD, and the causative agent spreads along visual pathways. A second case of CJD associated with a corneal transplant was reported without details. In 1977, CJD transmission caused by silver electrodes previously used in the brain of a person with CJD was first reported. Transmission occurred despite decontamination of the electrodes with ethanol and formaldehyde. Retrospective studies identified four other cases likely of similar cause. The rate of transmission from a single contaminated instrument is unknown, although it is not 100%. In some cases the exposure occurred weeks after the instruments were used on a person with CJD.

A review article published in 1979 indicated that 25 dura mater cases had occurred by that date in Australia, Canada, Germany, Italy, Japan, New Zealand, Spain, the United Kingdom, and the United States.

By 1985, a series of case reports in the United States showed that when injected, cadaver-extracted pituitary human growth hormone could transmit CJD to humans.

In 1992 it was recognized that human gonadotropin administered by injection could also transmit CJD from person to person.

In 2004, a report published by Edinburgh doctors in the *Lancet* medical journal demonstrated that vCJD was transmitted by blood transfusion.

Stanley B. Prusiner of the University of California, San Francisco (UCSF) was awarded the Nobel Prize in physiology or medicine in 1997 "for his discovery of Prions—a new biological principle of infection". However, Yale University neuropathologist Laura Manuelidis has challenged the prion protein (PrP) explanation for the disease. In January 2007, she and her colleagues reported that they had found a virus-like particle in naturally and experimentally infected animals. "The high infectivity of comparable, isolated virus-like particles that show no intrinsic PrP by antibody labeling, combined with their loss of infectivity when nucleic acid–protein complexes are disrupted, make it likely that these 25-nm particles are the causal TSE virions".

Australia

Four Australians had been reported with CJD following transfusion as of 1997. There have been ten cases of healthcare-acquired CJD in Australia. They consist of five deaths following treatment with pituitary extract hormone for either infertility or short stature, with no further cases since 1991. The five other deaths were caused by dura grafting during brain surgery, where the covering of the brain was repaired. There have been no other known healthcare-acquired CJD deaths in Australia.

New Zealand

A case was reported in 1989 in a 25-year-old man from New Zealand, who also received dura mater transplant. Five New Zealanders have been confirmed to have died of the sporadic form of Creutzfeldt–Jakob disease (CJD) in 2012.

United Kingdom

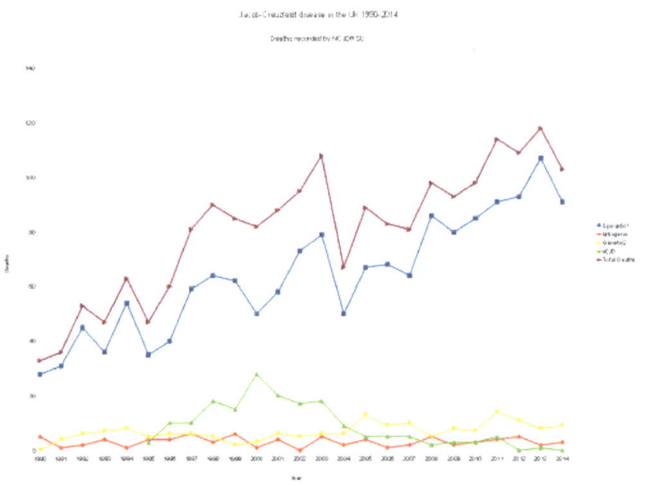

Deaths in the UK from Creutzfeldt–Jakob disease 1990–2014: while cases of vCJD have declined (green), reported cases of sporadic CJD continue to increase (blue).

Researchers believe one in 2,000 people in the UK is a carrier of the disease linked to eating contaminated beef (vCJD). The survey provides the most robust prevalence measure to date—and identifies abnormal prion protein across a wider age group than found previously and in all genotypes, indicating "infection" may be relatively common. This new study examined over 32,000 anonymous appendix samples. Of these, 16 samples were positive for abnormal prion protein, indicating an overall prevalence of 493 per million population, or one in 2,000 people are likely to be carriers. No difference was seen in different birth cohorts (1941–60 and 1961–85), in both sexes, and there was no apparent difference in abnormal prion prevalence in three broad geographical areas. Genetic testing of the 16 positive samples revealed a higher proportion of valine homozygous (VV) genotype on the codon 129 of the gene encoding the prion protein (PRNP) compared with the general UK population. This also differs from the 177 patients with vCJD, all of whom to date have been methionine homozygous (MM) genotype. The concern is that individuals with this VV genotype may be susceptible to developing the condition over longer incubation periods.

United States

In 1988, there was a confirmed death from CJD of a person from Manchester, New Hampshire. Massachusetts General Hospital believed the patient acquired the disease from a surgical instrument at a podiatrist's office. In September 2013, another patient in Manchester was posthumously determined to have died of the disease. The patient had undergone brain surgery at Catholic Medical Center three months before his death, and a surgical probe used in the procedure was subsequently reused in other operations. Public health officials identified thirteen patients at three hospitals who may have been exposed to the disease through the contaminated probe, but said the risk of anyone's contracting CJD is "extremely low." In January 2015, the former speaker of the Utah House of Representatives, Rebecca D. Lockhart, died of the disease within a few weeks of diagnosis. John Carroll, former editor of *The Baltimore Sun* and *Los Angeles Times*, died of CJD in Kentucky in June 2015, after having been diagnosed in January.

Gerstmann–Sträussler–Scheinker Syndrome

Gerstmann–Sträussler–Scheinker syndrome (GSS) is a very rare, usually familial, fatal neurodegenerative disease that affects patients from 20 to 60 years in age. Though exclusively heritable, this extremely rare disease is classified with the transmissible spongiform encephalopathies (TSE) due to the causative role played by PRNP, the human prion protein. The exact incidence of GSS is unknown, but is estimated to be between 1 and 10 per 100 million.

Familial cases are associated with autosomal-dominant inheritance. Gerstmann–Sträussler–Scheinker disease (GSS) is an extremely rare neurogenetic brain disorder. It is always inherited and is found in only a few families all over the world (NINDS ¶ 1). The trait is an autosomal-dominant trait caused by a gene mutation. It is also in a group of hereditary prion protein diseases or also known as TSEs. Many symptoms are associated with GSS, such as progressive ataxia, pyramidal signs, and even adult-onset dementia; they progress more as the disease progresses (Farlow, et al., Nov. 1989).

Eponym

GSS is named for Josef Gerstmann, Ernst Sträussler and Ilya Scheinker, the Austrian physicians who first described it in the mid-1930s.

Causes

GSS is one of a small number of diseases that are caused by prions, a class of pathogenic proteins highly resistant to proteases.

A change in codon 102 from proline to leucine has been found in the prion protein gene (*PRNP*, on chromosome 20) of most affected individuals. Therefore, it appears this genetic change is usually required for the development of the disease.

History

GSS is a disease that is very rare, making its history hard to track exactly where it descended from. Gerstmann–Sträussler–Scheinker syndrome (GSS) was first described as neurodegenerative diseases in the 1920s (Elsevier Science, 2002). Gerstmann–Sträussler–Scheinker (GSS) is called this because it was first reported in 1936 by Josef Gerstmann, Ernst Sträussler and Ilya Scheinker. In 1989, the first mutation of the prion protein gene was identified in a GSS family (Elsevier Science, 2002). Prion diseases (transmissible spongiform encephalopathies) are rare degenerative diseases of the brain thought to be caused by a protein that converts to an abnormal form called a prion (Gambetti Pierluigi, 2013). GSS was later realized to have many different gene mutation types, with some showing different symptoms first or having other symptoms worse than others. Doctors in different parts of the world are uncovering more generations and families that have the mutation. It is hard to discover GSS for two main reasons: (1) the disease has been reported in only a few countries; and (2) the disease may be underreported due to its clinical similarity to other diseases (Ghetti B, et al., 2003). The Indiana Kindred is the largest, spanning over 8 generations, and includes over 3,000 people with 57 individuals known to be affected (B. Ghetti, et al., 1996).

Symptoms

Symptoms start with slowly developing dysarthria (difficulty speaking) and cerebellar ataxia (unsteadiness) and then the progressive dementia becomes more evident. Loss of memory can be the first symptom of GSS. Extrapyramidal and pyramidal symptoms and signs may occur and the disease may mimic spinocerebellar ataxias in the beginning stages. Myoclonus (spasmodic muscle contraction) is less frequently seen than in Creutzfeldt–Jakob disease. Many patients also exhibit nystagmus (involuntary movement of the eyes), visual disturbances, and even blindness or deafness. The neuropathological findings of GSS include widespread deposition of amyloid plaques composed of abnormally folded prion protein.

Treatment and Testing

There is no cure for GSS, nor is there any known treatment to slow the progression of the disease. However, therapies and medication are aimed at treating or slowing down the effects of the symptoms. Their goal is to try to improve the patient's quality of life as much as possible. Despite there being no cure for GSS, it is possible to undergo testing for the presence of the underlying genetic mutation. Testing for GSS involves a blood and DNA examination in order to attempt to detect the mutated gene at certain codons. If the genetic mutation is present, the patient will eventually be afflicted by GSS, and, due to the genetic nature of the disease, the offspring of the patient are predisposed to a higher risk of inheriting the mutation.

Prognosis

There is no cure or treatment for GSS. It can, however, be identified through genetic testing. GSS is the slowest to progress among human prion diseases. Duration of illness can range from 3 months to 13 years, with an average duration of 5 or 6 years.

In Popular Culture

Several episodes of the television series *Pure Genius* feature characters with GSS.

Kuru (Disease)

Kuru is a rare, incurable neurodegenerative disorder which was prevalent among the Fore people of Papua New Guinea in the 1950s and 60s. Everyone has normal prion proteins, found mostly in the brain. However, infectious prions, which cause transmissible spongiform encephalopathies diseases such as kuru, can induce abnormal folding of normal prion proteins, which leads to symptoms such as coordination problems and neurodegeneration.

The term kuru derives from the Fore word kuria or guria ("to shake"), due to the body tremors that are a classic symptom of the disease and kúru itself means "trembling". It is now widely accepted that kuru was transmitted among members of the Fore tribe of Papua New Guinea via funerary cannibalism. Traditionally, deceased family members were cooked and eaten, which was thought to help free the spirit of the dead. Females and children usually consumed the brain, the organ in which infectious prions were most concentrated, thus allowing for transmission of kuru. Thus, the disease was more prevalent among women and children.

Due to kuru's long incubation period of anywhere from 10 to over 50 years, the disease has lingered. However, the epidemic has declined, from 200 deaths per year in 1957 to 1 or no deaths annually in 2005.

Signs and Symptoms

Kuru, a transmissible spongiform encephalopathy, is a disease of the nervous system that causes physiological and neurological effects which ultimately lead to death. It is characterized by progressive cerebellar ataxia, or loss of coordination and control over muscle movements.

The preclinical or asymptomatic phase, also called the incubation period, averages between 10–13 years, but can be as short as 5 and has been estimated to last as long as 50 years or more after initial exposure. The youngest individual recorded to have kuru was 12 years old.

The clinical stage, which begins at the first onset of symptoms, lasts an average of 12 months. The clinical progression of kuru is divided into three specific stages, the ambulant, sedentary and terminal stages. While there is some variation in these stages between individuals, they are highly conserved among the affected population. Before the onset of clinical symptoms, an individual can also present with prodromal symptoms including headache and joint pain in the legs.

In the first (ambulant) stage, the infected individual may exhibit unsteady stance and gait, decreased muscle control, tremors, difficulty pronouncing words (dysarthria), and titubation. This stage is named because the individual is still able to walk around despite symptoms.

In the second (sedentary) stage, the infected individual in is incapable of walking without support and suffers ataxia and severe tremors. Furthermore, the individual shows signs of emotional instability and depression, yet exhibits uncontrolled and sporadic laughter. Despite the other neurological symptoms, tendon reflexes are still intact at this stage of the disease.

In the third and final (terminal) stage, the infected individual's existing symptoms, like ataxia, progress to the point where they are no longer capable of sitting without support. New symptoms also emerge: the individual develops dysphagia, or difficulty swallowing, which can lead to severe malnutrition. They may also become incontinent, lose the ability to speak and become unresponsive to their surroundings, despite maintaining consciousness. Towards the end of the terminal stage patients often develop chronic ulcerated wounds that can be easily infected. An infected person usually dies within three months to two years after the first terminal stage symptoms, often because of pneumonia or infection.

Causes

Kuru is largely localized to the Fore people and people whom they intermarried, and was transmitted through ritualistic cannibalism. The Fore people ritualistically cooked and consumed body parts of their family members following their death to symbolize respect and mourning. Because the brain is the most infectious organ enriched in the infectious agent prion, women and children, who consumed brain and viscera, had much higher likelihood of being infected than men, who preferentially consumed muscles.

Prion

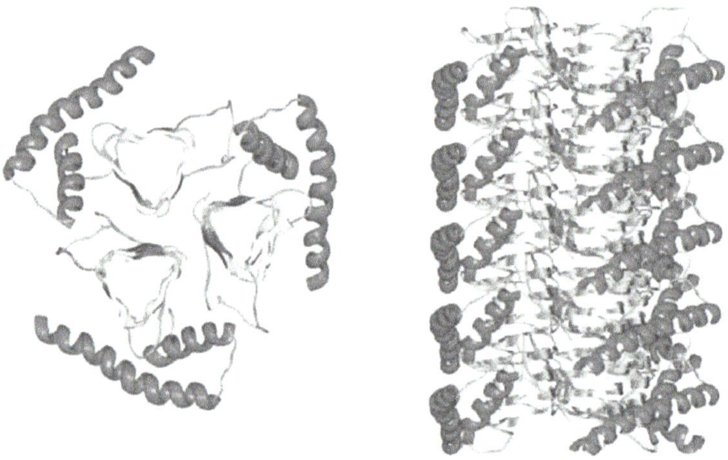

Cryoelectron Microscopy model of the misfolded PrP^{sc} protein, enriched in beta sheets (center).

The infectious agent is a misfolded form of a host-encoded protein called prion (PrP). Prion proteins are encoded by the Prion Protein Gene (PRNP). The two forms of prion are designated as PrP^{c}, which is a normally folded protein, and PrP^{sc}, a misfolded form which gives rise to the disease. The two forms do not differ in their amino acid sequence, however, the pathogenic PrP^{sc} isoform differs from the normal PrP^{c} form in its secondary and tertiary structure. The PrP^{sc} isoform is more enriched in beta sheets, while the normal PrP^{c} form is enriched in alpha helices. The differences in conformation allow PrP^{sc} to aggregate and be extremely resistant to protein degradation by enzymes or by other chemical and physical means. The normal form, on the other hand, is susceptible to complete proteolysis and soluble in non-denaturing detergents.

It has been suggested that pre-existing or acquired PrP^{sc} can promote the conversion of PrP^{c} into PrP^{sc}, which goes on to convert other PrP^{c}. This initiates a chain reaction that allows for its rapid propagation, resulting in the pathogenesis of prion diseases.

Transmission

In 1961, Australian Michael Alpers conducted extensive field studies among the Fore accompanied by anthropologist Shirley Lindenbaum. Their historical research suggested the epidemic may have originated around 1900 from a single individual who lived on the edge of Fore territory and who is thought to have spontaneously developed some form of CJD. Alpers and Lindenbaum's research conclusively demonstrated that kuru spread easily and rapidly in the Fore people due to their endocannibalistic funeral practices, in which relatives consumed the bodies of the deceased to return the "life force" of the deceased to the hamlet, a Fore societal subunit. Corpses of family members were often buried for days then exhumed once the corpses were infested with maggots at which point the corpse would be dismembered and served with the maggots as a side dish.

The sexual dimorphism evident in the infection rates — kuru was eight to nine times more prevalent in women and children than in men at its peak — is because Fore men considered consuming human flesh to weaken them in times of conflict or battle, while the women and children were more apt to eat the bodies of the deceased, including the brain, where the prion particles were particularly concentrated. Also, the strong possibility exists that it was passed on to women and children more easily because they took on the task of cleaning relatives after death and may have had open sores and cuts on their hands.

Although ingestion of the prion particles can lead to the disease, a high degree of transmission occurred if the prion particles could reach the subcutaneous tissue. With elimination of cannibalism because of Australian colonial law enforcement and the local Christian missionaries' efforts, Alpers' research showed that kuru was already declining among the Fore by the mid1960s. However, the mean incubation period of the disease is 14 years, and cases were reported with latencies of 40 years or more for those who were most genetically resilient, continuing to appear for several more decades. The last sufferer died in 2005.

Immunity

In 2009, researchers at the Medical Research Council discovered a naturally occurring variant of a prion protein in a population from Papua New Guinea that confers strong resistance to kuru. In the study, which began in 1996, researchers assessed over 3,000 people from the affected and surrounding Eastern Highland populations, and identified a variation in the prion protein G127. G127 polymorphism is the result of a missense mutation, and is highly geographically restricted to regions where the kuru epidemic was the most widespread. Researchers believe that the PrnP variant occurred very recently, estimating that the most recent common ancestor lived 10 generations ago.

Of the discovery, Professor John Collinge, director of the MRC's Prion Unit at University College London, has stated that:

It's absolutely fascinating to see Darwinian principles at work here. This community of people has developed their own biologically unique response to a truly terrible epidemic. The fact that this genetic evolution has happened in a matter of decades is remarkable.

—John Collinge, Medical Research Council

The findings of the study could help researchers better understand and develop treatments for other related prion diseases, such as Creutzfeldt-Jakob disease and Alzheimer's disease.

History

Prior to prions, the Fore people initially believed the causes of kuru to be sorcery or witchcraft. Meanwhile, patrol officers believed that kuru could be psychosomatic, or caused by a mental factor. The fore people believed that kuru was caused by witches, but the reasoning behind it and the witches who were causing it could not be explained. They also thought that the magic causing kuru was contagious. Another theory for what was causing kuru was cassowary disease, also called negi negi. This disease, the Fore people believed was caused by ghosts because of the shaking and strange behavior that comes with kuru. To attempt to cure this, they would feed victims pork and casuarinas bark. Prior to the late 1950s, patrol officers thought that kuru was psychosomatic and was caused by the trauma of western colonization and perpetuated by beliefs in sorcery and witchcraft. It was not until 1957 that cannibalism was investigated with data, by Gajdusek, to be the cause of kuru. However, it was not considered a priority because it was thought to be too strange or evidence that theorized cannibalism as a cause lacked proper evidence. Cannibalism, however, was a reasonable enough explanation for kuru that the Australian administration banned the practice of feasting on the dead, until it was nearly obsolete by 1960. As the number of cases of kuru decreased, those in medical research were able to properly investigate kuru, which then led to the modern proposition of prions being the cause of kuru.

Kuru was first described in official reports by Australian officers patrolling the Eastern Highlands of Papua New Guinea in the early 1950s. Some unofficial accounts place kuru in the region as early as 1910. In 1951, it was Arthur Carey who first used the term 'kuru' in his report to describe a new disease afflicting the Fore tribes of Papua New Guinea. In his report, Carey noted that kuru mostly afflicted Fore women, eventually killing them. In 1953, kuru was observed by patrol officer John McArthur who provided a description of the disease in his report. McArthur believed that kuru was merely a psychological episode resulting from the confirmed sorcery practices of the tribal people in the region.

It was not by the time that the Kuru disease had spread into an epidemic when Daniel Carleton Gajdusek, a virologist, and Vincent Zigas, a medical doctor, first started doing research on the disease in 1957. It was first noted in the Fore, Yate and Usurufa people in 1952-1953 by anthropologists Ronald Berndt and Catherine Berndt. After the disease had festered into a bigger epidemic the tribal people called to Charles Pfarr, a Lutheran Medical Officer to come to the area to report the disease to Australian authorities.

In effort to understand the pathology of Kuru disease, Gajdusek established the first experimental tests on chimpanzees for Kuru at the National Institutes of Health (NIH). The methods of the experiment would be to introduce the kuru brain material to the closest human relative, the chimpanzee, and to document the behaviors of until death or a negative outcome would occur. Michael Alpers, an Australian doctor, collaborated with Gajdusek in providing the samples of brain tissues he had taken from an 11-year-old Fore girl who had died of Kuru. In his work he was also the first to document the first bibliography of the Kuru disease. Gajdusek was joined by a man named Joe Gibbs to monitor and record the behavior of the apes and conduct autopsies. Within two years, one of the chimps, Daisy, had developed kuru, demonstrating that the unknown disease factor was transmitted through infected biomaterial and that it was capable of crossing the species barrier to other primates. After confirmation from Elisabeth Beck, this experiment brought about the first conducted transmission of Kuru and was deemed an very important finding in the advancement of human medicine leading to the award of a Nobel Prize to D. Carleton Gajdusek in 1976.

Subsequently, E. J. Field spent large parts of the late 1960s and early 1970s in New Guinea investigating the disease, connecting it to scrapie and multiple sclerosis. He noted similarities in the diseases interactions with glial cells, including the critical observation that the infectious process may depend on structural rearrangement of the host's molecules. This was an early observation of what was to later become the prion hypothesis.

Fatal Familial Insomnia

Fatal familial insomnia (FFI) is an extremely rare autosomal dominant inherited prion disease of the brain. It is almost always caused by a mutation to the protein PrP^{C}, but can also develop spontaneously in patients with a non-inherited mutation variant called sporadic fatal insomnia (sFI). FFI has no known cure and involves progressively worsening insomnia, which leads to hallucinations, delirium, confusional states like that of dementia, and eventually, death. The average survival span for patients diagnosed with FFI after the onset of symptoms is 18 months.

The mutated protein, called PrP^{Sc}, has been found in just 40 families worldwide, affecting about 100 people; if only one parent has the gene, the offspring have a 50% risk of inheriting it and developing the disease. With onset usually around middle age, it is essential that a potential patient be tested if they wish to avoid passing FFI on to their children. The first recorded case was an Italian man, who died in Venice in 1765.

Presentation

The age of onset is variable, ranging from 18 to 60, with an average of 50. The disease can be detected prior to onset by genetic testing. Death usually occurs between seven and 36 months from onset. The presentation of the disease varies considerably from person to person, even among patients from within the same family.

The disease has four stages:

1. The person has increasing insomnia, resulting in panic attacks, paranoia, and phobias. This stage lasts for about four months.
2. Hallucinations and panic attacks become noticeable, continuing for about five months.
3. Complete inability to sleep is followed by rapid loss of weight. This lasts for about three months.
4. Dementia, during which the patient becomes unresponsive or mute over the course of six months. This is the final progression of the disease, after which death follows.

Other symptoms include profuse sweating, pinpoint pupils, the sudden entrance into menopause for women and impotence for men, neck stiffness, and elevation of blood pressure and heart rate. Constipation is common as well. As the disease progresses, the patient is forever stuck in a state of pre-sleep limbo. During these stages, it is common for patients to repeatedly move their limbs as if dreaming.

The first reported case in the Netherlands was of a 57-year-old man of Egyptian descent. The man came in with symptoms of double vision and progressive memory loss, and his family also noted he had recently become disoriented, paranoid, and confused. While he tended to fall asleep during random daily activities, he experienced vivid dreams and random muscular jerks during normal slow wave sleep. After four months of these symptoms, he started having convulsions in the hands, trunk, and lower limbs while awake. The patient died at 58 (seven months after the onset of symptoms). An autopsy was completed post-mortem which revealed mild atrophy of the frontal cortex and moderate atrophy of the thalamus. The atrophy of the thalamus is one of the most common signs of fatal familial insomnia.

Effect on Sleep

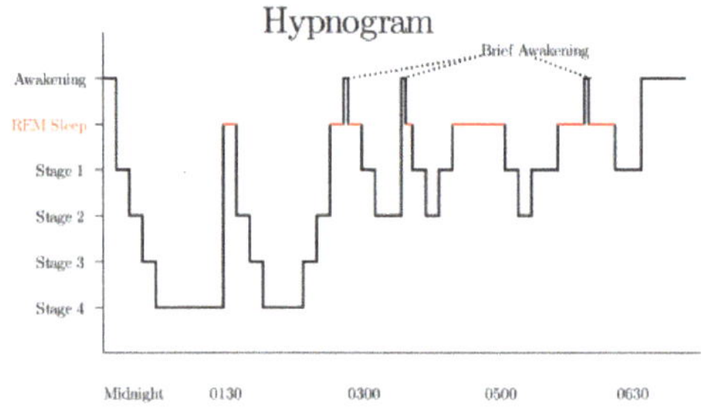

Normal sleep. FFI–patients cannot pass stage 1.

Normal sleep has different stages that together last 90 to 100 minutes:

- Non REM Stages 1 and 2: Light sleep NREM-sleep
- Non REM Stage 3 (previously 3 and 4): Deep slow wave sleep (SWS)
- REM-sleep when memorable dreams occur

FFI patients cannot go past stage 1 and thus their brains are not getting the rest they need to revive, as most reviving and repairing processes of the body are believed to happen during these deeper sleep stages. For example, psychiatrist Ian Oswald observed that during slow wave sleep (SWS), the pituitary gland increases its secretion of growth hormones. This discovery led Oswald to conclude that SWS restores the wear and tear bodily tissues gain throughout the day. Since a patient with FFI would be unable to reach SWS, and therefore the process of restoration during sleep, their body would become more worn each passing day.

Cause

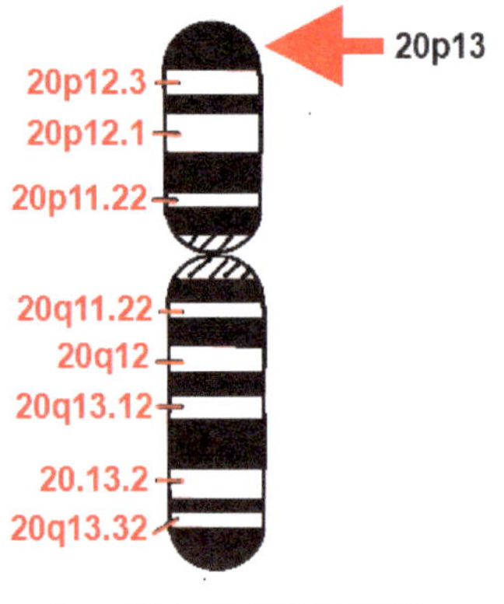

Location of *PRNP gene*

Idiogram of Chromosome 20 showing gene PRP location

Gene PRNP that provides instructions for making the prion protein PrP^C is located on the short (p) arm of chromosome 20 at position p13. Both FFI patients and those with familial Creutzfeldt–Jakob disease (fCJD) carry a mutation at codon 178 of the prion protein gene. FFI is also invariably linked to the presence of the methionine codon at position 129 of the mutant allele, whereas fCJD is linked to the presence of the valine codon at that position. "The disease is where there is a change of amino acid at position 178 when an asparagine (N) is found instead of the normal aspartic acid (D). This has to be accompanied with a methionine at position 129."

Treatment

In late 1983, Italian neurologist/sleep expert Dr. Ignazio Roiter received a patient at the University of Bologna hospital's sleep institute. The man, known only as Silvano, decided in a rare moment of consciousness to be recorded for future studies and to donate his brain for research in hopes of finding a cure for future victims. As of 2016, no cure or treatment has yet been found for FFI. Gene therapy has been thus far unsuccessful. While it is not currently possible to reverse the underlying illness, there is some evidence that treatments that focus solely upon the symptoms may improve quality of life.

It has been proven that sleeping pills and barbiturates are unhelpful; on the contrary, in 74% of cases, they have been shown to worsen the clinical manifestations and hasten the course of the disease.

One of the most notable cases is that of Michael (Michel A.) Corke, a music teacher from New Lenox, Illinois (born in Watseka, Illinois). He began to have trouble sleeping before his 40th birthday in 1991; following these first signs of insomnia, his health and state of mind quickly deteriorated as his condition worsened. Eventually, sleep became completely unattainable, and he was soon admitted to University of Chicago Hospital with a misdiagnosis of clinical depression due to multiple sclerosis. Medical professionals Dr. Raymond Roos and Dr. Anthony Reder, at first unsure of the nature of his illness, initially diagnosed multiple sclerosis; in a bid to provide temporary relief in the later stages of the disease, physicians induced a coma with the use of sedatives, to no avail as his brain still failed to shut down completely. Corke died in 1993, a month after his 42nd birthday, by which time he had been completely sleep-deprived for six months.

One person was able to exceed the average survival time by nearly one year with various strategies, including vitamin therapy and meditation, using different stimulants and hypnotics, and even complete sensory deprivation in an attempt to induce sleep at night and increase alertness during the day. He managed to write a book and drive hundreds of miles in this time but nonetheless, over the course of his trials, the person succumbed to the classic four-stage progression of the illness.

In the late 2000s, a mouse model was made for FFI. These mice expressed a humanized version of the PrP protein that also contains the D178N FFI mutation. These mice appear to have progressively fewer and shorter periods of uninterrupted sleep, damage in the thalamus, and early deaths, similar to humans with FFI.

As of 2016, studies suggest that doxycycline may be able to slow or even prevent the development of the disease.

Epidemiology

It was reported in 1998 that there were 25 families in the world known to carry the gene for FFI: eight German, five Italian, four American, two French, two Australian, two British, one Japanese, and one Austrian. In 2011, another family was added to the list when researchers found the first man in the Netherlands with FFI. While he had lived in the Netherlands for 19 years, he was of Egyptian descent. There are other prion diseases that are similar to FFI and could be related but are missing the D178N gene mutation.

Only nine cases of sporadic fatal insomnia have ever been diagnosed as of July 2005. In sFI, there is no mutation in *PRNP*-prion gene in D178N, but all have methionine homozygosity at codon 129.

Related Conditions

There are other diseases involving the mammalian prion protein. Some are transmissible (TSEs, including FFI) such as kuru, bovine spongiform encephalopathy (BSE, also known as "mad cow disease") in cows, and chronic wasting disease in American deer and American elk in some areas of the United States and Canada, as well as Creutzfeldt–Jakob disease (CJD). Until recently, prion diseases were only thought to be transmissible via direct contact with infected tissue, such as from eating infected tissue, transfusion, or transplantation; new research now suggests that prion diseases can be transmitted via aerosols, but that the general public is not at risk of airborne infection.

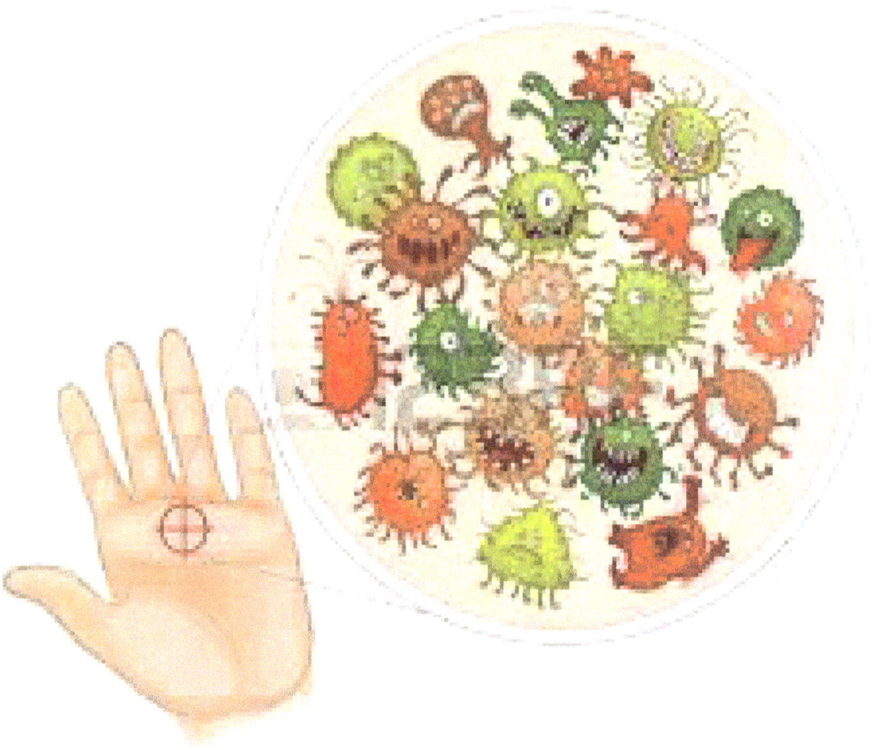

References

- Charles E. Rosenberg (2009). The Cholera Years the United States in 1832, 1849, and 1866. Chicago: University of Chicago Press. p. 74. ISBN 9780226726762.
- Haynes SW (1997). James K. Polk and the Expansionist Impulse. New York: Longman. p. 191. ISBN 978-0-673-99001-3.
- Schlossberg, David (2015). Clinical infectious disease (Second ed.). p. 334. ISBN 9781107038912.
- Ferri's Clinical Advisor 2015: 5 Books in 1. Elsevier Health Sciences. 2014. p. 479. ISBN 9780323084307.
- Shors, Teri (2013). The microbial challenge : a public health perspective (3rd ed.). Burlington, Mass.: Jones & Bartlett Learning. p. 457. ISBN 9781449673338.
- A. Helms, Richard (2006). Textbook of therapeutics : drug and disease management (8. ed.). Philadelphia, Pa. [u.a.]: Lippincott Williams & Wilkins. p. 2003. ISBN 9780781757348.
- Webber, Roger (2009). Communicable disease epidemiology and control : a global perspective (3rd ed.). Wallingford, Oxfordshire: Cabi. p. 79. ISBN 978-1-84593-504-7.
- Tintinalli, Judith E. (2010). Emergency Medicine: A Comprehensive Study Guide (Emergency Medicine (Tintinalli)). New York: McGraw-Hill Companies. pp. 830–839. ISBN 0-07-148480-9.
- Warrell D.A.; Cox T.M.; Firth J.D.; Benz E.J., eds. (2003). The Oxford Textbook of Medicine (4th ed.). Oxford University Press. ISBN 0-19-262922-0.
- Mandell, Gerald L.; Bennett, John E.; Dolin, Raphael (2004). Mandell's Principles and Practices of Infection Diseases (6th ed.). Churchill Livingstone. ISBN 0-443-06643-4.
- Feldman, Mark; Friedman, Lawrence S.; Sleisenger, Marvin H. (2002). Sleisenger & Fordtran's Gastrointestinal and Liver Disease (7th ed.). Saunders. ISBN 0-7216-8973-6.
- Charles E. Rosenberg (2009). The Cholera Years the United States in 1832, 1849, and 1866. Chicago: University of Chicago Press. p. 74. ISBN 9780226726762.
- Albert, edited by Neil S. Skolnik ; associate editor, Ross H. (2008). Essential infectious disease topics for primary care. Totowa, NJ: Humana Press. p. 66. ISBN 978-1-58829-520-0.
- Rousseaux, Wanda Haschek, Matthew Wallig, Colin (2009). Fundamentals of toxicologic pathology (2nd ed.). London: Academic. p. 182. ISBN 9780123704696.
- MacLachlan, edited by N. James; Dubovi, Edward J. (2009). Fenner's veterinary virology (4th ed.). Amsterdam: Elsevier Academic Press. p. 399. ISBN 9780123751584.
- Fox, James G.; et al., eds. (2002). Laboratory animal medicine (2nd ed.). Amsterdam: Academic Press. p. 649. ISBN 9780122639517.
- Zimmerman, Jeffrey; Karriker, Locke; Ramirez, Alejandro; Kent Schwartz; Gregory Stevenson (15 May 2012). Diseases of Swine (10th ed.). Chichester, West Sussex: John Wiley & Sons. p. 504. ISBN 978-0-8138-2267-9.
- Katzung, Bertram G. (2007). Basic and Clinical Pharmacology. New York, NY: McGraw Hill Medical. p. 733. ISBN 978-0-07-145153-6.
- Hof H (1996). Baron S; et al., eds. Listeria Monocytogenes in: Baron's Medical Microbiology (4th ed.). Univ of Texas Medical Branch. ISBN 0-9631172-1-1. (via NCBI Bookshelf).
- Swaminathan B, Gerner-Smidt P. 2007. The epidemiology of human listeriosis. Microbes In name="Mazza2002">Joseph Mazza (15 January 2002). Manual of clinical hematology. Lippincott Williams & Wilkins. pp. 127–. ISBN 978-0-7817-2980-2. Retrieved 29 June 2010.
- Connie R. Mahon; Donald C. Lehman; George Manuselis Jr. (25 March 2014). Textbook of Diagnostic Microbiology. Elsevier Health Sciences. pp. 357–. ISBN 978-0-323-29262-7.

- Franson JC, Friend M. "38: Avian Botulism". Field Manual of Wildlife Disease (PDF). U.S. Geological Survey. ISBN 978-0-607-88096-0. Retrieved 14 June 2016.
- Diamond JM (1997). Guns, germs, and steel: the fates of human societies. New York: W.W. Norton. p. 208. ISBN 0-393-03891-2.

5

Zoonotic Diseases that Spread through Food

The zoonotic diseases that spread through food are salmonellosis, bubonic plague, avian influenza, caliciviridae and trichinosis. Salmonellosis is an infection caused by bacterias, the symptoms of which vary from fever to abdominal cramps. The topics discussed in the chapter are of great importance to broaden the existing knowledge on zoonotic diseases.

Bubonic Plague

Bubonic plague is one of three types of bacterial infection caused by *Yersinia pestis*. Three to seven days after exposure to the bacteria flu like symptoms develop. This includes fever, headaches, and vomiting. Swollen and painful lymph nodes occur in the area closest to where the bacteria entered the skin. Occasionally the swollen lymph nodes may break open.

The three types of plague are the result of the route of infection: bubonic plague, septicemic plague, and pneumonic plague. Bubonic plague is mainly spread by infected fleas from small animals. It may also result from exposure to the body fluids from a dead plague infected animal. In the bubonic form of plague, the bacteria enter through the skin through a flea bite and travel via the lymphatic vessels to a lymph node, causing it to swell. Diagnosis is made by finding the bacteria in the blood, sputum, or fluid from lymph nodes.

Prevention is through public health measures such as not handling dead animals in areas where plague is common. Vaccines have not been found to be very useful for plague prevention. Several antibiotics are effective for treatment including streptomycin, gentamicin, and doxycycline. Without treatment it results in the death of 30% to 90% of those infected. Death if it occurs is typically within ten days. With treatment the risk of death is around 10%. Globally in 2013 there were about 750 documented cases which resulted in 126 deaths. The disease is most common in Africa.

Plague is believed to be the cause of the Black Death that swept through Asia, Europe, and Africa in the 14th century and killed an estimated 50 million people. This was about 25% to 60% of the European population. Because the plague killed so many of the working population, wages rose due to the demand for labor. Some historians see this as a turning point in European economic development.

Signs and Symptoms

The best-known symptom of bubonic plague is one or more infected, enlarged, and painful lymph nodes, known as buboes. After being transmitted via the bite of an infected flea, the *Y. pestis* bacteria become localized in an inflamed lymph node where they begin to colonize and reproduce. Buboes associated with the bubonic plague are commonly found in the armpits, upper femoral, groin and neck region. Acral gangrene (i.e., of the fingers, toes, lips and nose) is another common symptom.

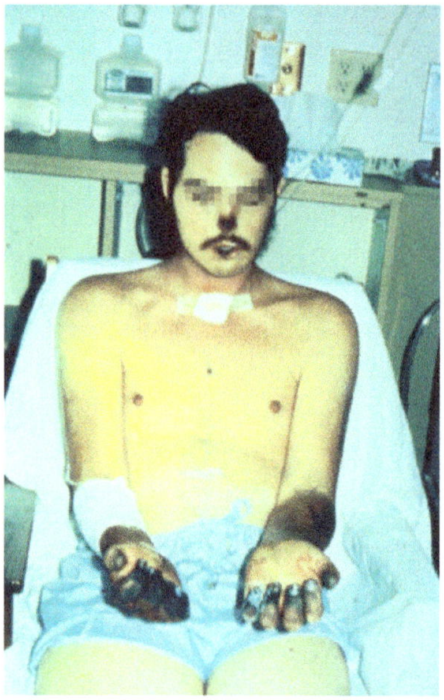

Acral necrosis of the nose, the lips, and the fingers and residual ecchymoses over both forearms in a patient recovering from bubonic plague that disseminated to the blood and the lungs. At one time, the patient's entire body was ecchymotic. Reprinted from *Textbook of Military Medicine*.

Because of its bite-based mode of transmission, the bubonic plague is often the first of a progressive series of illnesses. Bubonic plague symptoms appear suddenly a few days after exposure to the bacterium. Symptoms include:

- Chills
- General ill feeling (malaise)
- High fever (39 °C; 102 °F)
- Muscle cramps
- Seizures
- Smooth, painful lymph gland swelling called a bubo, commonly found in the groin, but may occur in the armpits or neck, most often near the site of the initial infection (bite or scratch)
- Pain may occur in the area before the swelling appears
- Gangrene of the extremities such as toes, fingers, lips and tip of the nose.

Other symptoms include heavy breathing, continuous vomiting of blood (hematemesis), aching limbs, coughing, and extreme pain caused by the decay or decomposition of the skin while the person is still alive. Additional symptoms include extreme fatigue, gastrointestinal problems, lenticulae (black dots scattered throughout the body), delirium, and coma.

Cause

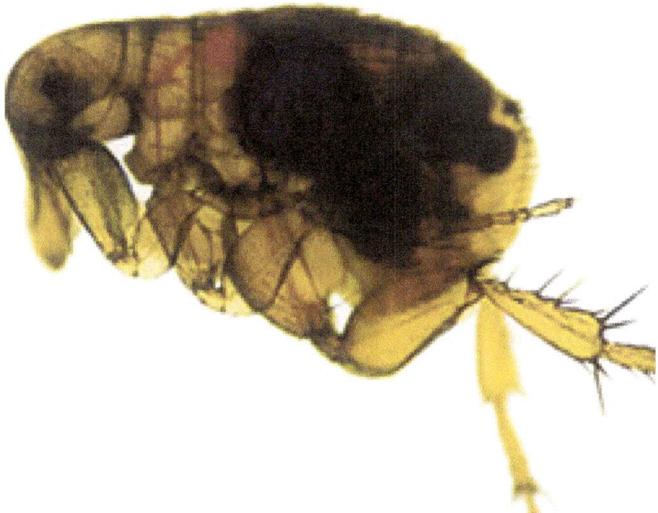

Oriental rat flea (*Xenopsylla cheopis*) infected with the *Yersinia pestis* bacterium which appears as a dark mass in the gut. The foregut of this flea is blocked by a *Y. pestis* biofilm; when the flea attempts to feed on an uninfected host, *Y. pestis* from the foregut is regurgitated into the wound, causing infection.

Bubonic plague is an infection of the lymphatic system, usually resulting from the bite of an infected flea, *Xenopsylla cheopis* (the rat flea). In very rare circumstances, as in the septicemic plague, the disease can be transmitted by direct contact with infected tissue or exposure to the cough of another human. The flea is parasitic on house and field rats, and seeks out other prey when its rodent hosts die. The bacteria remained harmless to the flea, allowing the new host to spread the bacteria. The bacteria form aggregates in the gut of infected fleas and this results in the flea regurgitating ingested blood, which is now infected, into the bite site of a rodent or human host. Once established, bacteria rapidly spread to the lymph nodes and multiply.

Y. pestis bacilli can resist phagocytosis and even reproduce inside phagocytes and kill them. As the disease progresses, the lymph nodes can haemorrhage and become swollen and necrotic. Bubonic plague can progress to lethal septicemic plague in some cases. The plague is also known to spread to the lungs and become the disease known as the pneumonic plague.

Diagnosis

Laboratory testing is required in order to diagnose and confirm plague. Ideally, confirmation is through the identification of *Y. pestis* culture from a patient sample. Confirmation of infection can be done by examining serum taken during the early and late stages of infection. To quickly screen for the *Y. pestis* antigen in patients, rapid dipstick tests have been developed for field use.

Treatment

Several classes of antibiotics are effective in treating bubonic plague. These include aminoglycosides such as streptomycin and gentamicin, tetracyclines (especially doxycycline), and the fluoroquinolone ciprofloxacin. Mortality associated with treated cases of bubonic plague is about 1–15%, compared to a mortality of 40–60% in untreated cases.

People potentially infected with the plague need immediate treatment and should be given antibiotics within 24 hours of the first symptoms to prevent death. Other treatments include oxygen, intravenous fluids, and respiratory support. People who have had contact with anyone infected by pneumonic plague are given prophylactic antibiotics. Using the broad-based antibiotic streptomycin has proven to be dramatically successful against the bubonic plague within 12 hours of infection.

History

First Outbreak

The first recorded epidemic affected the Eastern Roman Empire (Byzantine Empire) and was named the Plague of Justinian after emperor Justinian I, who was infected but survived through extensive treatment. The pandemic resulted in the deaths of an estimated 25 million (6th century outbreak) to 50 million people (two centuries of recurrence). The historian Procopius wrote, in Volume II of History of the Wars, of his personal encounter with the plague and the effect it had on the rising empire. In the spring of 542, the plague arrived in Constantinople, working its way from port city to port city and spreading around the Mediterranean Sea, later migrating inland eastward into Asia Minor and west into Greece and Italy. Because the infectious disease spread inland by the transferring of merchandise through Justinian's efforts in acquiring luxurious goods of the time and exporting supplies, his capital became the leading exporter of the bubonic plague. Procopius, in his work *Secret History*, declared that Justinian was a demon of an emperor who either created the plague himself or was being punished for his sinfulness.

Second Outbreak

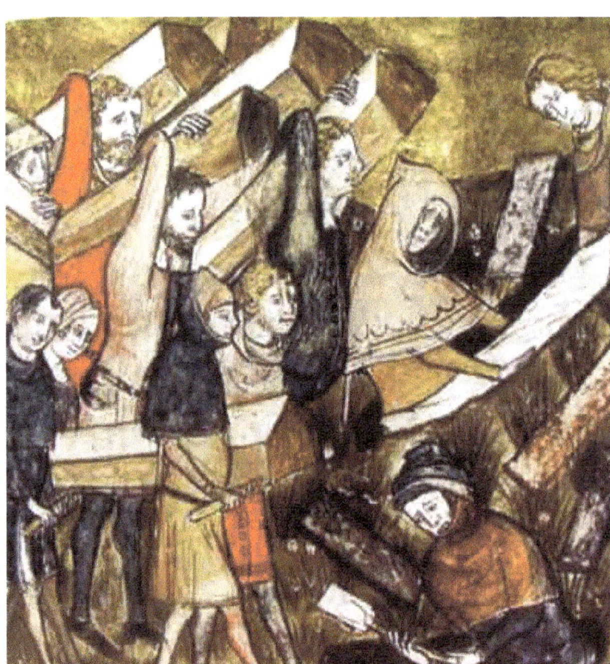

Citizens of Tournai bury plague victims. Miniature from *The Chronicles of Gilles Li Muisis* (1272–1352). Bibliothèque royale de Belgique, MS 13076-77, f. 24v.

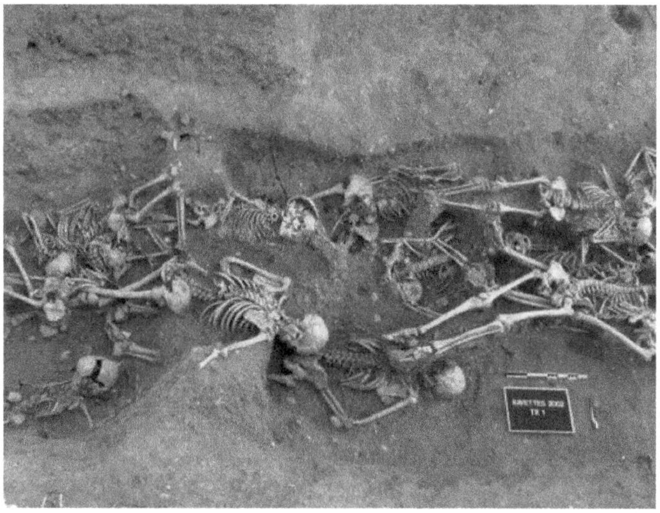

Bubonic plague victims in a mass grave from 1720–1721 in Martigues, France

In the Late Middle Ages (1340–1400) Europe experienced the most deadly disease outbreak in history when the Black Death, the infamous pandemic of bubonic plague, hit in 1347, killing a third of the human population. It is believed that society subsequently became more violent as the mass mortality rate cheapened life and thus increased warfare, crime, popular revolt, waves of flagellants, and persecution. The Black Death originated in or near China and spread from Italy and then throughout other European countries. Arab historians Ibn Al-Wardni and Almaqrizi believed the Black Death originated in Mongolia, and this was proven correct as Chinese records showed a huge outbreak in Mongolia in the early 1330s. Research published in 2002 suggests that it began in early 1346 in the steppe region, where a plague reservoir stretches from the northwestern shore of the Caspian Sea into southern Russia. The Mongols had cut off the trade route, the Silk Road, between China and Europe which halted the spread of the Black Death from eastern Russia to Western Europe. The epidemic began with an attack that Mongols launched on the Italian merchants' last trading station in the region, Caffa in the Crimea. In late 1346, plague broke out among the besiegers and from them penetrated into the town. When spring arrived, the Italian merchants fled on their ships, unknowingly carrying the Black Death. Carried by the fleas on rats, the plague initially spread to humans near the Black Sea and then outwards to the rest of Europe as a result of people fleeing from one area to another.

There were many ethno-medical beliefs for avoiding the Black Death. One of the most famous was that by walking around with flowers in or around their nose people would be able to "ward off the stench and perhaps the evil that afflicted them". People believed the plague to be a punishment from God, and that the only way to be rid of the plague was to be forgiven by God. One such method used was to carve the symbol of the cross onto the front door of a house with the words "Lord have mercy on us".

Pistoia, a city in Italy, went as far as enacting rules and regulations on the city and its inhabitants to keep it safe from the Black Death. The rules stated that no one was allowed to visit any plague-infected area and if they did they were not allowed back into the city. Some other rules were that no linen or woollen goods were to be imported into the city and no corpses were to be buried in the city. Despite strict enforcement of the rules, the city eventually became infected. People who were not infected with the plague gathered in groups and stayed away from the sick. They ate and drank with limited food and water and were not even allowed oral communication because it was believed that merely talking with one another increased the chance of passing on the disease.

While Europe was devastated by the disease, the rest of the world fared much better. In India, population rose from a population of 91 million in 1300, to 97 million in 1400, to 105 million in 1500. Sub-Saharan Africa remained largely unaffected by the plagues.

The next few centuries were marked by several localized or regional outbreaks of lesser severity. The Great Plague of Milan (1629-1631), the Great Plague of Seville (1647), the Great Plague of London (1665–1666), the Great Plague of Vienna (1679), Great Baltic plague (1708–1712), the Great Plague of Marseille (1720), the Great Plague of 1738 and Caragea's Plague (1813–1814) were the last major outbreaks of the bubonic plague in Europe.

Traditional Treatment

Medieval doctors thought the plague was created by air corrupted by humid weather, decaying unburied bodies, and fumes produced by poor sanitation. The recommended treatment of the plague was a good diet, rest, and relocating to a non-infected environment so the individual could get access to clean air. This did help, but not for the reasons the doctors of the time thought. In actuality, because they recommended moving away from unsanitary conditions, people were, in effect, getting away from the rodents that harbored the fleas carrying the infection. However, this also helped to spread the infection to new areas previously non-infected.

Third Outbreak

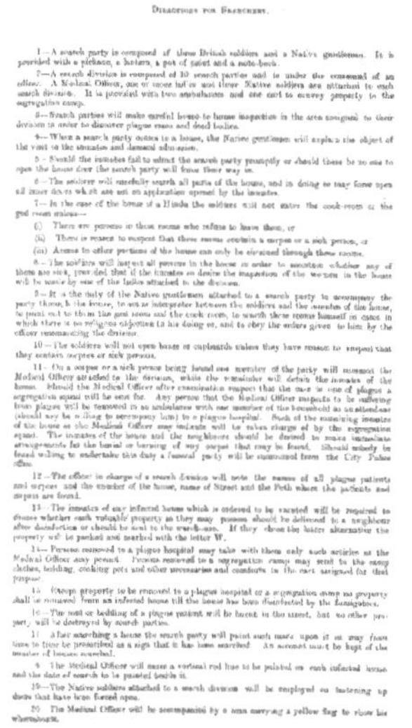
Directions for Searchers.

Directions for searchers, Poona (now Pune) plague of 1897

The plague resurfaced for a third time in the mid-19th century. Like the two previous outbreaks, this one also originated in Eastern Asia. The initial outbreak occurred in China's Yunnan province in 1855. The disease remained localized in Southwest China for several years before spreading. In the city of Canton, beginning in January 1894, the disease killed 80,000 people by June. Daily water-traffic with the nearby city of Hong Kong rapidly spread the plague there, killing over 2,400 within two months.

From China, the plague spread to the Indian subcontinent around 1896. Over the next thirty years, India would lose 12.5 million people to the bubonic plague. The disease was initially seen in port cities, beginning with Bombay (now Mumbai), but later emerged in Poona (now Pune), Kolkata, and Karachi (now in Pakistan). By 1899, the outbreak spread to smaller communities and rural areas in many regions of India. Overall, the impact of plague epidemics was greatest in western and northern India—in the provinces then designated as Bombay, Punjab, and the United Provinces—while eastern and southern India were not as badly affected. Ultimately, more than 12 million people died from the plague in India (including present day Pakistan and Bangladesh) and China alone.

In 1899, the plague reached the islands of Hawaii. The first evidence of the disease was found in Honolulu's Chinatown on Oahu. It was located very close to the island's piers, and rats in cargo ships from China were able to land on the Hawaiian islands unseen. As the rats, hosts for disease-carrying fleas, made their way deeper into the city, people started to fall ill. On December 12, 1899, the first case was confirmed. The Board of Health then quickly thought of ways to prevent the disease from spreading even further inland. Their solution was to burn down any buildings in Chinatown suspected of containing a source of the disease. On December 31, 1899, the board set the first fire. They had originally planned to burn only a few targeted buildings, and thought they could control the flames as each building was finished, but the fire got out of control, burning down untargeted neighboring buildings. The resulting fire caused many of Chinatown's homes to be destroyed and an estimated 4,000 people were left homeless.

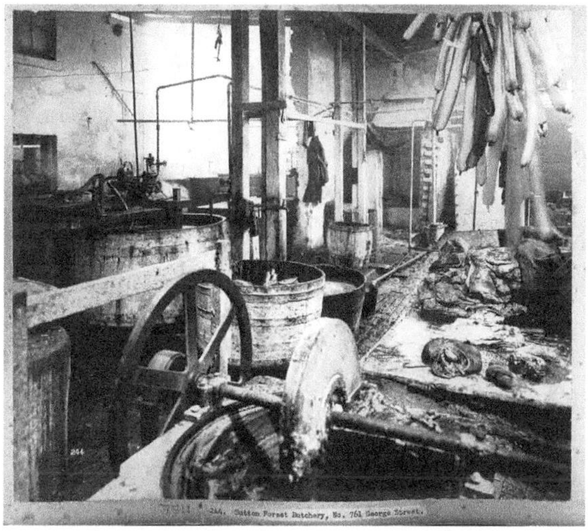

From a series of images depicting the state of houses and "slum" buildings in Sydney, Australia at the time of the 1900 outbreak and the cleansing and disinfecting operations which followed.

Australia suffered 12 major plague outbreaks between 1900 and 1925 originating from shipping. Research by Australian medical officers Thompson, Armstrong and Tidswell contributed to understanding the spread of *Yersinia pestis* to humans by fleas from infected rats.

According to the World Health Organization, the pandemic was considered active until 1959, when worldwide casualties dropped to 200 per year. In 1994, a plague outbreak in five Indian states caused an estimated 700 infections (including 52 deaths) and triggered a large migration of Indians within India as they tried to avoid the plague.

Biological Warfare

Some of the earliest instances of biological warfare were said to have been products of the plague, as armies of the 14th century were recorded catapulting diseased corpses over the walls of towns and villages to spread the pestilence.

Later, plague was used during the Second Sino-Japanese War as a bacteriological weapon by the Imperial Japanese Army. These weapons were provided by Shirō Ishii's units and used in experiments on humans before being used on the field. For example, in 1940, the Imperial Japanese Army Air Service bombed Ningbo with fleas carrying the bubonic plague. During the Khabarovsk War Crime Trials, the accused, such as Major General Kiyashi Kawashima, testified that, in 1941, some 40 members of Unit 731 air-dropped plague-contaminated fleas on Changde. These operations caused epidemic plague outbreaks.

Society and Culture

The scale of death and social upheaval associated with plague outbreaks has made the topic prominent in a number of historical and fictional accounts since the disease was first recognized. The Black Death in particular is described and referenced in numerous contemporary sources, some of which, including works by Chaucer, Boccaccio, and Petrarch, are considered part of the Western canon. The Decameron, by Boccaccio, is notable for its use of a frame story involving individuals who have fled Florence for a secluded villa to escape the Black Death. First person, sometimes sensationalized or fictionalized, accounts of living through plague years have also been popular across centuries and cultures.

Later works, such as Albert Camus's novel *The Plague* or Ingmar Bergman's film *The Seventh Seal* have used bubonic plague in settings, such quarantined cities in either medieval or modern times, as a backdrop to explore a variety of concepts. Common themes include the breakdown of society, institutions, and individuals during the plague, the cultural and psychological existential confrontation with mortality, and the allegorical use of the plague in reference to contemporary moral or spiritual questions.

Avian Influenza

Avian influenza — known informally as *avian flu* or bird flu — refers to "influenza caused by viruses adapted to birds." The type with the greatest risk is highly pathogenic avian influenza (HPAI).

"Bird flu" is a phrase similar to "swine flu," "dog flu," "horse flu," or "human flu" in that it refers to an illness caused by any of many different strains of influenza viruses that have adapted to a specific host. Out of the three types of influenza viruses (A, B, and C), influenza A virus is a zoonotic infection with a natural reservoir almost entirely in birds. Avian influenza, for most purposes, refers to the influenza A virus.

Though influenza A is adapted to birds, it can also stably adapt and sustain person-to person transmission. Recent influenza research into the genes of the Spanish flu virus shows it to have genes adapted from both human and avian strains. Pigs can also be infected with human, avian, and swine influenza viruses, allow for mixtures of genes (reassortment) to create a new virus, which can cause an antigenic shift to a new influenza A virus subtype which most people have little to no immune protection.

Avian influenza strains are divided into two types based on their pathogenicity: high pathogenicity (HP) or low pathogenicity (LP). The most well-known HPAI strain, H5N1, appeared in China in 1996, and also has low pathogenic strains found in North America. Companion birds in captivity are unlikely to contract the virus and there has been no report of a companion bird with avian influenza since 2003. Pigeons do not contract or spread the virus.

History

The most widely quoted date for the beginning of recorded history of avian influenza (initially known as fowl plague) was in 1878 when it was differentiated from other diseases that caused high mortality rates in birds. Fowl plague, however, also included Newcastle disease until as recently as the 1950s. Between 1959 and 1995, there were 15 recorded occasions of the emergence of HPAI viruses in poultry, but losses were minimal. Between 1996 and 2008 however, HPAI outbreaks in poultry have occurred at least 11 times and 4 of these outbreaks have involved millions of birds.

In the 1990s, the world's poultry population grew 76% in developing countries and 23% in developed countries, contributing to the increased prevalence of avian influenza. Before the 1990s, HPAI caused high mortality in poultry, but infections were sporadic and contained. Outbreaks have become more common due to the high density and frequent movement of flocks from intensive poultry production.

Influenza A/H5N1 was first isolated from a goose in China in 1996. Human infections were first reported in 1997 in Hong Kong. Since 2003, more than 700 human cases of Asian HPAI H5N1 have been reported to the WHO, primarily from 15 countries in Asia, Africa, the Pacific, Europe, and the Middle East, though over 60 countries have been affected.

Genetics

Genetic factors in distinguishing between "human flu viruses" and "avian flu viruses" include:

- PB2: (RNA polymerase): Amino acid (or residue) position 627 in the PB2 protein encoded by the PB2 RNA gene. Until H5N1, all known avian influenza viruses had a Glu at position 627, while all human influenza viruses had a Lys.
- HA: (hemagglutinin): Avian influenza HA viruses bind alpha 2-3 sialic acid receptors, while human influenza HA viruses bind alpha 2-6 sialic acid receptors. Swine influenza viruses have the ability to bind both types of sialic acid receptors. Hemagglutinin is the major antigen of the virus against which neutralizing antibodies are produced, and influenza virus epidemics are associated with changes in its antigenic structure. This was originally derived from pigs, and should technically be referred to as "pig flu".

Subtypes

There are many subtypes of avian influenza viruses, but only some strains of five subtypes have been known to infect humans: H5N1, H7N3, H7N7, H7N9, and H9N2. At least one person, an elderly woman in Jiangxi Province, China, died of pneumonia in December 2013 from the H10N8 strain, the first human fatality confirmed to be caused by that strain.

Most human cases of the avian flu are a result of either handling dead infected birds or from contact with infected fluids. It can also be spread through contaminated surfaces and droppings. While most wild birds mainly have only a mild form of the H5N1 strain, once domesticated birds such as chickens or turkeys are infected, it can become much more deadly because the birds are often in close contact. There is currently a large threat of this in Asia with infected poultry due to low hygiene conditions and close quarters. Although it is easy for humans to contract the infection from birds, human-to-human transmission is more difficult without prolonged contact. However, public health officials are concerned that strains of avian flu may mutate to become easily transmissible between humans. Some strains of avian influenza are present in the intestinal tract of large numbers of shore birds and water birds, but these strains rarely cause infection.

Spreading of H5N1 from Asia to Europe is much more likely caused by both legal and illegal poultry trades than dispersing through wild bird migrations, being that in recent studies, there were no secondary rises in infection in Asia when wild birds migrate south again from their breeding grounds. Instead, the infection patterns followed transportation such as railroads, roads, and country borders, suggesting poultry trade as being much more likely. While there have been strains of avian flu to exist in the United States, such as Texas in 2004, they have been extinguished and have not been known to infect humans.

Highly pathogenic strains spread quickly among flocks and can destroy a flock within 28 hours; the less pathogenic strains may affect egg production but are much less deadly.

Examples of Avian Influenza A Virus Strains:

HA subtype designation	NA subtype designation	Avian influenza A viruses
H1	N1	A/duck/Alberta/35/76(H1N1)
H1	N8	A/duck/Alberta/97/77(H1N8)
H2	N9	A/duck/Germany/1/72(H2N9)
H3	N8	A/duck/Ukraine/63(H3N8)
H3	N8	A/duck/England/62(H3N8)
H3	N2	A/turkey/England/69(H3N2)
H4	N6	A/duck/Czechoslovakia/56(H4N6)
H4	N3	A/duck/Alberta/300/77(H4N3)
H5	N3	A/tern/South Africa/300/77(H4N3)
H5	N4	A/Ethiopia/300/77(H6N6)
H5	N8	H5N8
H5	N9	A/turkey/Ontario/7732/66(H5N9)
H5	N1	A/chick/Scotland/59(H5N1)

H6	N2	A/turkey/ Massachusetts/3740/65(H6N2)
H6	N8	A/turkey/Canada/63(H6N8)
H6	N5	A/shearwater/Australia/72(H6N5)
H6	N6	A/jyotichinara/Ehiopia/73(H6N6)
H6	N1	A/duck/Germany/1868/68(H6N1)
H7	N7	A/fowl plague virus/Dutch/27(H7N7)
H7	N1	A/chick/Brescia/1902(H7N1)
H7	N9	A/chick/China/2013(H7N9)
H7	N3	A/turkey/England/639H7N3)
H7	N1	A/fowl plague virus/ Rostock/34(H7N1)
H8	N4	A/turkey/Ontario/6118/68(H8N4)
H9	N2	A/turkey/Wisconsin/1/66(H9N2)
H9	N6	A/duck/Hong Kong/147/77(H9N6)
H9	N6	A/duck/Hong Kong/147/77(H9N6)
H9	N8	A/manishsurpur/ Malawi/149/77(H9N8)
H9	N7	A/turkey/Scotland/70(H9N7)
H10	N8	A/quail/Italy/1117/65(H10N8)
H11	N6	A/duck/England/56(H11N6)
H11	N9	A/duck/Memphis/546/74(H11N9)
H12	N5	A/duck/Alberta/60/76/(H12N5)
H13	N6	A/gull/Maryland/704/77(H13N6)
H14	N4	A/duck/Gurjev/263/83(H14N4)
H15	N9	A/shearwater/ Australia/2576/83(H15N9)

Spread

Avian influenza is most often spread by contact between infected and healthy birds, though can also be spread indirectly through contaminated equipment. The virus is found in secretions from the nostrils, mouth, and eyes of infected birds as well as their droppings. HPAI infection is spread to people often through direct contact with infected poultry, such as during slaughter or plucking. Though the virus can spread through airborne secretions, the disease itself is not an airborne disease. Highly pathogenic strains spread quickly among flocks and can destroy a flock within 28 hours; the less pathogenic strains may affect egg production but are much less deadly.

Although it is possible for humans to contract the avian influenza virus from birds, human-to-human contact is much more difficult without prolonged contact. However, public health officials are concerned that strains of avian flu may mutate to become easily transmissible between humans. Some strains of avian influenza are present in the intestinal tract of large numbers of shore birds and water birds, but these strains rarely cause human infection.

Five manmade ecosystems have contributed to modern avian influenza virus ecology: integrated indoor commercial poultry, range-raised commercial poultry, live poultry markets, backyard and hobby flocks, and bird collection and trading systems including cockfighting. Indoor commercial poultry has had the largest impact on the spread of HPAI, with the increase in HPAI outbreaks largely the result of increased commercial production since the 1990s.

Village Poultry

In the early days of the HPAI H5N1 pandemic, village poultry and their owners were frequently implicated in disease transmission. Village poultry, also known as backyard and hobby flocks, are small flocks raised under extensive conditions and often allowed free range between multiple households. However, research has shown that these flocks pose less of a threat than intensively raised commercial poultry with homogenous genetic stock and poor biosecurity. Backyard and village poultry also do not travel great distances compared to transport of intensively raised poultry and contribute less to the spread of HPAI. This initial implication of Asian poultry farmers as one broad category presented challenges to prevention recommendations as commercial strategies did not necessarily apply to backyard poultry flocks.

H5N1

The highly pathogenic influenza A virus subtype H5N1 is an emerging avian influenza virus that is causing global concern as a potential pandemic threat. It is often referred to simply as "bird flu" or "avian influenza", even though it is only one of many subtypes.

H5N1 has killed millions of poultry in a growing number of countries throughout Asia, Europe, and Africa. Health experts are concerned that the coexistence of human flu viruses and avian flu viruses (especially H5N1) will provide an opportunity for genetic material to be exchanged between species-specific viruses, possibly creating a new virulent influenza strain that is easily transmissible and lethal to humans. The mortality rate for humans with H5N1 is 60%.

Since first human H5N1 outbreak occurred in 1997, there has been an increasing number of HPAI H5N1 bird-to-human transmissions, leading to clinically severe and fatal human infections. Because a significant species barrier exists between birds and humans, the virus does not easily spread to humans, however some cases of infection are being researched to discern whether human-to-human transmission is occurring. More research is necessary to understand the pathogenesis and epidemiology of the H5N1 virus in humans. Exposure routes and other disease transmission characteristics, such as genetic and immunological factors that may increase the likelihood of infection, are not clearly understood.

The first known transmission of H5N1 to a human occurred in Hong Kong in 1997, when there was an outbreak of 18 human cases; 6 deaths were confirmed. None of the infected people worked with poultry. After culling all of the poultry in the area, no more cases were diagnosed. In 2006, the first human-to-human transmission likely occurred when 7 members of a family in Sumatra became infected after contact with a family member who had worked with infected poultry.

Although millions of birds have become infected with the virus since its discovery, 359 people have died from the H5N1 in twelve countries according to World Health Organization reports as of August 10, 2012.

As an example, the H5N1 outbreak in Thailand caused massive economic losses, especially among poultry workers. Infected birds were culled and slaughtered. The public lost confidence with the poultry products, thus decreasing the consumption of chicken products. This also elicited a ban from importing countries. There were, however, factors which aggravated the spread of the virus, including bird migration, cool temperature (increases virus survival) and several festivals at that time.

Controversial Research

A study published in 2012 in Science Magazine reported on research findings that allowed for the airborne transmission of H5N1 in laboratory ferrets. The study identified the 5 mutations necessary for the virus to become airborne and immediately spiked controversy over the ethical implications of making such potentially dangerous information available to the general public. The study was allowed to remain available in its entirety, though remains a controversial topic within the scientific community.

The study in question, however, created airborne H5N1 via amino acid substitutions that largely mitigated the devastating effects of the disease. This fact was underscored by the 0% fatality rate among the ferrets infected via airborne transmission, as well as the fundamental biology underlying the substitutions. Flu viruses attach to host cells via the hemagluttinin proteins on their envelope. These hemagluttinin proteins bind to sialic acid receptors on host cells, which can fall into two categories. The sialic acid receptors can be either 2,3 or 2,6-linked, with the species of origin largely deciding receptor preference. In influenzas of avian origin 2,3-linkage is preferred, vs. influenzas of human origin in which 2,6-linkage is preferable. 2,3-linked SA receptors in humans are found predominantly in the lower respiratory tract, a fact that is the primary foundation for the deadliness of avian influenzas in humans, and also the key to their lack of airborne transmission. In the study that created an airborne avian influenza among ferrets it was necessary to switch the receptor preference of the host cells to those of 2,6-linkage, found predominantly in humans' upper respiratory tract, in order to create an infection that could shed aerosolized virus particles. Such an infection, however, must occur in the upper respiratory tract of humans, thus fundamentally undercutting the fatal trajectory of the disease.

H7N9

Influenza A virus subtype H7N9 is a novel avian influenza virus first reported to have infected humans in 2013 in China. Most of the reported cases of human infection have resulted in severe respiratory illness. In the month following the report of the first case, more than 100 people had been infected, an unusually high rate for a new infection; a fifth of those patients had died, a fifth had recovered, and the rest remained critically ill. The World Health Organization (WHO) has identified H7N9 as "...an unusually dangerous virus for humans." As of June 30, 133 cases have been reported, resulting in the deaths of 43.

Research regarding background and transmission is ongoing. It has been established that many of the human cases of H7N9 appear to have a link to live bird markets. As of July 2013, there had been no evidence of sustained human-to-human transmission, however a study group headed by one of the world's leading experts on avian flu reported that several instances of human-to-human infection were suspected. It has been reported that H7N9 virus does not kill poultry, which will make surveillance much more difficult. Researchers have commented on the unusual prevalence of older males among H7N9-infected patients. While several environmental, behavioral, and biological explanations for this pattern have been proposed, as yet, the reason is unknown. Currently no vaccine exists, but the use of influenza antiviral drugs known as neuraminidase inhibitors in cases of early infection may be effective.

The number of cases detected after April fell abruptly. The decrease in the number of new human H7N9 cases may have resulted from containment measures taken by Chinese authorities, including closing live bird markets, or from a change in seasons, or possibly a combination of both factors. Studies indicate that avian influenza viruses have a seasonal pattern, thus it is thought that infections may pick up again when the weather turns cooler in China.

In Domestic Animals

Several domestic species have been infected with and shown symptoms of H5N1 viral infection, including cats, dogs, ferrets, pigs, and birds.

Birds

Attempts are made in the United States to minimize the presence of HPAI in poultry through routine surveillance of poultry flocks in commercial poultry operations. Detection of a HPAI virus may result in immediate culling of the flock. Less pathogenic viruses are controlled by vaccination, which is done primarily in turkey flocks (ATCvet codes: QI01AA23 (WHO) for the inactivated fowl vaccine, QI01CL01 (WHO) for the inactivated turkey combination vaccine).

Seals

A recent strain of the virus is able to infect the lungs of seals.

Cats

Avian influenza in cats can show a variety of symptoms and usually lead to death. Cats are able to get infected by either consuming an infected bird or by contracting the virus from another infected cat.

Global Impact

In 2005, the formation of the International Partnership on Avian and Pandemic Influenza was announced in order to elevate the importance of avian flu, coordinate efforts, and improve disease reporting and surveillance in order to better respond to future pandemics. New networks of laboratories have emerged to detect and respond to avian flu, such as the Crisis Management Center for Animal Health, the Global Avian Influenza Network for Surveillance, OFFLU, and the Global Early Warning System for major animal diseases. After the 2003 outbreak, WHO member states have also recognized the need for more transparent and equitable sharing of vaccines and other benefits from these networks. Cooperative measures created in response to HPAI have served as a basis for programs related to other emerging and re-emerging infectious diseases.

HPAI control has also been used for political ends. In Indonesia, negotiations with global response networks were used to recentralize power and funding to the Ministry of Health. In Vietnam policymakers, with the support of the Food and Agriculture Organization of the United Nations (FAO), used HPAI control to accelerate the industrialization of livestock production for export by proposing to increase the portion of large-scale commercial farms and reducing the number of poultry keepers from 8 to 2 million by 2010.

Stigma

Backyard poultry production was viewed as "traditional Asian" agricultural practices that contrasted with modern commercial poultry production and seen as a threat to biosecurity. Backyard production appeared to hold greater risk than commercial production due to lack of biosecurity and close contact with humans, though HPAI spread in intensively raised flocks was greater due to high density rearing and genetic homogeneity. Asian culture itself was blamed as the reason why certain interventions, such as those that only looked at placed-based interventions, would fail without looking for a multifaceted solutions.

Indonesia

Press accounts of avian flu in Indonesia were seen by poultry farmers as conflating suspected cases while the public did see the accounts as informative, though many became de-sensitized to the idea of impending danger or only temporarily changed their poultry-related behavior. Rumors also circulated in Java in 2006. These tended to focus on bird flu being linked to big businesses in order to drive small farmers out of the market by exaggerating the danger of avian influenza, avian flu being introduced by foreigners to force Indonesians to purchase imported chicken and keep Indonesian chicken off the world market, and the government using avian flu as a ploy to attract funds from wealthy countries. Such rumors reflected concerns about big businesses, globalization, and a distrust of the national government in a country where "the amount of decentralization here is breathtaking" according to Steven Bjorge, a WHO epidemiologist in Jakarta in 2006.

In the context a decentralized national government that the public did not completely trust, Indonesian Health Minister Siti Fadilah Supari announced in December 2006 that her government would no longer be sharing samples of H5N1 collected from Indonesian patients. This decision came as a shock to the international community as it disrupted the Global Influenza Surveillance Network (GISN) coordinated by the WHO for managing seasonal and pandemic influenza. GISN is based on countries sharing virus specimens freely with the WHO which assesses and eventually sends these samples to pharmaceutical companies in order to produce vaccines that are sold back to these countries. Though this was initially seen as an attempt to protect national sovereignty at all costs, it was instead used for a domestic political struggle. Prior to Indonesia's dispute with the GISN, the Ministry of Health, already weak due to the decentralized nature the government, was experiencing further leakage of funding to state and non-state agencies due to global health interventions. By reasserting control over public health issues and funding by setting itself up as the sole Indonesian representative to the WHO, the Ministry of Health made itself a key player in the management of future international funds relating vaccine production and renegotiated benefits from global surveillance networks.

Economic

Approximately 20% of the protein consumed in developing countries come from poultry. In the wake of the H5N1 pandemic, millions of poultry were killed. In Vietnam alone, over 50 million domestic birds were killed due to HPAI infection and control attempts. A 2005 report by the FAO totaled economic losses in South East Asia around US$10 billion. This had the greatest impact on small scale commercial and backyard producers relative to total assets compared to industrial chains which primarily experience temporary decreases in exports and loss of consumer confidence. Some governments did provide compensation for culled poultry, it was often far below market value (close to 30% of market value in Vietnam), while others such as Cambodia provide no compensation to farmers at all.

As poultry serves as a source of food security and liquid assets, the most vulnerable populations were poor small scale farmers. The loss of birds due to HPAI and culling in Vietnam led to an average loss of 2.3 months of production and US$69–108 for households where many have an income of $2 a day or less. The loss of food security for vulnerable households can be seen in the stunting of children under 5 in Egypt. Women are another population at risk as in most regions of the world, small flocks are tended to by women. Widespread culling also resulted in the decreased enrollment of girls in school in Turkey.

Prevention

People who do not regularly come into contact with birds are not at high risk for contracting avian influenza. Those at high risk include poultry farm workers, animal control workers, wildlife biologists, and ornithologists who handle live birds. Organizations with high-risk workers should have an avian influenza response plan in place before any cases have been discovered. Biosecurity of poultry flocks is also important for prevention. Flocks should be isolated from outside birds, especially wild birds, and their waste; vehicles used around the flock should be regularly disinfected and not shared between farms; and birds from slaughter channels should not be returned to the farm.

With proper infection control and use of personal protective equipment (PPE), the chance for infection is low. Protecting the eyes, nose, mouth, and hands is important for prevention because these are the most common ways for the virus to enter the body. Appropriate personal protective equipment includes aprons or coveralls, gloves, boots or boot covers, and a head cover or hair cover. Disposable PPE is recommended. An N-95 respirator and unvented/indirectly vented safety goggles are also part of appropriate PPE. A powered air purifying respirator (PAPR) with hood or helmet and face shield is also an option.

Proper reporting of an isolated case can help to prevent spread. The Centers for Disease Control and Prevention (US) recommendation is that if a worker develops symptoms within 10 days of working with infected poultry or potentially contaminated materials, they should seek care and notify their employer, who should notify public health officials.

For future avian influenza threats, the WHO suggests a 3 phase, 5 part plan.

- Phase: Pre-pandemic
    - Reduce opportunities for human infection
    - Strengthen the early warning system
- Phase: Emergence of a pandemic virus
    - Contain or delay spread at the source
- Phase: Pandemic declared and spreading internationally
    - Reduce morbidity, mortality, and social disruption
    - Conduct research to guide response measures

Vaccines for poultry have been formulated against several of the avian H5N1 influenza varieties. Control measures for HPAI encourage mass vaccinations of poultry though The World Health Organization has compiled a list of known clinical trials of pandemic influenza prototype vaccines, including those against H5N1. In some countries still at high risk for HPAI spread, there is compulsory strategic vaccination though vaccine supply shortages remain a problem.

For Village Poultry Farmers

Initial response to H5N1, a one size fits all recommendation was used for all poultry production systems, though measures for intensively raised birds were not necessarily appropriate for extensively raised birds. When looking at village poultry, it was first assumed that the household was the unit and that flocks did not make contact with other flocks, though more effective measures came into use when the epidemiological unit was the village.

Recommendations also involve restructuring commercial markets to improve biosecurity against avian influenza. Poultry production zoning is used to limit poultry farming to specific areas outside of urban environments while live poultry markets improve biosecurity by limiting the number of traders holding licenses and subjecting producers and traders to more stringent inspections. These recommendations in combination with requirements to fence and house all poultry, and limit free ranging flocks will eventually lead to fewer small commercial producers and backyard producers, costing livelihoods as they are unable to meet the conditions needed to participate.

A summary of reports to the World Organisation for Animal Health in 2005 and 2010 suggest that surveillance and under-reporting in developed and developing countries is still a challenge. Often, donor support can focus on HPAI control alone, while similar diseases such as Newcastle disease, acute fowl cholera, infectious laryngotracheitis, and infectious bursal disease still affect poultry populations. When HPAI tests come back negative, a lack of funded testing for differential diagnoses can leave farmers wondering what killed their birds.

Since traditional production systems require little investment and serve as a safety net for lower income households, prevention and treatment can been seen as less cost effective than letting a few birds die. Effective control not only requires prior agreements to be made with relevant government agencies, such as seen with Indonesia, they must also not unduly threaten food security.

Culling

Culling is used in order to decrease the threat of avian influenza transmission by killing potentially infected birds. The FAO manual on HPAI control recommends a zoning strategy which begins with the identification of an infected area (IA) where sick or dead birds have tested positive. All poultry in this zone are culled while the area 1 to 5 km from the outer boundary of the IA is considered the restricted area (RA) placed under strict surveillance. 2 to 10 km from the RA is the control area (CA) that serves as a buffer zone in case of spread. Culling is not recommended beyond the IA unless there is evidence of spread. The manual, however, also provides examples of how control was carried out between 2004 and 2005 to contain H5N1 where all poultry was to be stamped out in a 3 km radius beyond the infected point and beyond that a 5 km radius where all fowl was to be vaccinated. This culling method was indiscriminate as a large proportion of the poultry inside these areas were small backyard flocks which did not travel great enough distances to carry infection to adjacent villages without human effort and may have not been infected at all. Between 2004 and 2005, over 100 million chickens were culled in Asia to contain H5N1.

The risk of mass culling of birds and the resulting economic impact led farmers who were reluctant to report sick poultry. The culls often preempted actual lab testing for H5N1 as avian flu policy justified sacrificing poultry as a safeguard against HPAI spread. In response to these policies, farmers in Vietnam between 2003 and 2004 became more and more unwilling to surrender apparently healthy birds to authorities and stole poultry destined for culls as it stripped poultry of their biosocial and economic worth. By the end of 2005, the government implemented a new policy that targeted high-risk flock in the immediate vicinity of infected farms and instituted voluntary culling with compensation in the case of a local outbreak.

Not only did culling result in severe economic impacts especially for small scale farmers, culling itself may be an ineffective preventative measure. In the short-term, mass culling achieves it goals of limiting the immediate spread of HPAI, it has been found to impede the evolution of host resistance which is important for the long-term success of HPAI control. Mass culling also selects for elevated influenza virulence and results in the greater mortality of birds overall. Effective culling strategies must be selective as well as considerate of economic impacts to optimize epidemiological control and minimize economic and agricultural destruction.

People-poultry Relations

Prevention and control programs must take into account local understandings of people-poultry relations. In the past, programs that have focused on singular, place-based understandings of disease transmission have been ineffective. In the case of Northern Vietnam, health workers saw poultry as commodities with an environment that was under the control of people. Poultry existed in the context of farms, markets, slaughterhouses, an roads while humans were indirectly the primary transmitters of avian flu, placing the burden of disease control on people. However, farmers saw their free ranging poultry in an environment dominated by nonhuman forces that they could not exert control over. There were a host of nonhuman actors such as wild birds and weather patterns whose relationships with the poultry fostered the disease and absolved farmers of complete responsibility for disease control.

Attempts at singular, place-based controls sought to teach farmers to identify areas where their behavior could change without looking at poultry behaviors. Behavior recommendations by Vietnam's National Steering Committee for Avian Influenza Control and Prevention (NSCAI) were drawn from the FAO Principles of Biosecurity. These included restrictions from entering areas where poultry are kept by erecting barriers to segregate poultry from non-human contact, limits on human movement of poultry and poultry-related products ideally to transporters, and recommendations for farmers to wash hands and footwear before and after contact with poultry. Farmers, pointed to wind and environmental pollution as reasons poultry would get sick. NSCAI recommendations also would disrupt longstanding livestock production practices as gates impede sales by restricting assessment of birds by appearance and offend customers by limiting outside human contact. Instead of incorporating local knowledge into recommendations, cultural barriers were used as scapegoats for failed interventions. Prevention and control methods have been more effective when also considering the social, political, and ecological agents in play.

Escherichia Coli O157:H7

Escherichia coli O157:H7 is a serotype of the bacterial species *Escherichia coli* and is one of the Shiga toxin–producing types of *E. coli*. It is a cause of disease, typically foodborne illness of the "colonic escherichiosis" type, through consumption of contaminated and raw food, including raw milk. Infection with this type of pathogenic bacteria may lead to hemorrhagic diarrhea, and to kidney failure; these have been reported to cause the deaths of children younger than five years of age, of elderly patients, and of patients whose immunologies are otherwise compromised.

Transmission is via the fecal–oral route, and most illness has been through distribution of contaminated raw leaf green vegetables, undercooked meat and raw milk.

Signs and Symptoms

E. coli O157:H7 infection often causes severe, acute hemorrhagic diarrhea (although nonhemorrhagic diarrhea is also possible) and abdominal cramps. Usually little or no fever is present, and the illness resolves in five to 10 days. It can also be asymptomatic.

In some people, particularly children under five years of age, persons whose immunologies are otherwise compromised, and the elderly, the infection can cause hemolytic uremic syndrome (HUS), in which the red blood cells are destroyed and the kidneys fail. About 2–7% of infections lead to this complication. In the United States, HUS is the principal cause of acute kidney failure in children, and most cases of HUS are caused by *E. coli* O157:H7.

Bacteriology

Strains of *E. coli* that express Shiga and Shiga-like toxins gained this ability due to infection with a prophage containing the structural coding for the toxin, and nonproducing strains may become infected and produce shiga-like toxins after incubation with shiga toxin positive strains. The prophage responsible seems to have infected the strain's ancestors fairly recently, as viral particles have been observed to replicate in the host if it is stressed in some way (e.g. antibiotics).

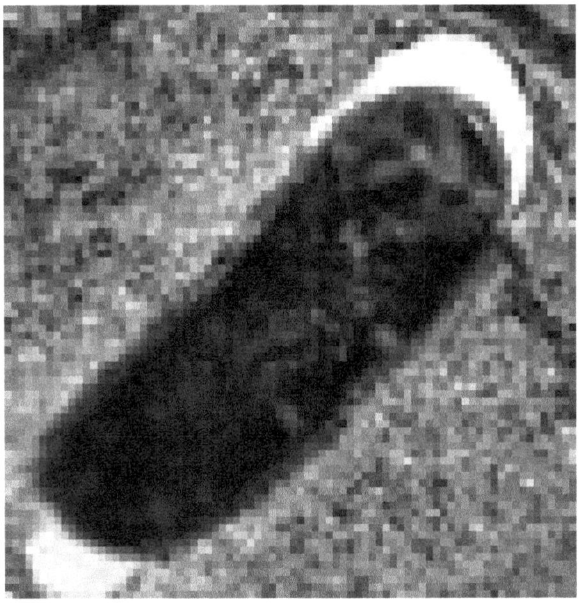

E. coli O157:H7

All clinical isolates of *E. coli* O157:H7 possess the plasmid pO157. The periplasmic catalase is encoded on pO157 and may enhance the virulence of the bacterium by providing additional oxidative protection when infecting the host. *E. coli* O157:H7 non-hemorrhagic strains are converted to hemorrhagic strains by lysogenic conversion after a bacteriophage infection to non-hemorrhagic cells.

Natural Habitat

While it is relatively uncommon, the *E. coli* serotype O157:H7 can naturally be found in the intestinal contents of some cattle, goats, and even sheep. The digestive tract of cattle lack the Shiga toxin receptor globotriaosylceramide, and thus, these can be asymptomatic carriers of the bacterium. The prevalence of *E. coli* O157:H7 in North American feedlot cattle herds ranges from 0 to 60%. Some cattle may also be so-called "super-shedders" of the bacterium. Super-shedders may be defined as cattle exhibiting rectoanal junction colonization and excreting $>10^{3\text{ to }4}$ CFU g^{-1} feces. Super-shedders have been found to constitute a small proportion of the cattle in a feedlot (<10%) but they may account for >90% of all *E. coli* O157:H7 excreted.

Transmission

Infection with *E. coli* O157:H7 follows ingestion of contaminated food or water, or oral contact with contaminated surfaces. It is highly virulent, with a low infectious dose: an inoculation of fewer than 10 to 100 CFU of *E. coli* O157:H7 is sufficient to cause infection, compared to over one-million CFU for other pathogenic *E. coli* strains.

Diagnosis

A stool culture can detect the bacterium, although it is not a routine test and so must be specifically requested. The sample is cultured on sorbitol-MacConkey (SMAC) agar, or the variant cefixime potassium tellurite sorbitol-MacConkey agar (CT-SMAC). On SMAC agar O157 colonies appear clear due to their inability to ferment sorbitol, while the colonies of the usual sorbitol-fermenting serotypes of *E. coli* appear red. Sorbitol nonfermenting colonies are tested for the somatic O157 antigen before being confirmed as *E. coli* O157. Like all cultures, diagnosis is time-consuming with this method; swifter diagnosis is possible using quick *E. coli* DNA extraction method plus PCR techniques. Newer technologies using fluorescent and antibody detection are also under development.

Surveillance

E. coli O157:H7 infection is nationally reportable in the USA and Great Britain, and is reportable in most US states. It is also reportable in most states of Australia including Queensland.

Treatment

While fluid replacement and blood pressure support may be necessary to prevent death from dehydration, most victims recover without treatment in five to 10 days. There is no evidence that antibiotics improve the course of disease, and treatment with antibiotics may precipitate hemolytic uremic syndrome. Antidiarrheal agents, such as loperamide (imodium), should also be avoided as they may prolong the duration of the infection.

Certain novel treatment strategies, such as the use of anti-induction strategies to prevent toxin production and the use of anti-Shiga toxin antibodies, have also been proposed.

Costs

The pathogen results in an estimated 2,100 hospitalizations annually in the United States. The illness is often misdiagnosed; therefore, expensive and invasive diagnostic procedures may be performed. Patients who develop HUS often require prolonged hospitalization, dialysis, and long-term followup.

Prevention

Proper hand washing after using the lavatory or changing a diaper, especially among children or those with diarrhea, reduces the risk of transmission. Anyone with a diarrheal illness should avoid swimming in public pools or lakes, sharing baths with others, and preparing food for others and even avoiding raw milk.

United States

The U.S.D.A. banned the sale of ground beef contaminated with the O157:H7 strain in 1994.

Campylobacteriosis

Campylobacteriosis is an infection by the *Campylobacter* bacterium, most commonly *C. jejuni*. It is among the most common bacterial infections of humans, often a foodborne illness. It produces an inflammatory, sometimes bloody, diarrhea or dysentery syndrome, mostly including cramps, fever and pain.

Cause

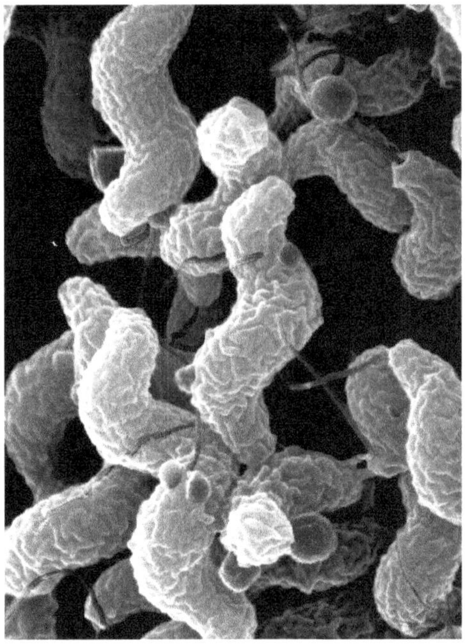

Campylobacter bacteria are the number-one cause of food-related gastrointestinal illness in the United States. This scanning electron microscope image shows the characteristic spiral, or corkscrew, shape of *C. jejuni* cells and related structures.

Campylobacteriosis is caused by *Campylobacter* bacteria (curved or spiral, motile, non–spore-forming, Gram-negative rods). The disease is usually caused by *C. jejuni*, a spiral and comma shaped bacterium normally found in cattle, swine, and birds, where it is nonpathogenic, but the illness can also be caused by *C. coli* (also found in cattle, swine, and birds), *C. upsaliensis* (found in cats and dogs) and *C. lari* (present in seabirds in particular).

One effect of campylobacteriosis is tissue injury in the gut. The sites of tissue injury include the jejunum, the ileum, and the colon. *C jejuni* appears to achieve this by invading and destroying epithelial cells.

C. jejuni can also cause a latent autoimmune effect on the nerves of the legs, which is usually seen several weeks after a surgical procedure of the abdomen. The effect is known as an acute idiopathic demyelinating polyneuropathy (AIDP), i.e. Guillain–Barré syndrome, in which one sees symptoms of ascending paralysis, dysaesthesias usually below the waist, and, in the later stages, respiratory failure.

Some strains of *C jejuni* produce a cholera-like enterotoxin, which is important in the watery diarrhea observed in infections. The organism produces diffuse, bloody, edematous, and exudative enteritis. In a small number of cases, the infection may be associated with hemolytic uremic syndrome and thrombotic thrombocytopenic purpura through a poorly understood mechanism.

Transmission

The common routes of transmission for the disease-causing bacteria are fecal-oral, person-to-person sexual contact, ingestion of contaminated food (generally unpasteurized (raw) milk and undercooked or poorly handled poultry), and waterborne (i.e., through contaminated drinking water). Contact with contaminated poultry, livestock, or household pets, especially puppies, can also cause disease.

Animals farmed for meat are the main source of campylobacteriosis. A study published in PLoS Genetics (September 26, 2008) by researchers from Lancashire, England, and Chicago, Illinois, found that 97 percent of campylobacteriosis cases sampled in Lancashire were caused by bacteria typically found in chicken and livestock. In 57 percent of cases, the bacteria could be traced to chicken, and in 35 percent to cattle. Wild animal and environmental sources were accountable for just three percent of disease.

The infectious dose is 1000–10,000 bacteria (although ten to five hundred bacteria can be enough to infect humans). *Campylobacter* species are sensitive to hydrochloric acid in the stomach, and acid reduction treatment can reduce the amount of inoculum needed to cause disease.

Exposure to bacteria is often more common during travelling, and therefore campylobacteriosis is a common form of travelers' diarrhea.

Epidemiology

Campylobacter is one of the most common causes of human bacterial gastroenteritis. For instance, an estimated 2 million cases of *Campylobacter* enteritis occur annually in the U.S., accounting for 5–7% of cases of gastroenteritis. Furthermore, in the United Kingdom during 2000, *Campylobacter jejuni* was involved in 77.3% in all cases of laboratory confirmed foodborne illness. About 15 of every 100,000 people are diagnosed with campylobacteriosis every year, and with many cases going unreported, up to 0.5% of the general population may unknowingly harbor *Campylobacter* in their gut.

A large animal reservoir is present as well, with up to 100% of poultry, including chickens, turkeys, and waterfowl, having asymptomatic infections in their intestinal tracts. Infected chicken feces may contain up to 10^9 bacteria per 25 grams, and due to the installations, the bacteria are rapidly spread to other chickens. This vastly exceeds the infectious dose of 1000–10,000 bacteria for humans.

In January 2013, the UK's Food Standards Agency warned that two-thirds of all raw chicken bought from UK shops was contaminated with campylobacter, affecting an estimated half a million people annually and killing approximately 100.

Symptoms

The prodromal symptoms are fever, headache, and myalgia, which can be severe, lasting as long as 24 hours. After 1 – 5 days, typically, these are followed by diarrhea (as many as 10 watery, frequently bloody, bowel movements per day) or dysentery, cramps, abdominal pain, and fever as high as 40 °C (104 °F). In most people, the illness lasts for 2–10 days. It is classified as invasive/inflammatory diarrhea, also described as bloody diarrhea or dysentery.

There are other diseases showing similar symptoms. For instance, abdominal pain and tenderness may be very localized, mimicking acute appendicitis. Furthermore, *Helicobacter pylori* is closely related to Campylobacter and causes peptic ulcer disease.

Other Factors

In patients with HIV, infections may be more frequent, may cause prolonged bouts of dirty brown diarrhea, and may be more commonly associated with bacteremia and antibiotic resistance. In participants of unprotected anal intercourse, campylobacteriosis is more localized to the distal end of the colon and may be termed a proctocolitis. The severity and persistence of infection in patients with AIDS and hypogammaglobulinemia indicates that both cell-mediated and humoral immunity are important in preventing and terminating infection.

Diagnosis

Campylobacter organisms can be detected by performing a Gram stain of a stool sample with high specificity and a sensitivity of ~60%, but are most often diagnosed by stool culture. Fecal leukocytes should be present and indicate the diarrhea to be inflammatory in nature. Methods currently being developed to detect the presence of campylobacter organisms include antigen testing via an EIA or PCR.

Treatment

The infection is usually self-limiting, and in most cases, symptomatic treatment by liquid and electrolyte replacement is enough in human infections.

Antibiotics

Antibiotic treatment only has a marginal effect on the duration of symptoms, and its use is not recommended except in high-risk patients with clinical complications.

Erythromycin can be used in children, and tetracycline in adults. Some studies show, however, that erythromycin rapidly eliminates *Campylobacter* from the stool without affecting the duration of illness. Nevertheless, children with dysentery due to *C. jejuni* benefit from early treatment with erythromycin. Treatment with antibiotics, therefore, depends on the severity of symptoms. Quinolones are effective if the organism is sensitive, but high rates of quinolone use in livestock means that quinolones are now largely ineffective.

Antimotility agents, such as loperamide, can lead to prolonged illness or intestinal perforation in any invasive diarrhea, and should be avoided. Trimethoprim/sulfamethoxazole and ampicillin are ineffective against *Campylobacter*.

In Animals

In the past, poultry infections were often treated by mass administration of enrofloxacin and sarafloxacin for single instances of infection. The FDA banned this practice, as it promoted the development of fluoroquinolone-resistant populations. A major broad-spectrum fluoroquinolone used in humans is ciprofloxacin.

Currently growing resistance of the *Campylobacter* to fluoroquinolones and macrolides is of a major concern.

Prognosis

Campylobacteriosis is usually self-limited without any mortality (assuming proper hydration is maintained). However, there are several possible complications.

Complications

Complications include toxic megacolon, dehydration and sepsis. Such complications generally occur in young children (< 1 year of age) and immunocompromised people. A chronic course of the disease is possible; this disease process is likely to develop without a distinct acute phase. Chronic campylobacteriosis features a long period of sub-febrile temperature and asthenia; eye damage, arthritis, endocarditis may develop if infection is untreated.

Occasional deaths occur in young, previously healthy individuals because of blood volume depletion (due to dehydration), and in persons who are elderly or immunocompromised.

Some individuals (1–2 in 100,000 cases) develop Guillain–Barré syndrome, in which the nerves that join the spinal cord and brain to the rest of the body are damaged, sometimes permanently. This occurs only with infection of *C. jejuni* and *C. upsaliensis*.

Prevention

- Pasteurization of milk and chlorination of drinking water destroy the organism.
- Treatment with antibiotics can reduce fecal excretion.
- Infected health care workers should not provide direct patient care.
- Separate cutting boards should be used for foods of animal origin and other foods. After preparing raw food of animal origin, all cutting boards and countertops should be carefully cleaned with soap and hot water.
- Contact with pet saliva and feces should be avoided.

The World Health Organization recommends the following:

- Food should be properly cooked and hot when served.
- Consume only pasteurized or boiled milk and milk products, never raw milk products.
- Make sure that ice is from safe water.
- If you are not sure of the safety of drinking water, boil it, or disinfect it with chemical disinfectant.
- Wash hands thoroughly and frequently with soap, especially after using the toilet and after contact with pets and farm animals.
- Wash fruits and vegetables thoroughly, especially if they are to be eaten raw. Peel fruits and vegetables whenever possible.
- Food handlers, professionals and at home, should observe hygienic rules during food preparation.

- Professional food handlers should immediately report to their employer any fever, diarrhea, vomiting or visible infected skin lesions.

Caliciviridae

Caliciviridae is a family of viruses, members of Class IV of the Baltimore scheme. They are positive-sense, single stranded RNA which is non-segmented. There are currently seven species in this family, divided among 5 genera. Diseases associated with this family include: feline calicivirus: respiratory disease; rabbit hemorrhagic disease virus: often-fatal hemorrhages; norwalk group of viruses: gastroenteritis. Caliciviruses naturally infect vertebrates, and have been found in a number of organisms such as humans, cattle, pigs, cats, chickens, reptiles, dolphins and amphibians. The caliciviruses have a simple construction and are not enveloped. The capsid appears hexagonal/spherical and has icosahedral symmetry (T=1 or T=3) with a diameter of 35–39 nm.

Caliciviruses are not very well studied because until recently they could not be grown in culture, and there is no suitable animal model. However, the recent application of modern genomic technologies has led to an increased understanding of the virus family. A recent isolate from rhesus monkeys—Tulane virus—can be grown in culture and this system promises to increase our understanding of these viruses.

Taxonomy

The *Caliciviridae* family includes the following genera:

- Genus *Lagovirus*; type species: *Rabbit hemorrhagic disease virus*
- Genus *Nebovirus*; type species: *Newbury-1 virus*
- Genus *Norovirus*; type species: *Norwalk virus*
- Genus *Sapovirus*; type species: *Sapporo virus*
- Genus *Vesivirus*; type species: *Vesicular exanthema of swine virus*

Group: ssRNA(+)

Two additional genera have been proposed: *Recovirus* for a novel calicivirus detected in stool specimens from rhesus monkeys and *Valovirus*—for a novel group of swine caliciviruses known as the St-Valérien-like viruses. These genera have yet to be officially approved. There are a number of other unclassified caliciviruses including the chicken calicivirus.

Virology

All viruses in this family possess a non-segmented, polyadenylated, positive sense single stand RNA genome of ~7.5–8.5 kilobases in length, enclosed in an icosahedral capsid of 27–40 nanometers in diameter.

Genus	Structure	Symmetry	Capsid	Genomic Arrangement	Genomic Segmentation
Nebovirus	Icosahedral	T=1, T=3	Non-Enveloped	Linear	Monopartite
Lagovirus	Icosahedral	T=1, T=3	Non-Enveloped	Linear	Monopartite
Sapovirus	Icosahedral	T=3	Non-Enveloped	Linear	Monopartite
Norovirus	Icosahedral	T=1, T=3	Non-Enveloped	Linear	Monopartite
Vesivirus	Icosahedral	T=1, T=3	Non-Enveloped	Linear	Monopartite

Life Cycle

Viral replication is cytoplasmic. Entry into the host cell is achieved by attachment to host receptors, which mediates endocytosis. Replication follows the positive stranded RNA virus replication model. Positive stranded RNA virus transcription is the method of transcription. Translation takes place by leaky scanning, and RNA termination-reinitiation. Vertebrates serve as the natural host. Transmission routes are fecal-oral.

Genus	Host Details	Tissue Tropism	Entry Details	Release Details	Replication Site	Assembly Site	Transmission
Nebovirus	Bovine	Liver	Cell receptor endocytosis	Lysis	Cytoplasm	Cytoplasm	Unknown
Lagovirus	Lagomorphs	Liver	Cell receptor endocytosis	Lysis	Cytoplasm	Cytoplasm	Contact
Sapovirus	Humans; swine	Intestinal epithelium	Cell receptor endocytosis	Lysis	Cytoplasm	Cytoplasm	Oral-fecal
Norovirus	Humans; mammals	Intestinal epithelium	Cell receptor endocytosis	Lysis	Cytoplasm	Cytoplasm	Oral-fecal
Vesivirus	Felines	Upper respiratory	Cell receptor endocytosis	Lysis	Cytoplasm	Cytoplasm	Aerosol

Human Disease

Calicivirus infections commonly cause acute gastroenteritis, which is the inflammation of the stomach and intestines (e.g. the Norwalk Virus). Symptoms can include vomiting and diarrhea. These symptoms emerge after an incubation time of 2 days and the symptoms only generally last for 3 days. Most calicivirus infections do not call for medical attention, but those who are immunocompromised may need to be hospitalized for rehydration therapy.

Animal Viruses

Feline calicivirus (FCV)—a member of the *Vesivirus*—represents an important pathogen of cats.

Sapovirus, *Norovirus* and *Vesivirus* have been detected in pigs, making this animal species of particular interest in the study of calicivirus pathogenesis and host range.

The first mouse norovirus, murine norovirus 1 (MNV-1), was discovered in 2003. Since then, numerous murine norovirus strains have been identified and they were assigned a new genogroup in the genus *Norovirus*.

Rabbit hemorrhagic disease virus (RHDV) is a pathogen of rabbits that causes major problems throughout the world where rabbits are reared for food and clothing, make a significant contribution to ecosystem ecology, and where they support valued wildlife as a food source.

Trichinosis

Trichinosis is a parasitic disease caused by roundworms of the *Trichinella* type. During the initial infection invasion of the intestines can result in diarrhea, abdominal pain, and vomiting. Migration of larvae to muscle, which occurs about a week after being infected, can cause swelling of the face, inflammation of the whites of the eyes, fever, muscle pains, and a rash. Minor infection may be without symptoms. Complications may include inflammation of heart muscle, central nervous system involvement, and inflammation of the lungs.

Trichinosis is mainly spread when undercooked meat containing *Trichinella* cysts is eaten. Most often this is pork but can also occur from bear and dog meat. Several subtypes of *Trichinella* can cause disease with *T. spiralis* being the most common. After being eaten the larvae are released from their cysts in the stomach. They then invade the wall of the small intestine, where they develop into adult worms. After 1 week, the females release new larvae that migrate to voluntarily controlled muscles where they form cyst. The diagnosis is usually based on symptoms and confirmed by finding specific antibodies in the blood or larvae on tissue biopsy.

The best way to prevent trichinellosis is to fully cook meat. A food thermometer can verify that the temperature inside the meat is high enough. Infection is typically treated with antiparasitic medication such as albendazole or mebendazole. Rapid treatment may kill adult worms and thereby stop further worsening of symptoms. Both medications are considered safe but have been associated with side effects such as bone marrow suppression. Their use during pregnancy or in children under the age of 2 years is poorly studied but appears to be safe. Treatment with steroids is sometimes also required in severe cases. Without treatment symptoms typically resolve within three months.

About 10,000 infections occur a year. At least 55 countries including the United States, China, Argentina, and Russia have had recently documented cases. While the disease occurs in the tropics it is less common there. Rates of trichinosis in the United States have decreased from about 400 cases per year in the 1940s to 20 per year in the 2000s. The risk of death from infection is low.

Signs and Symptoms

The great majority of trichinosis infections have either minor or no symptoms and no complications. There are two main phases for the infection: enteral (affecting the intestines) and parenteral (outside the intestines). The symptoms vary depending on the phase, species of *Trichinella*, amount of encysted larvae ingested, age, sex, and host immunity.

Enteral Phase

A large burden of adult worms in the intestines promote symptoms such as nausea, heartburn, dyspepsia, and diarrhea from two to seven days after infection, while small worm burdens generally are asymptomatic. Eosinophilia presents early and increases rapidly.

Parenteral Phase

The severity of symptoms caused by larval migration from the intestines depends on the number of larvae produced. As the larvae migrate through tissue and vessels, the body's inflammatory response results in edema, muscle pain, fever, and weakness. A classic sign of trichinosis is periorbital edema, swelling around the eyes, which may be caused by vasculitis. Splinter hemorrhage in the nails is also a common symptom.

They may very rarely cause enough damage to produce serious neurological deficits (such as ataxia or respiratory paralysis) from worms entering the central nervous system. The CNS is compromised by trichinosis in 10–24% of reported cases of cerebral venous sinus thrombosis, a very rare form of stroke (3-4 cases per million annual incidence in adults). Trichinosis can be fatal depending on the severity of the infection; death can occur 4–6 weeks after the infection, and is usually caused by myocarditis, encephalitis, or pneumonia.

Cause

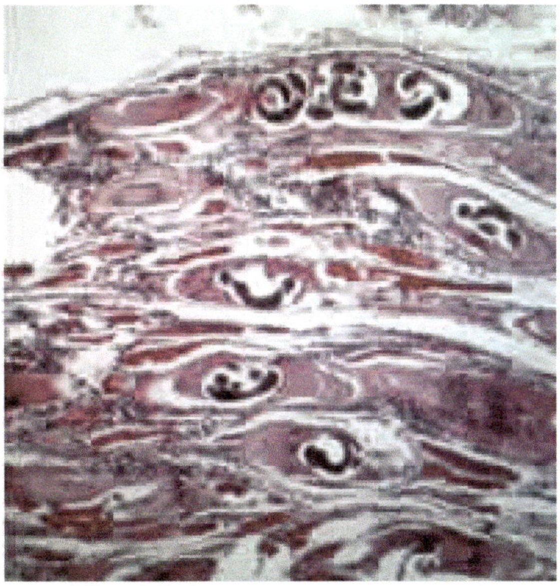

Trichinella spiralis larvae in muscle tissue but some randomly appear in long section.

The classical agent is *T. spiralis* (found worldwide in many carnivorous and omnivorous animals), but there are several other species of *Trichinella* now recognized, including *T. pseudospiralis* (mammals and birds worldwide), *T. nativa* (Arctic bears), *T. nelsoni* (African predators and scavengers), *T. britovi* (carnivores of Europe and western Asia), and *T. papuae* (wild and domestic pigs, Papua New Guinea and Thailand). *Trichinella zimbabwensis* is found in crocodiles in Africa but to date there are no known associations of this species with human disease.

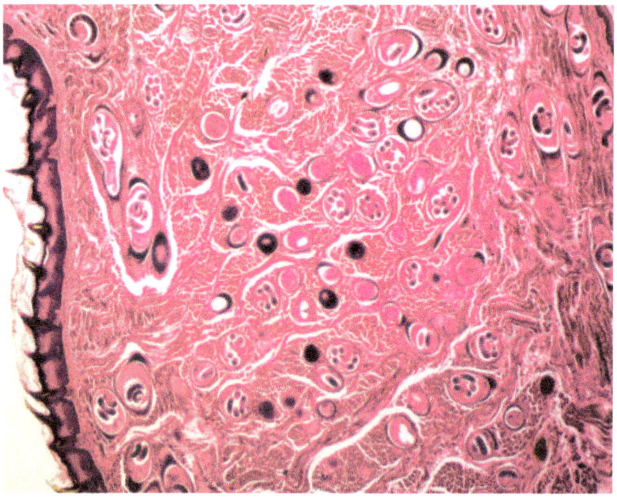

Animal tissue infected with the parasite that causes the disease trichinosis. Most parasites are shown in cross section

Species and characteristics

- *T. spiralis* is most adapted to swine, most pathogenic in humans and is cosmopolitan in distribution.
- *T. britovi* is the second most common species to infect humans; it is distributed throughout Europe, Asia, and northern and western Africa usually in wild boar and domesticated pigs.
- *T. nativa*, which has a high resistance to freezing, is found in the Arctic and subarctic regions; reservoir hosts include polar bears, Arctic foxes, walruses and other wild game.
- *T. pseudospiralis* infects birds and mammals, and has demonstrated infection in humans; it is a nonencapsulated species.
- *T. papuae* infects both mammals and reptiles, including crocodiles, humans, and pigs; this species, found in Papua New Guinea and Thailand, is also nonencapsulated.
- *T. nelsoni*, found in eastern Africa, has been documented to cause a few human cases.
- *T. murrelli* also infects humans, especially from black bear meat; it is distributed among wild carnivores in North America.
- *T. zimbabwensis* can infect mammals and possibly humans; this nonencapsulated species was detected in reptiles of Africa.

Taxonomy

- Kingdom: Animalia
- Phylum: Nematoda
- Class: Adenophorea
- Order: Trichurida

- Family: Trichinellidae
- Genus: *Trichinella*

Life Cycle

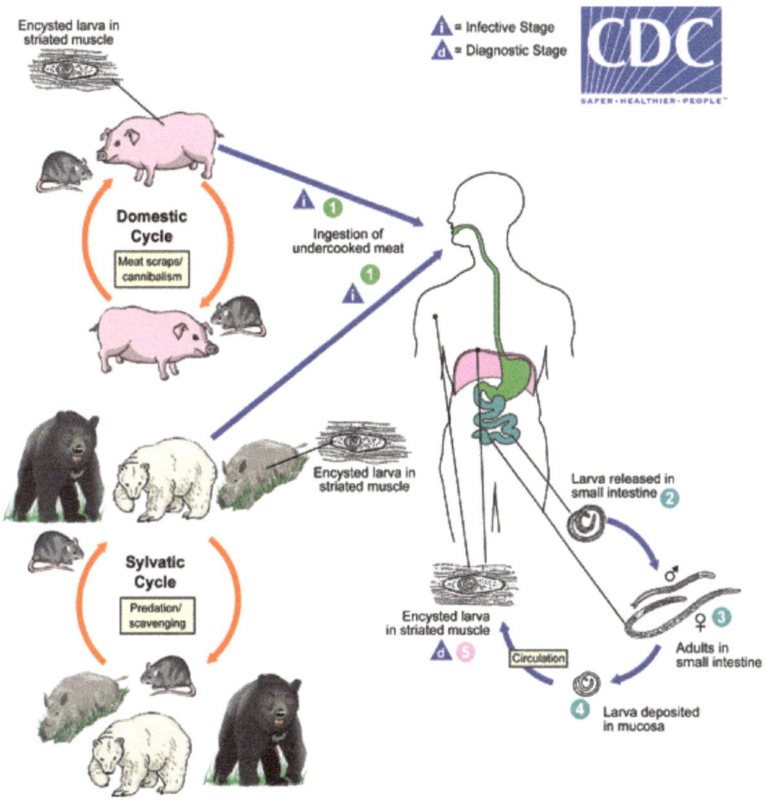

Life cycle of *Trichinella spiralis*

The typical life cycle for *T. spiralis* involves humans, pigs, and rodents. Pigs become infected when they eat infectious cysts in raw meat, often pork or rats (sylvatic cycle). Humans become infected when they eat raw or undercooked infected pork (domestic cycle). After humans ingest the cysts from infected undercooked meat, pepsin and hydrochloric acid help free the larvae in the cysts in the stomach. The larvae then migrate to the small intestine, where they molt four times before becoming adults.

Thirty to 34 hours after the cysts were originally ingested, the adults mate, and within five days produce larvae. The worms can only reproduce for a limited time because the immune system will eventually expel them from the small intestine. The larvae then use their piercing mouthpart, called the "stylet", to pass through the intestinal mucosa and enter the lymphatic vessels, and then enter the bloodstream.

The larvae travel by capillaries to various organs, such as the retina, myocardium, or lymph nodes; however, only larvae that migrate to skeletal muscle cells survive and encyst. The larval host cell becomes a nurse cell in which the larvae will be encapsulated. The development of a capillary network around the nurse cell completes encystation of the larvae. It is not soil-transmitted.

Diagnosis

Diagnosis of trichinosis is confirmed by a combination of exposure history, clinical diagnosis, and laboratory testing.

Exposure History

An epidemiological investigation can be done to determine a patient's exposure to raw infected meat. Often, an infection arises from home-preparation of contaminated meat, in which case microscopy can be used to determine the infection. However, exposure does not have to be directly from an infected animal. Other exposure includes the consumption of products from a laboratory-confirmed infected animal or by sharing a common exposure as a laboratory-confirmed infected human.

Clinical Diagnosis

Clinical presentation of the common trichinosis symptoms may also suggest infection. These symptoms include circumorbital edema, splinter hemorrhage, nonspecific gastroenteritis, and muscle pain. The case definition for trichinosis at the European Center for Disease Control states "at least three of the following six: fever, muscle soreness and pain, gastrointestinal symptoms, facial edema, eosinophilia, and subconjuctival, subungual, and retinal hemorrhages."

Laboratory Testing

Blood tests and microscopy can be used to aid in the diagnosis of trichinosis. Blood tests include a complete blood count for eosinophilia, creatine phosphokinase activity, and various immunoassays such as ELISA for larval antigens.

Prevention

Legislation

Laws and rules required of food producers may improve food safety for consumers, such as the rules established by the European Commission for inspections, rodent control, and improved hygiene. Similar protocol exists in the United States in the USDA guidelines for establishment responsibilities in inspecting pork.

Education and Training

Public education about the dangers of consuming raw and undercooked meat, especially pork, may reduce infection rates. Hunters are also an at-risk population due to their contact and consumption of wild game, including bear. As such, many states, such as New York, require the completion of a course in such matters before a hunting license can be obtained.

Food Preparation

Larvae may be killed by the heating or irradiation of raw meat. Freezing is only usually effective for *T. spiralis*, since other species, such as *T. nativa*, are freeze resistant and can survive long-term freezing.

- All meat (including pork) can be safely prepared by cooking to an internal temperature of 165 °F (74 °C) or higher for 15 seconds or more.
- Wild game: Wild game meat must be cooked thoroughly. Freezing wild game does not kill all trichinosis larval worms. This is because the worm species that typically infests wild game can resist freezing.
- Pork: Freezing cuts of pork less than 6 inches thick for 20 days at 5 °F (−15 °C) or three days at −4 °F (−20 °C) kills *T. spiralis* larval worms; but this will not kill other trichinosis larval worm species, such as *T. nativa*, if they have infested the pork food supply (which is unlikely).

Pork can be safely cooked to a slightly lower temperature provided that the internal meat temperature is at least as hot for at least as long as listed in the USDA table below. Nonetheless, it is prudent to allow a margin of error for variation in internal temperature within a particular cut of pork, which may have bones that affect temperature uniformity. In addition, your thermometer has measurement error that must be considered. Pork may be cooked for significantly longer and at a higher uniform internal temperature than listed here to be safe.

Internal Temperature	**Internal Temperature**	**Minimum Time**
(°F)	(°C)	(minutes)
120	49	1260
122	50.0	570
124	51.1	270
126	52.2	120
128	53.4	60
130	54.5	30
132	55.6	15
134	56.7	6
136	57.8	3
138	58.9	2
140	60.0	1
142	61.1	1
144	62.2	Instant

Unsafe and unreliable methods of cooking meat include the use of microwave ovens, curing, drying, and smoking, as these methods are difficult to standardize and control.

Pig Farming

- Keeping pigs in clean pens with floors that can be washed (such as concrete)
- Not allowing hogs to eat carcasses of other animals, including rats, which may be infected with *Trichinella*

- Cleaning meat grinders thoroughly when preparing ground meats
- Control and destruction of meat containing trichinae, e.g., removal and proper disposal of porcine diaphragms prior to public sale of meat

The Centers for Disease Control and Prevention makes the following recommendation: "Curing (salting), drying, smoking, or microwaving meat does not consistently kill infective worms." However, under controlled commercial food processing conditions, some of these methods are considered effective by the United States Department of Agriculture (USDA).

The USDA Animal and Plant Health Inspection Service (APHIS) is responsible for the regulations concerning the importation of swine from foreign countries. The Foreign Origin Meat and Meat Products, Swine section covers swine meat (cooked, cured and dried, and fresh). APHIS developed the National Trichinae Certification Program; this is a voluntary "preharvest" program for U.S. swine producers "that will provide documentation of swine management practices" to reduce the incidence of *Trichinella* in swine. The CDC reports 0.013% of U.S. swine is infected with *Trichinella*.

Treatment

As is desirable with most diseases, early treatment is better and decreases the risk of developing disease. If larvae do encyst in skeletal muscle cells, they can remain infectious for months to years.

Primary Treatment

Early administration of anthelmintics, such as mebendazole or albendazole, decreases the likelihood of larval encystation, particularly if given within three days of infection. However, most cases are diagnosed after this time.

Mebendazole (200–400 mg three times a day for three days) or albendazole (400 mg twice a day for 8–14 days) are given to treat trichinosis. These drugs prevent newly hatched larvae from developing, but should not be given to pregnant women or children under two years of age.

Secondary Treatment

After infection, steroids, such as prednisone may be used to relieve muscle pain associated with larval migration.

Vaccine Research

There are currently no vaccines for trichinosis, although experimental mice studies have suggested a possibility. In one study, microwaved *Trichinella* larvae were used to immunize mice, which were subsequently infected. Depending on dosage and the frequency of immunization, results ranged from a decreased larval count to complete protection from trichinosis.

Another study, Dea-Ayuela et al. (2006) used extracts and excretory-secretory products from first stage larvae to produce an oral vaccine. To prevent the gastric acids from dissolving the antigens before reaching the small intestine, scientists encapsulated the antigens in a microcapsule made of copolymers. This vaccine significantly increased CD4+ cells and increased antigen-specific serum IgGq and IgA, resulting in a statistically significant reduction in the average number of adult worms in the small intestine of mice. The significance of this approach is that if the white blood cells in the small intestine have been exposed to *Trichinella* antigens (through vaccination) then, when an individual gets infected, the immune system will respond to expel the worms from the small intestine fast enough to prevent the female worms from releasing their larvae. Yuan Gu et al. (2008) tested a DNA vaccine on mice which "induced a muscle larvae burden reduction in BALB/c mice by 29% in response to T. spiralis infection". Researchers trying to develop a vaccine for *Trichinella* have tried to using either "larval extracts, excretory-secretory antigen, DNA vaccine, or recombinant antigen protein."

Epidemiology

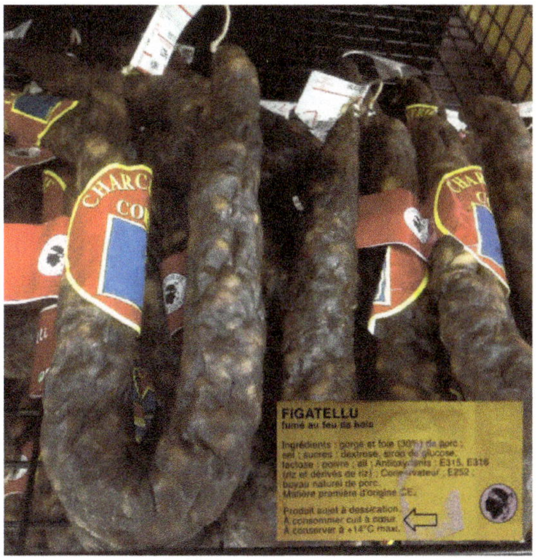

Pork sausages eaten raw by consumers caused an outbreak of trichinellosis in 2015 in France

About 11 million individuals are infected with *Trichinella*; *Trichinella spiralis* is the species responsible for most of these infections. Infection was once very common, but is now rare in the developed world.There were however two known outbreaks in 2015. The most recent one happened in France being associated with pork sausages from Corsica which were eaten raw. Around 40 people were also infected in Liguria, Italy during a New Year's Eve a few months earlier. The incidence of trichinosis in the U.S. has decreased dramatically in the past century. From 1997 to 2001, an annual average of 12 cases per year were reported in the United States. The number of cases has decreased because of legislation prohibiting the feeding of raw meat garbage to hogs, increased commercial and home freezing of pork, and the public awareness of the danger of eating raw or undercooked pork products.

In the developing world, most infections are associated with undercooked pork. For example, in Thailand, between 200 and 600 cases are reported annually around the Thai New Year. This is mostly attributable to a particular delicacy, *larb*, which calls for undercooked pork as part of the recipe. In parts of Eastern Europe, the World Health Organization (WHO) reports some swine herds have trichinosis infection rates above 50%, and there are correspondingly large numbers of human infections.

United States

Historically, pork products were thought to have the most risk of infecting humans with Trichinella spiralis. However, a trichinosis surveillance conducted between 1997-2001 showed a higher percentage of cases caused by consumption of wild game. This is thought to be due to the Federal Swine Health Protection Act (Public Law 96-468) that was passed by Congress in 1980. Before this act swine were fed garbage that could potentially be infected by Trichinella spiralis. This act was put in place to prevent contaminated food from being given to swine. Additionally, other regulations were put in place such as rodent control, limiting commercial swines contact with wildlife, maintaining good hygiene, and removing dead pigs from pens immediately.

Between 2002 and 2007, 11 cases were reported to CDC each year on average in the United States; these were mostly the result of eating undercooked game, bear meat, or home-reared pigs. It is common in developing countries where meat fed to pigs is raw or undercooked, but many cases also come from developed countries in Europe and North America, where raw or undercooked pork and wild game may be consumed as delicacies.

Reemergence

The disappearance of the pathogen from domestic pigs has led to a relaxation of legislation and control efforts by veterinary public health systems. It has since been thought of as a reemerging zoonosis supplemented by the increased distribution of meat products, political changes, a changing climate, and increasing sylvatic transmission.

It is also important to keep in mind major socio-political changes can produce conditions that favor the resurgence of *Trichinella* infections in swine and, consequently, humans. For instance, "the overthrow of the social and political structures in the 1990s" in Romania led to an increase in the incidence rate of trichinosis. There is also a high incidence of trichinosis among refugees from Southeast Asia. China reports approximately 10,000 cases every year, and is therefore the country with the highest numbers of cases. In China, between 1964 and 1998, over 20,000 people were infected with Trichinosis and more than 200 people died.

The kashrut and halal dietary laws of Judaism and Islam prohibit eating pork. In the 19th century, when the association between trichinosis and undercooked pork was first established, it was suggested that this association was the reason for the prohibition, reminiscent of the earlier opinion of the medieval Jewish philosopher Maimonides that food forbidden by Jewish law was "unwholesome". This theory was controversial and eventually fell out of favor.

History

As early as 1835, trichinosis was known to have been caused by a parasite, but the mechanism of infection was unclear at the time. A decade later, American scientist Joseph Leidy pinpointed undercooked meat as the primary vector for the parasite, and it was not until two decades afterwards that this hypothesis was fully accepted by the scientific community.

History

Parasite

The circumstances surrounding the first observation and identification of *Trichinella spiralis* are controversial due to a lack of medical records. In 1835, James Paget, a first-year medical student, first observed the larval form of *T. spiralis* while witnessing an autopsy at St. Bartholomew's Hospital in London. Paget took special interest in the presentation of muscle with white flecks, described as a "sandy diaphragm".

Although Paget is most likely the first person to have noticed and recorded these findings, the parasite was named and published in a report by his professor, Richard Owen, who is now credited for the discovery of the *T. spiralis* larval form.

Life Cycle

A series of experiments conducted between 1850 and 1870 by the German researchers Rudolf Virchow, Rudolf Leuckart and Friedrich Albert von Zenker, which involved feeding infected meat to a dog and performing the subsequent necropsy, led to the discovery of the life cycle of *Trichinella*. Through these experiments, Virchow was able to describe the development and infectivity of *T. spiralis*.

Research

The International Commission on Trichinellosis (ICT) was created in 1958 in Budapest and is aiming to exchange information on the biology, the physiopathology, the epidemiology, the immunology, and the clinical aspects of trichinosis in humans and animals. Prevention is a primary goal. Since the creation of the ICT, its members (more than 110 from 46 countries) have regularly gathered and worked together during meetings held every four years : the International Conference on Trichinellosis.

References

- Echenberg, Myron J. (2007). Plague Ports: The Global Urban Impact of Bubonic Plague, 1894–1901. New York, NY: New York Unive rsity Press. ISBN 0-8147-2232-6. OCLC 70292105.
- Keyes, Daniel C. (2005). Medical response to terrorism : preparedness and clinical practice. Philadelphia [u.a.]: Lippincott Williams & Wilkins. p. 74. ISBN 9780781749862.
- LeRoux, Neil (2007). Martin Luther As Comforter: Writings on Death Volume 133 of Studies in the History of Christian Traditions. BRILL. p. 247. ISBN 9789004158801.
- Edman, Bruce F. Eldridge, John D. (2004). Medical Entomology a Textbook on Public Health and Veterinary Problems Caused by Arthropods (Rev. edition. ed.). Dordrecht: Springer Netherlands. p. 390. ISBN 9789400710092.
- Rosen, William (2007), Justinian's Flea: Plague, Empire, and the Birth of Europe. Viking Adult; pg 3; ISBN 978-0-670-03855-8.
- Cohn, Samuel K. (2003). The Black Death Transformed: Disease and Culture in Early Renaissance Europe. A Hodder Arnold. p. 336. ISBN 0-340-70646-5.
- Cox, N.; Kawaoka (1998). "22". In Mahy B. and Collier L. Topley and Wilson's Microbiology and Microbial Infections. 1 Virology. Y. (9 ed.). Arnold. p. 415. ISBN 0-340-61470-6.
- Tamparo, Carol (2011). Fifth Edition : Diseases of the Human Body. Philadelphia, PA: F.A. Davis Company. p.61. ISBN 978-0-8036-2505-1
- Hansman, GS (editor) (2010). Caliciviruses: Molecular and Cellular Virology. Caister Academic Press. ISBN 978-1-904455-63-9.

- Cook, Gordon Charles; Zumla, Alimuddin (2009). Manson's Tropical Diseases. Elsevier Health Sciences. p. 325. ISBN 1416044701.
- Farrar, Jeremy (2013). Manson's tropical diseases. (23 ed.). Philadelphia: Saunders [Imprint]. pp. 791–794. ISBN 978-0-7020-5101-2.
- pp. 67–70, chapter 4, Good to Eat: Riddles of Food and Culture, Marvin Harris, New York: Simon and Schuster, 1985, ISBN 0-671-50366-9.
- "Transmission of Influenza Viruses from Animals to People". www.cdc.gov. Retrieved 2016-05-12.
- "Trichinellosis Fact Sheet – Division of Parasitic Diseases". Centre for Disease Control, US Government. August 2012. Retrieved 2016-06-05.
- "Relazione dei nas - Genova, allarme carne cruda: decine di intossicati dopo Capodanno". Retrieved 2016-09-16.
- "Avian Influenza Low Pathogenic H5N1 vs. Highly Pathogenic H5N1". United States Department of Agriculture. 23 July 2015
- "Recommendations for Worker Protection and Use of Personal Protective Equipment (PPE) to Reduce Exposure to Highly Pathogenic Avian Influenza A H5 Viruses : Avian Influenza (Flu)". www.cdc.gov. Retrieved 2015-07-25.
- "CDC - NIOSH Publications and Products - Protecting Poultry Workers from Avian Influenza (Bird Flu) (2008-128)". www.cdc.gov. Retrieved 2015-07-31.
- "Relazione annuale al PNI 2015 Trichine - Prevenzione e controllo" – via Ministero della Salute www.salute.gov.it.
- Rudi Hendrikx, DVM. "Avian Influenza in Pigeons" (PDF). Archived from the original (PDF) on 2014-02-22. Retrieved 2014-02-06.
- Alders, R., Awuni, J. A., Bagnol, B., Farrell, P., & Haan, N. (2014). Impact of avian influenza on village poultry production globally. EcoHealth, 11 (1): 63-72.
- Hameiri, S. (2014). Avian influenza, 'viral sovereignty', and the politics of health security in Indonesia. The Pacific Review, 27 (3): 333-356.
- "Transmission of Influenza Viruses from Animals to People". Centers for Disease Control and Prevention. 19 Aug 2014.
- "Symptoms of Plague". Brief Overview of Plague. iTriage. Healthagen, LLC. Retrieved November 26, 2014.
- World Health Organization (November 2014). "Plague Fact sheet N°267". Retrieved 10 May 2015.

6

Food Safety: An Integrated Study

Food safety is the handling and storing of food in ways that helps in preventing foodborne illnesses. The aspects elucidated are food processing, food preservation, food storage and calcium propanoate. The major categories of food safety are dealt with great details in the chapter.

Food Safety

Food safety is a scientific discipline describing handling, preparation, and storage of food in ways that prevent foodborne illness. This includes a number of routines that should be followed to avoid potentially severe health hazards. In this way food safety often overlaps with food defense to prevent harm to consumers. The tracks within this line of thought are safety between industry and the market and then between the market and the consumer. In considering industry to market practices, food safety considerations include the origins of food including the practices relating to food labeling, food hygiene, food additives and pesticide residues, as well as policies on biotechnology and food and guidelines for the management of governmental import and export inspection and certification systems for foods. In considering market to consumer practices, the usual thought is that food ought to be safe in the market and the concern is safe delivery and preparation of the food for the consumer.

Food can transmit disease from person to person as well as serve as a growth medium for bacteria that can cause food poisoning. In developed countries there are intricate standards for food preparation, whereas in lesser developed countries the main issue is simply the availability of adequate safe water, which is usually a critical item. In theory, food poisoning is 100% preventable. The five key principles of food hygiene, according to WHO, are:

1. Prevent contaminating food with pathogens spreading from people, pets, and pests.
2. Separate raw and cooked foods to prevent contaminating the cooked foods.
3. Cook foods for the appropriate length of time and at the appropriate temperature to kill pathogens.
4. Store food at the proper temperature.
5. Do use safe water and safe raw materials.

Issues

Food safety issues and regulations concern:

- Agriculture and animal husbandry practices

- Food manufacturing practices
- Food additives
- Novel foods
- Genetically modified foods
- Food labels

ISO 22000

ISO 22000 is a standard developed by the International Organization for Standardization dealing with food safety. This is a general derivative of ISO 9000. ISO 22000 standard: The ISO 22000 international standard specifies the requirements for a food safety management system that involves interactive communication, system management, prerequisite programs, HACCP principles.

Incidence

A 2003 World Health Organization (WHO) report concluded that about 30% of reported food poisoning outbreaks in the WHO European Region occur in private homes. According to the WHO and CDC, in the USA alone, annually, there are 76 million cases of foodborne illness leading to 325,000 hospitalizations and 5,000 deaths.

Regulations by Jurisdiction and Agency

WHO and FAO

In 1963, the WHO and FAO published the Codex Alimentarius which serves as an guideline to food safety.

However, according to Unit 04 - Communication of Health & Consumers Directorate-General of the European Commission (SANCO): "The Codex, while being recommendations for voluntary application by members, Codex standards serve in many cases as a basis for national legislation. The reference made to Codex food safety standards in the World Trade Organizations' Agreement on Sanitary and Phytosanitary measures (SPS Agreement) means that Codex has far reaching implications for resolving trade disputes. WTO members that wish to apply stricter food safety measures than those set by Codex may be required to justify these measures scientifically." So, an agreement made in 2003, signed by all member states, inclusive all EU, in the codex Stan Codex 240 – 2003 for coconut milk, sulphite containing additives like E223 and E 224 are allowed till 30 mg/kg, does NOT mean, they are allowed into the EU, see RASFF entries from Denmark: 2012.0834; 2011.1848; en 2011.168, "sulphite unauthorised in coconut milk from Thailand ". Same for polysorbate E 435: see 2012.0838 from Denmark, unauthorised polysorbates in coconut milk and, 2007.AIC from France. Only for the latter the EU amended its regulations with (EU) No 583/2012 per 2 July 2012 to allow this additive, already used for decades and absolutely necessary.

Australia

Food Standards Australia New Zealand requires all food businesses to implement food safety systems. These systems are designed to ensure food is safe to consume and halt the increasing incidence of food poisoning, and they include basic food safety training for at least one person in each business. Food safety training is delivered in various forms by, among other organisations, Registered Training Organizations (RTOs), after which staff are issued a nationally recognised unit of competency code on their certificate. Basic food safety training includes:

- Understanding the hazards associated with the main types of food and the conditions to prevent the growth of bacteria which can cause food poisoning and to prevent illness.
- Potential problems associated with product packaging such as leaks in vacuum packs, damage to packaging or pest infestation, as well as problems and diseases spread by pests.
- Safe food handling. This includes safe procedures for each process such as receiving, re-packing, food storage, preparation and cooking, cooling and re-heating, displaying products, handling products when serving customers, packaging, cleaning and sanitizing, pest control, transport and delivery. Also covers potential causes of cross contamination.
- Catering for customers who are particularly at risk of food-borne illness, as well as those with allergies or intolerance.
- Correct cleaning and sanitizing procedures, cleaning products and their correct use, and the storage of cleaning items such as brushes, mops and cloths.
- Personal hygiene, hand washing, illness, and protective clothing.

Food safety standards and requirements are set out at the national level in the Food Standards Code, and brought Into force in each state by state-based Acts and Regulations. Legislation means that people responsible for selling or serving unsafe food may be liable for heavy fines.

China

Food safety is a growing concern in Chinese agriculture. The Chinese government oversees agricultural production as well as the manufacture of food packaging, containers, chemical additives, drug production, and business regulation. In recent years, the Chinese government attempted to consolidate food regulation with the creation of the State Food and Drug Administration in 2003, and officials have also been under increasing public and international pressure to solve food safety problems. However, it appears that regulations are not well known by the trade. Labels used for "green" food, "organic" food and "pollution-free" food are not well recognized by traders and many are unclear about their meaning. A survey by the World Bank found that supermarket managers had difficulty in obtaining produce that met safety requirements and found that a high percentage of produce did not comply with established standards.

Traditional marketing systems, whether in China or the rest of Asia, presently provide little motivation or incentive for individual farmers to make improvements to either quality or safety as their produce tends to get grouped together with standard products as it progresses through the marketing channel. Direct linkages between farmer groups and traders or ultimate buyers, such as supermarkets, can help avoid this problem. Governments need to improve the condition of many markets through upgrading management and reinvesting market fees in physical infrastructure. Wholesale markets need to investigate the feasibility of developing separate sections to handle fruits and vegetables that meet defined safety and quality standards.

European Union

The parliament of the European Union (EU) makes legislation in the form of directives and regulations, many of which are mandatory for member states and which therefore must be incorporated into individual countries' national legislation. As a very large organisation that exists to remove barriers to trade between member states, and into which individual member states have only a proportional influence, the outcome is often seen as an excessively bureaucratic 'one size fits all' approach. However, in relation to food safety the tendency to err on the side of maximum protection for the consumer may be seen as a positive benefit. The EU parliament is informed on food safety matters by the European Food Safety Authority.

Individual member states may also have other legislation and controls in respect of food safety, provided that they do not prevent trade with other states, and can differ considerably in their internal structures and approaches to the regulatory control of food safety.

From 13 December 2014, new legislation - the EU Food Information for Consumers Regulation 1169/2011 - require food businesses to provide allergy information on food sold unpackaged, in for example catering outlets, deli counters, bakeries and sandwich bars.

France

Agence nationale de sécurité sanitaire de l'alimentation, de l'environnement et du travail (anses) is a French governmental agency dealing with food safety.

Germany

The Federal Ministry of Food, Agriculture and Consumer Protection (BMEL) is a Federal Ministry of the Federal Republic of Germany. History: Founded as Federal Ministry of Food, Agriculture and Foresting in 1949, this name did not change until 2001. Then the name changed to Federal Ministry of Consumer Protection, Food and Agriculture. At the 22nd of November 2005, the name got changed again to its current state: Federal Ministry of Food, Agriculture and Consumer Protection. The reason for this last change was that all the resorts should get equal ranking which was achieved by sorting the resorts alphabetically. Vision: A balanced and healthy diet with safe food, distinct consumer rights and consumer information for various areas of life, and a strong and sustainable agriculture as well as perspectives for our rural areas are important goals of the Federal Ministry of Food, Agriculture and Consumer Protection (BMELV). The Federal Office of Consumer Protection and Food Safety is under the control of the Federal Ministry of Food, Agriculture and Consumer Protection. It exercises several duties, with which it contributes to safer food and thereby intensifies health-based consumer protection in Germany. Food can be manufactured and sold within Germany without a special permission, as long as it does not cause any damage on consumers' health and meets the general standards set by the legislation. However, manufacturers, carriers, importers and retailers are responsible for the food they pass into circulation. They are obliged to ensure and document the safety and quality of their food with the use of in-house control mechanisms.

Hong Kong

In Hong Kong SAR, the Centre for Food Safety is in charge of ensuring food sold is safe and fit for consumption.

India

Food Safety and Standards Authority of India, established under the Food Safety and Standards Act, 2006, is the regulating body related to food safety and laying down of standards of food in India.

New Zealand

The New Zealand Food Safety Authority (NZFSA), or Te Pou Oranga Kai O Aotearoa is the New Zealand government body responsible for food safety. NZFSA is also the controlling authority for imports and exports of food and food-related products. The NZFSA as of 2012 is now a division of the Ministry for Primary Industries (MPI) and is no longer its own organization.

Pakistan

Pakistan does not have an integrated legal framework but has a set of laws, which deals with various aspects of food safety. These laws, despite the fact that they were enacted long time ago, have tremendous capacity to achieve at least minimum level of food safety. However, like many other laws, these laws remain very poorly enforced. There are four laws that specifically deal with food safety. Three of these laws directly focus issues related to food safety, while the fourth, the Pakistan Standards and Quality Control Authority Act, is indirectly relevant to food safety.

The Pure Food Ordinance 1960 consolidates and amends the law in relation to the preparation and the sale of foods. All provinces and some northern areas have adopted this law with certain amendments. Its aim is to ensure purity of food being supplied to people in the market and, therefore, provides for preventing adulteration. The Pure Food Ordinance 1960 does not apply to cantonment areas. There is a separate law for cantonments called "The Cantonment Pure Food Act, 1966". There is no substantial difference between the Pure Food Ordinance 1960 and The Cantonment Pure Food Act. Even the rules of operation are very much similar.

Pakistan Hotels and Restaurant Act, 1976 applies to all hotels and restaurants in Pakistan and seeks to control and regulate the rates and standard of service(s) by hotels and restaurants. In addition to other provisions, under section 22(2), the sale of food or beverages that are contaminated, not prepared hygienically or served in utensils that are not hygienic or clean is an offense. There are no express provisions for consumer complaints in the Pakistan Restaurants Act, 1976, Pakistan Penal Code, 1860 and Pakistan Standards and Quality Control Authority Act, 1996. The laws do not prevent citizens from lodging complaints with the concerned government officials; however, the consideration and handling of complaints is a matter of discretion of the officials.

South Korea

Korea Food & Drug Administration

Korea Food & Drug Administration (KFDA) is working for food safety since 1945. It is part of the Government of South Korea.

IOAS-Organic Certification Bodies Registered in KFDA: "Organic" or related claims can be labelled on food products when organic certificates are considered as valid by KFDA. KFDA admits organic certificates which can be issued by 1) IFOAM (International Federation of Organic Agriculture Movement) accredited certification bodies 2) Government accredited certification bodies – 328 bodies in 29 countries have been registered in KFDA.

Food Import Report: According to Food Import Report, it is supposed to report or register what you import. Competent authority is as follows:

Product	Authority
Imported Agricultural Products, Processed Foods, Food Additives, Utensils, Containers & Packages or Health Functional Foods	KFDA (Korea Food and Drug Administration)
Imported Livestock, Livestock products (including Dairy products)	NVRQS (National Veterinary Research and Quarantine Service)
Packaged meat, milk & dairy products (butter, cheese), hamburger patties, meat ball and other processed products which are stipulated by Livestock Sanitation Management Act	NVRQS (National Veterinary Research and Quarantine Service)
Imported Marine products; fresh, chilled, frozen, salted, dehydrated, eviscerated marine produce which can be recognized its characteristics	NFIS (National Fisheries Products Quality Inspection Service)

National Institute of Food and Drug Safety Evaluation

National Institute of Food and Drug Safety Evaluation (NIFDS) is functioning as well. The National Institute of Food and Drug Safety Evaluation is a national organization for toxicological tests and research. Under the Korea Food & Drug Administration, the Institute performs research on toxicology, pharmacology, and risk analysis of foods, drugs, and their additives. The Institute strives primarily to understand important biological triggering mechanisms and improve assessment methods of human exposure, sensitivities, and risk by (1) conducting basic, applied, and policy research that closely examines biologically triggering harmful effects on the regulated products such as foods, food additives, and drugs, and operating the national toxicology program for the toxicological test development and inspection of hazardous chemical substances assessments. The Institute ensures safety by investigation and research on safety by its own researchers, contract research by external academicians and research centers.

Taiwan

In Taiwan, the Ministry of Health and Welfare in charge of Food and Drug Safety, also evaluate the catering industry to maintenance the food product quality. Currently, US$29.01 million of budget is allocated each year for food safety-related efforts.

United Kingdom

In the UK the Food Standards Agency is an independent government department responsible for food safety and hygiene across the UK. They work with businesses to help them produce safe food, and with local authorities to enforce food safety regulations. In 2006 food hygiene legislation changed and new requirements came into force. The main requirement resulting from this change is that if you own or run a food business in the UK, you must have a documented Food Safety Management System, which is based on the principles of Hazard Analysis Critical Control Point HACCP.

United States

The US food system is regulated by numerous federal, state and local officials. It has been criticized as lacking in "organization, regulatory tools, and not addressing food borne illness."

Federal Level Regulation

The Food and Drug Administration publishes the Food Code, a model set of guidelines and procedures that assists food control jurisdictions by providing a scientifically sound technical and legal basis for regulating the retail and food service industries, including restaurants, grocery stores and institutional foodservice providers such as nursing homes. Regulatory agencies at all levels of government in the United States use the FDA Food Code to develop or update food safety rules in their jurisdictions that are consistent with national food regulatory policy. According to the FDA, 48 of 56 states and territories, representing 79% of the U.S. population, have adopted food codes patterned after one of the five versions of the Food Code, beginning with the 1993 edition.

In the United States, federal regulations governing food safety are fragmented and complicated, according to a February 2007 report from the Government Accountability Office. There are 15 agencies sharing oversight responsibilities in the food safety system, although the two primary agencies are the U.S. Department of Agriculture (USDA) Food Safety and Inspection Service (FSIS), which is responsible for the safety of meat, poultry, and processed egg products, and the Food and Drug Administration (FDA), which is responsible for virtually all other foods.

The Food Safety and Inspection Service has approximately 7,800 inspection program personnel working in nearly 6,200 federally inspected meat, poultry and processed egg establishments. FSIS is charged with administering and enforcing the Federal Meat Inspection Act, the Poultry Products Inspection Act, the Egg Products Inspection Act, portions of the Agricultural Marketing Act, the Humane Slaughter Act, and the regulations that implement these laws. FSIS inspection program personnel inspect every animal before slaughter, and each carcass after slaughter to ensure public health requirements are met. In fiscal year (FY) 2008, this included about 50 billion pounds of livestock carcasses, about 59 billion pounds of poultry carcasses, and about 4.3 billion pounds of processed egg products. At U.S. borders, they also inspected 3.3 billion pounds of imported meat and poultry products.

Industry Pressure

There have been concerns over the efficacy of safety practices and food industry pressure on U.S. regulators. A study reported by Reuters found that "the food industry is jeopardizing U.S. public health by withholding information from food safety investigators or pressuring regulators to withdraw or alter policy designed to protect consumers". A survey found that 25% of U.S. government inspectors and scientists surveyed have experienced during the past year corporate interests forcing their food safety agency to withdraw or to modify agency policy or action that protects consumers. Scientists have observed that management undercuts field inspectors who stand up for food safety against industry pressure. According to Dr. Dean Wyatt, a USDA veterinarian who oversees federal slaughter house inspectors, "Upper level management does not adequately support field inspectors and the actions they take to protect the food supply. Not only is there lack of support, but there's outright obstruction, retaliation and abuse of power." A growing number of food and beverage manufacturers are improving food safety standards by incorporating a food safety management system which automates all steps in the food quality management process.

State and Local Regulation

A number of U.S. states have their own meat inspection programs that substitute for USDA inspection for meats that are sold only in-state. Certain state programs have been criticized for undue leniency to bad practices.

However, other state food safety programs supplement, rather than replace, Federal inspections, generally with the goal of increasing consumer confidence in the state's produce. For example, state health departments have a role in investigating outbreaks of food-borne disease bacteria, as in the case of the 2006 outbreak of *Escherichia coli* O157:H7 (a pathogenic strain of the ordinarily harmless bacteria, *E. coli*) from processed spinach. Health departments also promote better food processing practices to eliminate these threats.

In addition to the US Food and Drug Administration, several states that are major producers of fresh fruits and vegetables (including California, Arizona and Florida) have their own state programs to test produce for pesticide residues.

Restaurants and other retail food establishments fall under state law and are regulated by state or local health departments. Typically these regulations require official inspections of specific design features, best food-handling practices, and certification of food handlers. In some places a letter grade or numerical score must be prominently posted following each inspection. In some localities, inspection deficiencies and remedial action are posted on the Internet.

Vietnam

The Vietnam Food Administration is responsible for managing food hygiene, safety, and quality and has made significant progress since its establishment in 1999. Food safety remains a high priority in Vietnam with the growth of export markets and increasing food imports raising the need to rapidly build capacity of the Food Administration in order to reduce threats of foodborne disease. The Food Administration has demonstrated commitment to the food safety challenges it faces, and has embarked on an innovative capacity building activity with technical assistance from the World Health Organization.

Manufacturing Control

United Kingdom

Foodstuffs in the UK have one of two labels to indicate the nature of the deterioration of the product and any subsequent health issues. EHO Food Hygiene certification is required to prepare and distribute food. While there is no specified expiry date of such a qualification the changes in legislation it is suggested to update every five years.

Best before indicates a future date beyond which the food product *may* lose quality in terms of taste or texture amongst others, but does not imply any serious health problems if food is consumed beyond this date (within reasonable limits).

Use by indicates a legal date beyond which it is not permissible to sell a food product (usually one that deteriorates fairly rapidly after production) due to the potential serious nature of consumption of pathogens. Leeway is sometimes provided by producers in stating display until dates so that products are not at their limit of safe consumption on the actual date stated (this latter is voluntary and not subject to regulatory control). This allows for the variability in production, storage and display methods.

United States

With the exception of infant formula and baby foods which must be withdrawn by their expiration date, Federal law does not require expiration dates. For all other foods, except dairy products in some states, freshness dating is strictly voluntary on the part of manufacturers. In response to consumer demand, perishable foods are typically labelled with a Sell by date. It is up to the consumer to decide how long after the Sell by date a package is usable. Other common dating statements are Best if used by, Use-by date, Expiration date, Guaranteed fresh <date>, and Pack date.

Australia and New Zealand

Guide to Food Labelling and Other Information Requirements: This guide provides background information on the general labelling requirements in the Code. The information in this guide applies both to food for retail sale and to food for catering purposes. Foods for catering purposes means those foods for use in restaurants, canteens, schools, caterers or self-catering institutions, where food is offered for immediate consumption. Labelling and information requirements in the new Code apply both to food sold or prepared for sale in Australia and New Zealand and food imported into Australia and New Zealand. Warning and Advisory Declarations, Ingredient Labelling, Date Marking, Nutrition Information Requirements, Legibility Requirements for Food Labels, Percentage Labelling, Information Requirements for Foods Exempt from Bearing a Label.

Food Processing

Food processing is the transformation of raw ingredients, by physical or chemical means into food, or of food into other forms. Food processing combines raw food ingredients to produce marketable food products that can be easily prepared and served by the consumer. Food processing typically involves activities such as mincing and macerating, liquefaction, emulsification, and cooking (such as boiling, broiling, frying, or grilling); pickling, pasteurization, and many other kinds of preservation; and canning or other packaging. (Primary-processing such as dicing or slicing, freezing or drying when leading to secondary products are also included.)

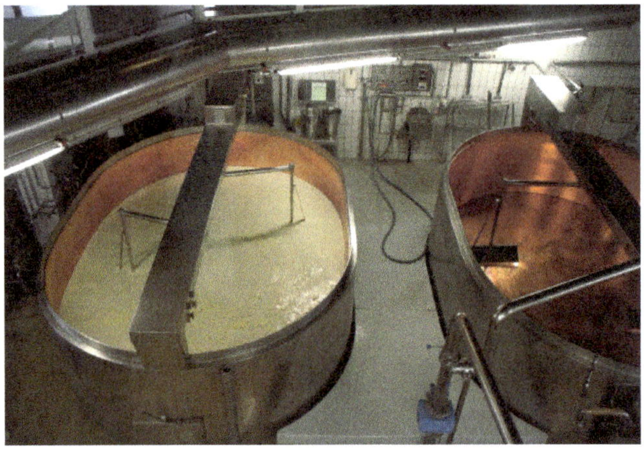

Industrial cheese production

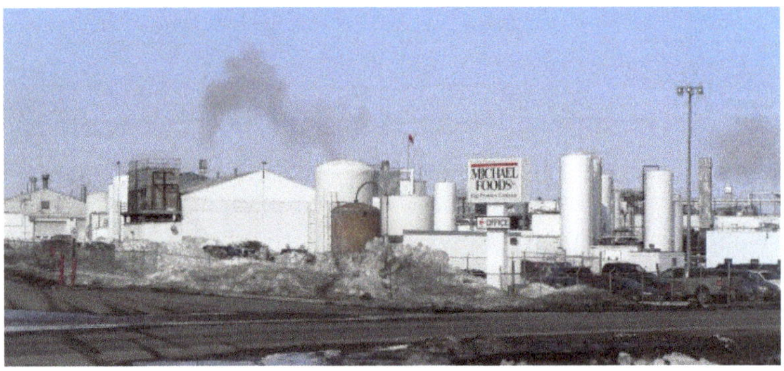

Michael Foods egg-processing plant in Wakefield, Nebraska

History

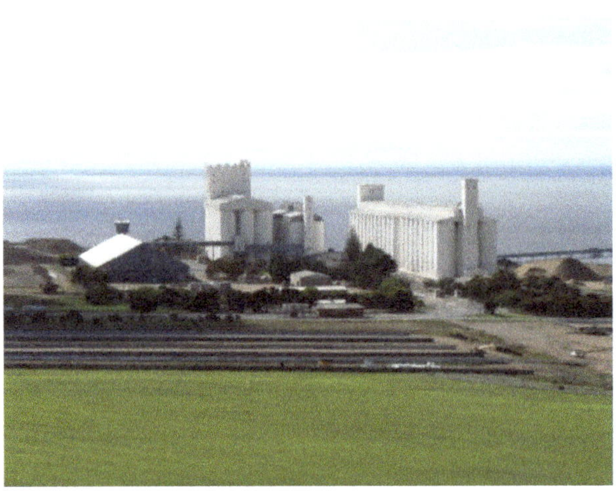

Grain silos in Ardrossan, Scotland

Food processing dates back to the prehistoric ages when crude processing incorporated fermenting, sun drying, preserving with salt, and various types of cooking (such as roasting, smoking, steaming, and oven baking), Such basic food processing involved chemical enzymatic changes to the basic structure of food in its natural form, as well served to build a barrier against surface microbial activity that caused rapid decay. Salt-preservation was especially common for foods that constituted warrior and sailors' diets until the introduction of canning methods. Evidence for the existence of these methods can be found in the writings of the ancient Greek, Chaldean, Egyptian and Roman civilizations as well as archaeological evidence from Europe, North and South America and Asia. These tried and tested processing techniques remained essentially the same until the advent of the industrial revolution. Examples of ready-meals also date back to before the preindustrial revolution, and include dishes such as Cornish pasty and Haggis. Both during ancient times and today in modern society these are considered processed foods.

Modern food processing technology developed in the 19th and 20th centuries was developed in a large part to serve military needs. In 1809 Nicolas Appert invented a hermetic bottling technique that would preserve food for French troops which ultimately contributed to the development of tinning, and subsequently canning by Peter Durand in 1810. Although initially expensive and somewhat hazardous due to the lead used in cans, canned goods would later become a staple around the world. Pasteurization, discovered by Louis Pasteur in 1864, improved the quality of preserved foods and introduced the wine, beer, and milk preservation.

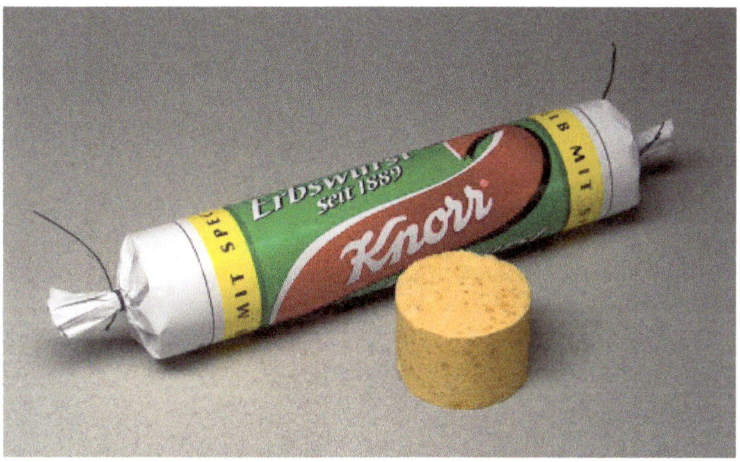

A form of pre-made split-pea soup that has become traditional

In the 20th century, World War II, the space race and the rising consumer society in developed countries (including the United States) contributed to the growth of food processing with such advances as spray drying, evaporation, juice concentrates, freeze drying and the introduction of artificial sweeteners, colouring agents, and such preservatives as sodium benzoate. In the late 20th century, products such as dried instant soups, reconstituted fruits and juices, and self cooking meals such as MRE food ration were developed.

In western Europe and North America, the second half of the 20th century witnessed a rise in the pursuit of convenience. Food processing companies marketed their products especially towards middle-class working wives and mothers. Frozen foods (often credited to Clarence Birdseye) found their success in sales of juice concentrates and "TV dinners". Processors utilised the perceived value of time to appeal to the postwar population, and this same appeal contributes to the success of convenience foods today.

Benefits and Drawbacks

Benefits

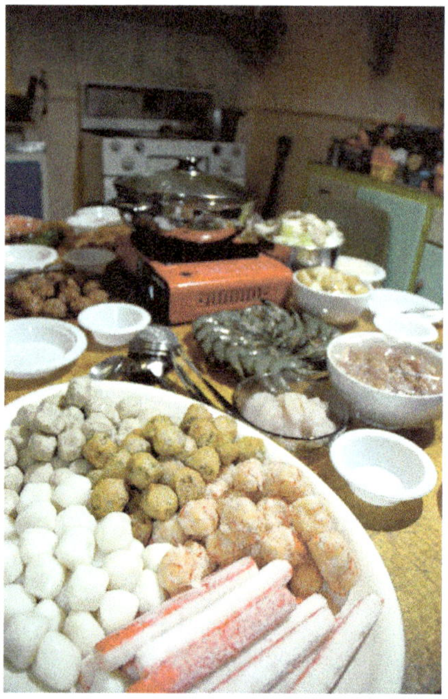

Processed seafood - fish, squid, prawn balls and simulated crab sticks (surimi)

Benefits of food processing include toxin removal, preservation, easing marketing and distribution tasks, and increasing food consistency. In addition, it increases yearly availability of many foods, enables transportation of delicate perishable foods across long distances and makes many kinds of foods safe to eat by de-activating spoilage and pathogenic micro-organisms. Modern supermarkets would not exist without modern food processing techniques, and long voyages would not be possible.

Processed foods are usually less susceptible to early spoilage than fresh foods and are better suited for long distance transportation from the source to the consumer. When they were first introduced, some processed foods helped to alleviate food shortages and improved the overall nutrition of populations as it made many new foods available to the masses.

Processing can also reduce the incidence of food borne disease. Fresh materials, such as fresh produce and raw meats, are more likely to harbour pathogenic micro-organisms (e.g. Salmonella) capable of causing serious illnesses.

The extremely varied modern diet is only truly possible on a wide scale because of food processing. Transportation of more exotic foods, as well as the elimination of much hard labour gives the modern eater easy access to a wide variety of food unimaginable to their ancestors.

The act of processing can often improve the taste of food significantly.

Mass production of food is much cheaper overall than individual production of meals from raw ingredients. Therefore, a large profit potential exists for the manufacturers and suppliers of processed food products. Individuals may see a benefit in convenience, but rarely see any direct financial cost benefit in using processed food as compared to home preparation.

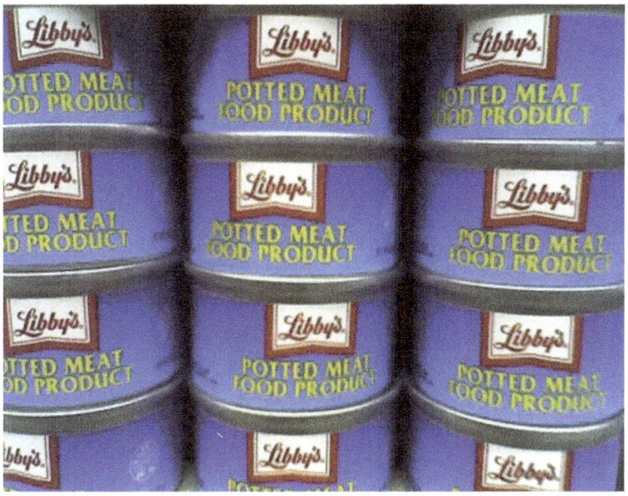

Libby's brand 'Potted Meat Food Product'

Processed food freed people from the large amount of time involved in preparing and cooking "natural" unprocessed foods. The increase in free time allows people much more choice in life style than previously allowed. In many families the adults are working away from home and therefore there is little time for the preparation of food based on fresh ingredients. The food industry offers products that fulfill many different needs: e.g. fully prepared ready meals that can be heated up in the microwave oven within a few minutes.

Modern food processing also improves the quality of life for people with allergies, diabetics, and other people who cannot consume some common food elements. Food processing can also add extra nutrients such as vitamins.

Drawbacks

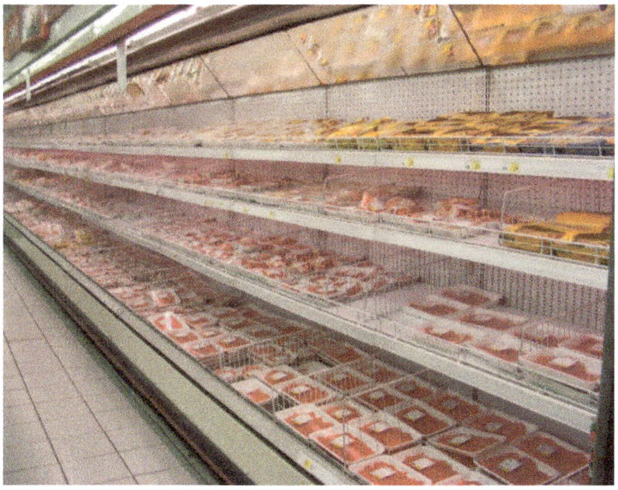

Meat packages in a Roman supermarket

Any processing of food can affect its nutritional density. The amount of nutrients lost depends on the food and processing method. For example, heat destroys vitamin C. Therefore, canned fruits possess less vitamin C than their fresh alternatives. The USDA conducted a study in 2004, creating a nutrient retention table for several foods.

New research highlighting the importance to human health of a rich microbial environment in the intestine indicates that abundant food processing (not fermentation of foods) endangers that environment.

Using food additives represents another safety concern. The health risks of any given additive vary greatly from person to person; for example using sugar as an additive endangers diabetics. In the European Union, only European Food Safety Authority (EFSA) approved food additives (e.g., sweeteners, preservatives, stabilizers) are permitted at specified levels for use in food products. Approved additives receive an E number (E for Europe), simplifying communication about food additives included in the ingredients' list for all the different languages spoken in the EU. As effects of chemical additives are learnt, changes to laws and regulatory practices are made to make such processed foods more safe.

Food processing is typically a mechanical process that utilizes large mixing, grinding, chopping and emulsifying equipment in the production process. These processes inherently introduce a number of contamination risks. As a mixing bowl or grinder is used over time the food contact parts will tend to fail and fracture. This type of failure will introduce into the product stream small to large metal contaminants. Further processing of these metal fragments will result in downstream equipment failure and the risk of ingestion by the consumer. Food manufacturers utilize industrial metal detectors to detect and reject automatically any metal fragment. Large food processors will utilize many metal detectors within the processing stream to reduce both damage to processing machinery as well as risk to consumer health.

Performance Parameters for Food Processing

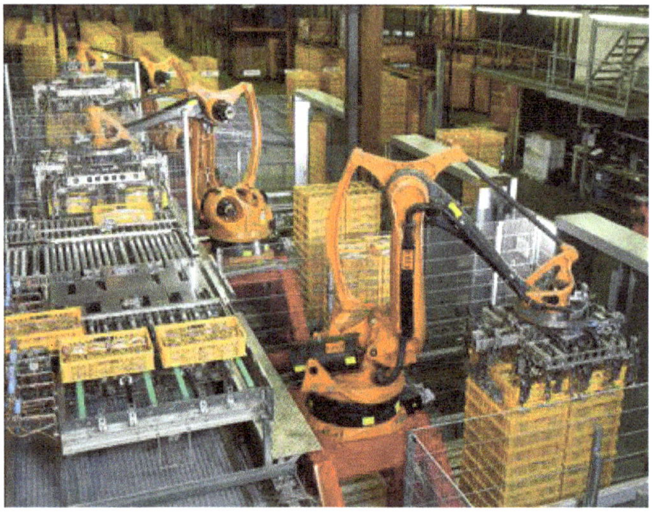

Factory automation - robotics palettizing bread

When designing processes for the food industry the following performance parameters may be taken into account:

- Hygiene, e.g. measured by number of micro-organisms per mL of finished product
- Energy efficiency measured e.g. by "ton of steam per ton of sugar produced"
- Minimization of waste, measured e.g. by "percentage of peeling loss during the peeling of potatoes"

- Labour used, measured e.g. by "number of working hours per ton of finished product"
- Minimization of cleaning stops measured e.g. by "number of hours between cleaning stops"

De-agglomerating Batter Mixes in Food Processing

Problems often occur during preparation of batter mixes because flour and other powdered ingredients tend to form lumps or agglomerates as they are being mixed during production. A conventional mixer/agitator cannot break down these agglomerates, resulting in a lumpy batter. If lumpy batter is used to enrobe products, it causes an unsatisfactory appearance with misshapen or oversize products that do not fit properly into packaging. This can force production to a standstill. Furthermore, batter mix is generally recirculated from an enrobing system back to a holding vessel; lumps then have a tendency to build up, reducing the flow of material and raising potential sanitation issues.

Using a high shear in-line mixer in place of a conventional agitator or mixer can quickly solve problems of agglomeration with dry ingredients. A single pass through a self-pumping, in-line mixer adds high shear to batter, which de-agglomerates the mix, resulting in a homogeneous, smooth batter. With a consistent, smooth batter, finished product appearance is improved; the effectiveness and hygiene of the recirculation system is increased; and a better yield of raw materials is achieved. By increasing overall product quality, the amount of raw materials needed is decreased, thereby lowering manufacturing costs and increasing shelf life. Increased shelf life is achieved by creating and maintaining an emulsion, often by adding a food stabilizer.

High shear in-line mixers process food to be made faster and cheaper while increasing consistency of the finished food. Powder and liquid mixing systems are capable of rapidly incorporating large quantities of powders at high concentrations – agglomerate free and fully hydrated. Advances in technology have made processing equipment easy to clean, leading to a much safer processed food.

Trends in Modern Food Processing

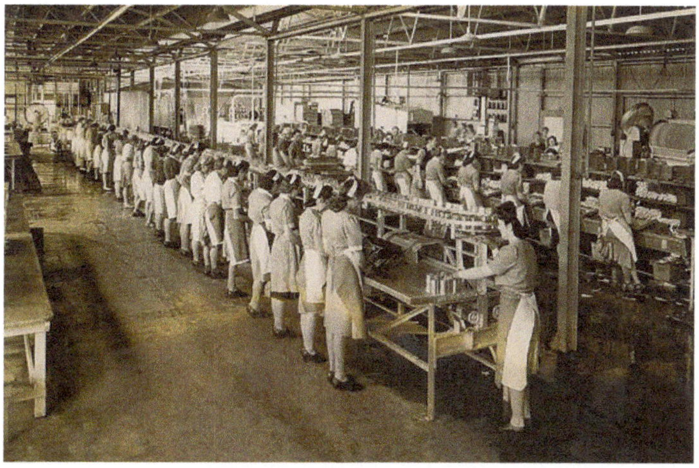

Women working in a cannery

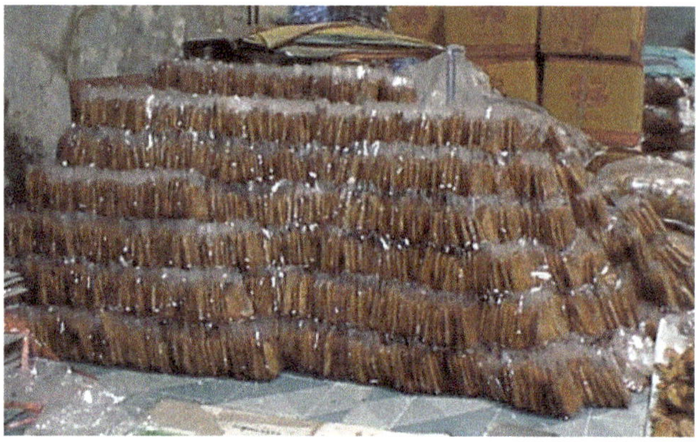

Dried bananas packaged in Ban Bang Krathum, Bang Krathum, Phitsanulok, Thailand

Health

- Reduction of fat content in final product by using baking instead of deep-frying in the production of potato chips, another processed food.
- Maintaining the natural taste of the product by using less artificial sweetener than was used before.

Hygiene

The rigorous application of industry and government endorsed standards to minimise possible risk and hazards. The international standard adopted is HACCP.

Efficiency

- Rising energy costs lead to increasing usage of energy-saving technologies, e.g. frequency converters on electrical drives, heat insulation of factory buildings and heated vessels, energy recovery systems, keeping a single fish frozen all the way from China to Switzerland.
- Factory automation systems (often Distributed control systems) reduce personnel costs and may lead to more stable production results.

Industries

Food processing industries and practices include the following:

- Cannery
- Fish processing
- Food packaging plant
- Industrial rendering
- Meat packing plant
- Slaughterhouse
- Sugar industry

Food Preservation

Food preservation involves preventing the growth of bacteria, fungi (such as yeasts), or other micro-organisms (although some methods work by introducing benign bacteria or fungi to the food), as well as slowing the oxidation of fats that cause rancidity. Food preservation may also include processes that inhibit visual deterioration, such as the enzymatic browning reaction in apples after they are cut during food preparation.

Many processes designed to preserve food will involve a number of food preservation methods. Preserving fruit by turning it into jam, for example, involves boiling (to reduce the fruit's moisture content and to kill bacteria, etc.), sugaring (to prevent their re-growth) and sealing within an airtight jar (to prevent recontamination). Some traditional methods of preserving food have been shown to have a lower energy input and carbon footprint, when compared to modern methods.

Some methods of food preservation are known to create carcinogens. In 2015, the International Agency for Research on Cancer of the World Health Organization classified processed meat, i.e. meat that has undergone salting, curing, fermenting, and smoking, as "carcinogenic to humans".

Maintaining or creating nutritional value, texture and flavor is an important aspect of food preservation, although, historically, some methods drastically altered the character of the food being preserved. In many cases these changes have come to be seen as desirable qualities – cheese, yogurt and pickled onions being common examples.

Traditional Techniques

New techniques of food preservation became available to the home chef from the dawn of agriculture until the Industrial Revolution.

Drying

Drying is one of the oldest techniques used to hamper the decomposition of food products. As early as 12,000 B.C., Middle Eastern and Oriental cultures were drying foods using the power of the sun. Vegetables and fruits are naturally dried by the sun and wind, but "still houses" were built in areas that did not have enough sunlight to dry things. A fire would be built inside the building to provide the heat to dry the various fruits, vegetables, and herbs.

Cooling

Cooling preserves food by slowing down the growth and reproduction of micro-organisms and the action of enzymes that cause food to rot. The introduction of commercial and domestic refrigerators drastically improved the diets of many in the Western world by allowing foods such as fresh fruit, salads and dairy products to be stored safely for longer periods, particularly during warm weather.

Freezing

Freezing is also one of the most commonly used processes, both commercially and domestically, for preserving a very wide range of foods, including prepared foods that would not have required freezing in their unprepared state. For example, potato waffles are stored in the freezer, but potatoes themselves require only a cool dark place to ensure many months' storage. Cold stores provide large-volume, long-term storage for strategic food stocks held in case of national emergency in many countries.

Boiling

Boiling liquid food items can kill any existing microbes. Milk and water are often boiled to kill any harmful microbes that may be present in them.

Heating

Heating to temperatures which are sufficient to kill microorganisms inside the food is a method used with perpetual stews. Milk is also boiled before storing to kill many microorganisms.

Salting

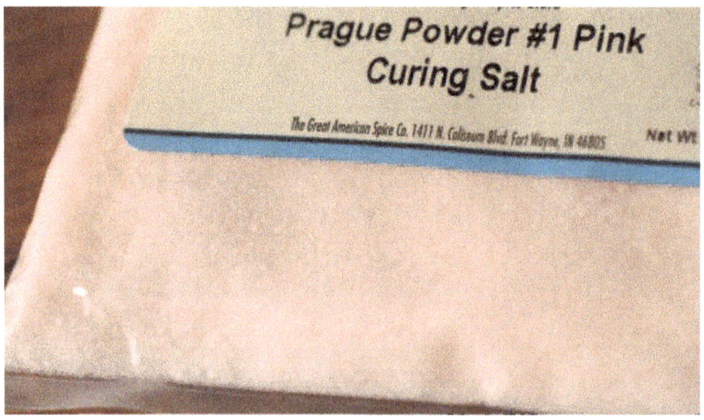

Bag of Prague powder #1, also known as "curing salt" or "pink salt". It is typically a combination of salt and sodium nitrite, with the pink color added to distinguish it from ordinary salt.

Salting or curing draws moisture from a substance through a process of osmosis. substances are cured with salt or sugar, or a combination of the two. Nitrates and nitrites are also often used to cure meat and contribute the characteristic pink colour. It was a main method of preservation in medieval times and around the 1700s.

Sugaring

The earliest cultures have used sugar as a preservative, and it was commonplace to store fruit in honey. Similar to pickled foods, sugar cane was brought to Europe through the trade routes. In northern climates without sufficient sun to dry foods, preserves are made by heating the fruit with sugar. "Sugar tends to draw water from the microbes (plasmolysis). This process leaves the microbial cells dehydrated, thus killing them. In this way, the food will remain safe from microbial spoilage." Sugar is used to preserve fruits, either in an anti-microbial syrup with fruit such as apples, pears, peaches, apricots and plums, or in crystallized form where the preserved material is cooked in sugar to the point of crystallization and the resultant product is then stored dry. This method is used for the skins of citrus fruit (candied peel), angelica and ginger. Also sugaring can be used in jam jellies.

Smoking

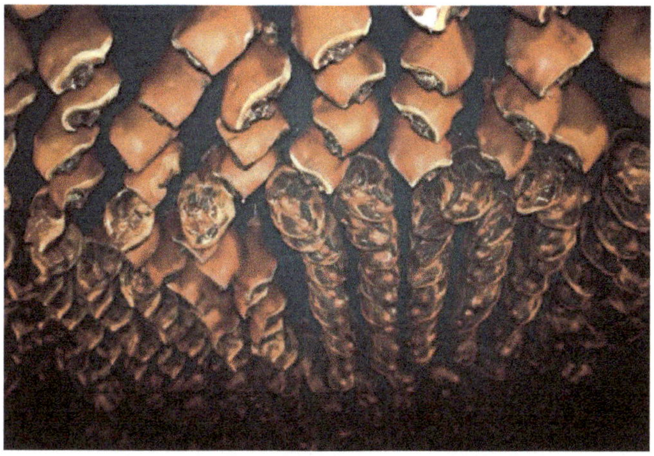

Smoked ham in a smokehouse in Schleswig-Holstein, Germany

Smoking is used to lengthen the shelf life of perishable food items. This effect is achieved by exposing the food to smoke from burning plant materials such as wood. Smoke deposits a number of pyrolysis products onto the food, including the phenols syringol, guaiacol and catechol. These compounds aid in the drying and preservation of meats and other foods. Most commonly subjected to this method of food preservation are meats and fish that have undergone curing. Fruits and vegetables like paprika, cheeses, spices, and ingredients for making drinks such as malt and tea leaves are also smoked, but mainly for cooking or flavoring them. It is one of the oldest food preservation methods, which probably arose after the development of cooking with fire.

Pickling

Pickling is a method of preserving food in an edible anti-microbial liquid. Pickling can be broadly classified into two categories: chemical pickling and fermentation pickling.

In chemical pickling, the food is placed in an edible liquid that inhibits or kills bacteria and other micro-organisms. Typical pickling agents include brine (high in salt), vinegar, alcohol, and vegetable oil, especially olive oil but also many other oils. Many chemical pickling processes also involve heating or boiling so that the food being preserved becomes saturated with the pickling agent. Common chemically pickled foods include cucumbers, peppers, corned beef, herring, and eggs, as well as mixed vegetables such as piccalilli.

In fermentation pickling, the food itself produces the preservation agent, typically by a process that produces lactic acid. Fermented pickles include sauerkraut, nukazuke, kimchi, surströmming,

Lye

Sodium hydroxide (lye) makes food too alkaline for bacterial growth. Lye will saponify fats in the food, which will change its flavor and texture. Lutefisk uses lye in its preparation, as do some olive recipes. Modern recipes for century eggs also call for lye.

Canning

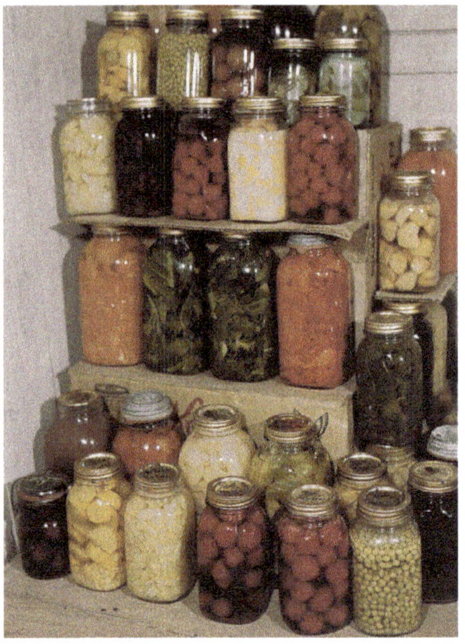

Preserved food

Canning involves cooking food, sealing it in sterile cans or jars, and boiling the containers to kill or weaken any remaining bacteria as a form of sterilization. It was invented by the French confectioner Nicolas Appert. By 1806, this process was used by the French Navy to preserve meat, fruit, vegetables, and even milk. Although Appert had discovered a new way of preservation, it wasn't understood until 1864 when Louis Pasteur found the relationship between microorganisms, food spoilage, and illness.

Foods have varying degrees of natural protection against spoilage and may require that the final step occur in a pressure cooker. High-acid fruits like strawberries require no preservatives to can and only a short boiling cycle, whereas marginal vegetables such as carrots require longer boiling and addition of other acidic elements. Low-acid foods, such as vegetables and meats, require pressure canning. Food preserved by canning or bottling is at immediate risk of spoilage once the can or bottle has been opened.

Lack of quality control in the canning process may allow ingress of water or micro-organisms. Most such failures are rapidly detected as decomposition within the can causes gas production and the can will swell or burst. However, there have been examples of poor manufacture (underprocessing) and poor hygiene allowing contamination of canned food by the obligate anaerobe *Clostridium botulinum*, which produces an acute toxin within the food, leading to severe illness or death. This organism produces no gas or obvious taste and remains undetected by taste or smell. Its toxin is denatured by cooking, however. Cooked mushrooms, handled poorly and then canned, can support the growth of Staphylococcus aureus, which produces a toxin that is not destroyed by canning or subsequent reheating.

Jellying

Food may be preserved by cooking in a material that solidifies to form a gel. Such materials include gelatin, agar, maize flour, and arrowroot flour. Some foods naturally form a protein gel when cooked, such as eels and elvers, and sipunculid worms, which are a delicacy in Xiamen, in the Fujian province of the People's Republic of China. Jellied eels are a delicacy in the East End of London, where they are eaten with mashed potatoes. Potted meats in aspic (a gel made from gelatine and clarified meat broth) were a common way of serving meat off-cuts in the UK until the 1950s. Many jugged meats are also jellied.

A traditional British way of preserving meat (particularly shrimp) is by setting it in a pot and sealing it with a layer of fat. Also common is potted chicken liver; compare pâté.

Jugging

Meat can be preserved by jugging. Jugging is the process of stewing the meat (commonly game or fish) in a covered earthenware jug or casserole. The animal to be jugged is usually cut into pieces, placed into a tightly-sealed jug with brine or gravy, and stewed. Red wine and/or the animal's own blood is sometimes added to the cooking liquid. Jugging was a popular method of preserving meat up until the middle of the 20th century.

Burial

Burial of food can preserve it due to a variety of factors: lack of light, lack of oxygen, cool temperatures, pH level, or desiccants in the soil. Burial may be combined with other methods such as salting or fermentation. Most foods can be preserved in soil that is very dry and salty (thus a desiccant) such as sand, or soil that is frozen.

Many root vegetables are very resistant to spoilage and require no other preservation than storage in cool dark conditions, for example by burial in the ground, such as in a storage clamp. Century eggs are created by placing eggs in alkaline mud (or other alkaline substance), resulting in their "inorganic" fermentation through raised pH instead of spoiling. The fermentation preserves them and breaks down some of the complex, less flavorful proteins and fats into simpler, more flavorful ones. Cabbage was traditionally buried in the fall in northern farms in the U.S. for preservation. Some methods keep it crispy while other methods produce sauerkraut. A similar process is used in the traditional production of kimchi. Sometimes meat is buried under conditions that cause preservation. If buried on hot coals or ashes, the heat can kill pathogens, the dry ash can desiccate, and the earth can block oxygen and further contamination. If buried where the earth is very cold, the earth acts like a refrigerator.

In Orissa, India, it is practical to store rice by burying it underground. This method helps to store for three to six months during the dry season.

Curing

The earliest form of curing was dehydration. To accelerate this process, salt is usually added. In the culinary world, it was common to choose raw salts from various sources (rock salt, sea salt, etc.). More modern "examples of salts that are used as preservatives include sodium chloride (NaCl), sodium nitrate ($NaNO_3$) and sodium nitrite ($NaNO_2$). Even at mild concentrations (up to 2%), sodium chloride, found in many food products, is capable of neutralizing the antimicrobial character of natural compounds."

Fermentation

Some foods, such as many cheeses, wines, and beers, use specific micro-organisms that combat spoilage from other less-benign organisms. These micro-organisms keep pathogens in check by creating an environment toxic for themselves and other micro-organisms by producing acid or alcohol. Methods of fermentation include, but are not limited to, starter micro-organisms, salt, hops, controlled (usually cool) temperatures and controlled (usually low) levels of oxygen. These methods are used to create the specific controlled conditions that will support the desirable organisms that produce food fit for human consumption.

Fermentation is the microbial conversion of starch and sugars into alcohol. Not only can fermentation produce alcohol, but it can also be a valuable preservation technique. Fermentation can also make foods more nutritious and palatable. For example, drinking water in the Middle Ages was dangerous because it often contained pathogens that could spread disease. When the water is made into beer, the boiling during the brewing process kills any bacteria in the water that could make people sick. Additionally, the water now has the nutrients from the barley and other ingredients, and the microorganisms can also produce vitamins as they ferment.

Industrial/modern Techniques

Techniques of food preservation were developed in research laboratories for commercial applications.

Pasteurization

Pasteurization is a process for preservation of liquid food. It was originally applied to combat the souring of young local wines. Today, the process is mainly applied to dairy products. In this method, milk is heated at about 70 °C for 15 to 30 seconds to kill the bacteria present in it and cooling it quickly to 10 °C to prevent the remaining bacteria from growing. The milk is then stored in sterilized bottles or pouches in cold places. This method was invented by Louis Pasteur, a French chemist, in 1862.

Vacuum Packing

Vacuum-packing stores food in a vacuum environment, usually in an air-tight bag or bottle. The vacuum environment strips bacteria of oxygen needed for survival. Vacuum-packing is commonly used for storing nuts to reduce loss of flavor from oxidization. A major drawback to vacuum packaging, at the consumer level, is that vacuum sealing can deform contents and rob certain foods, such as cheese, of its flavor.

Artificial Food Additives

Preservative food additives can be *antimicrobial*, which inhibit the growth of bacteria or fungi, including mold, or *antioxidant*, such as oxygen absorbers, which inhibit the oxidation of food constituents. Common antimicrobial preservatives include calcium propionate, sodium nitrate, sodium nitrite, sulfites (sulfur dioxide, sodium bisulfite, potassium hydrogen sulfite, etc.) and disodium EDTA. Antioxidants include BHA and BHT. Other preservatives include formaldehyde (usually in solution), glutaraldehyde (kills insects), ethanol, and methylchloroisothiazolinone.

Radiation

Irradiation of food is the exposure of food to ionizing radiation. The two types of ionizing radiation used are beta particles (high-energy electrons) and gamma rays (emitted from radioactive sources as cobalt-60 or cesium-137). Treatment effects include killing bacteria, molds, and insect pests, reducing the ripening and spoiling of fruits, and at higher doses inducing sterility. The technology may be compared to pasteurization; it is sometimes called "cold pasteurization", as the product is not heated.

The irradiation process is not directly related to nuclear energy, but does use radioactive isotopes produced in nuclear reactors. Cobalt-60, for example does not occur naturally and can only be produced through neutron bombardment of cobalt-59. Ionizing radiation at high energy levels is hazardous to life (hence its usefulness in sterilisation); for this reason, irradiation facilities have a heavily shielded irradiation room where the process takes place. Radiation safety procedures are used to ensure that neither the workers in such facilities nor the environment receives any radiation dose above administrative limits. Irradiated food does not and cannot become radioactive, and national and international expert bodies have declared food irradiation as wholesome. However, the wholesomeness of consuming such food is disputed by opponents and consumer organizations. National and international expert bodies have declared food irradiation as "wholesome"; organizations of the United Nations, such as the World Health Organization and Food and Agriculture Organization, endorse food irradiation. International legislation on whether food may be irradiated or not varies worldwide from no regulation to full banning. Irradiation may allow lower-quality or contaminated foods to be rendered marketable.

Approximately 500,000 tons of food items are irradiated per year worldwide in over 40 countries. These are mainly spices and condiments with an increasing segment of fresh fruit irradiated for fruit fly quarantine.

Pulsed Electric Field Electroporation

Pulsed electric field (PEF) electroporation is a method for processing cells by means of brief pulses of a strong electric field. PEF holds potential as a type of low-temperature alternative pasteurization process for sterilizing food products. In PEF processing, a substance is placed between two electrodes, then the pulsed electric field is applied. The electric field enlarges the pores of the cell membranes, which kills the cells and releases their contents. PEF for food processing is a developing technology still being researched. There have been limited industrial applications of PEF processing for the pasteurization of fruit juices. To date, several PEF treated juices are available on the market in Europe. Furthermore, for several years a juice pasteurization application in the US has used PEF. For cell disintegration purposes especially potato processors show great interest in PEF technology as an efficient alternative for their preheaters. Potato applications are already operational in the US and Canada. There are also commercial PEF potato applications in various countries in Europe, as well as in Australia, India and China.

Modified Atmosphere

Modifying atmosphere is a way to preserve food by operating on the atmosphere around it. Salad crops that are notoriously difficult to preserve are now being packaged in sealed bags with an atmosphere modified to reduce the oxygen (O_2) concentration and increase the carbon dioxide (CO_2) concentration. There is concern that, although salad vegetables retain their appearance and texture in such conditions, this method of preservation may not retain nutrients, especially vitamins. There are two methods for preserving grains with carbon dioxide. One method is placing a block of dry ice in the bottom and filling the can with the grain. Another method is purging the container from the bottom by gaseous carbon dioxide from a cylinder or bulk supply vessel.

Carbon dioxide prevents insects and, depending on concentration, mold and oxidation from damaging the grain. Grain stored in this way can remain edible for approximately five years.

Nitrogen gas (N_2) at concentrations of 98% or higher is also used effectively to kill insects in the grain through hypoxia. However, carbon dioxide has an advantage in this respect, as it kills organisms through hypercarbia and hypoxia (depending on concentration), but it requires concentrations of above 35%, or so. This makes carbon dioxide preferable for fumigation in situations where a hermetic seal cannot be maintained.

Controlled Atmospheric Storage (CA): "CA storage is a non-chemical process. Oxygen levels in the sealed rooms are reduced, usually by the infusion of nitrogen gas, from the approximate 21 percent in the air we breathe to 1 percent or 2 percent. Temperatures are kept at a constant 0 to 2 °C (32 to 36 °F). Humidity is maintained at 95 percent and carbon dioxide levels are also controlled. Exact conditions in the rooms are set according to the apple variety. Researchers develop specific regimens for each variety to achieve the best quality. Computers help keep conditions constant." "Eastern Washington, where most of Washington's apples are grown, has enough warehouse storage for 181 million boxes of fruit, according to a report done in 1997 by managers for the Washington State Department of Agriculture Plant Services Division. The storage capacity study shows that 67 percent of that space —enough for 121,008,000 boxes of apples — is CA storage."

Air-tight storage of grains (sometimes called hermetic storage) relies on the respiration of grain, insects, and fungi that can modify the enclosed atmosphere sufficiently to control insect pests. This is a method of great antiquity, as well as having modern equivalents. The success of the method relies on having the correct mix of sealing, grain moisture, and temperature.

A patented process uses fuel cells to exhaust and automatically maintain the exhaustion of oxygen in a shipping container, containing, for example, fresh fish.

Nonthermal Plasma

This process subjects the surface of food to a "flame" of ionized gas molecules, such as helium or nitrogen. This causes micro-organisms to die off on the surface.

High-pressure Food Preservation

High-pressure food preservation or pascalization refers to the use of a food preservation technique that makes use of high pressure. "Pressed inside a vessel exerting 70,000 pounds per square inch (480 MPa) or more, food can be processed so that it retains its fresh appearance, flavor, texture and nutrients while disabling harmful microorganisms and slowing spoilage." By 2005, the process was being used for products ranging from orange juice to guacamole to deli meats and widely sold.

Biopreservation

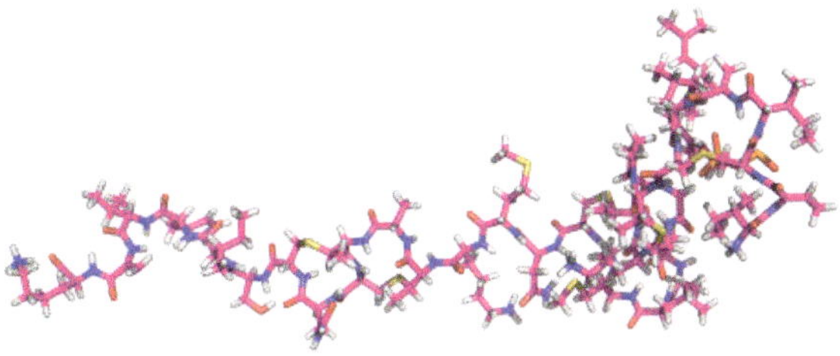

3D stick model of nisin. Some lactic acid bacteria manufacture nisin. It is a particularly effective preservative.

Biopreservation is the use of natural or controlled microbiota or antimicrobials as a way of preserving food and extending its shelf life. Beneficial bacteria or the fermentation products produced by these bacteria are used in biopreservation to control spoilage and render pathogens inactive in food. It is a benign ecological approach which is gaining increasing attention.

Of special interest are lactic acid bacteria (LAB). Lactic acid bacteria have antagonistic properties that make them particularly useful as biopreservatives. When LABs compete for nutrients, their metabolites often include active antimicrobials such as lactic acid, acetic acid, hydrogen peroxide, and peptide bacteriocins. Some LABs produce the antimicrobial nisin, which is a particularly effective preservative.

These days, LAB bacteriocins are used as an integral part of hurdle technology. Using them in combination with other preservative techniques can effectively control spoilage bacteria and other pathogens, and can inhibit the activities of a wide spectrum of organisms, including inherently resistant Gram-negative bacteria.

Hurdle Technology

Hurdle technology is a method of ensuring that pathogens in food products can be eliminated or controlled by combining more than one approach. These approaches can be thought of as "hurdles" the pathogen has to overcome if it is to remain active in the food. The right combination of hurdles can ensure all pathogens are eliminated or rendered harmless in the final product.

Hurdle technology has been defined by Leistner (2000) as an intelligent combination of hurdles that secures the microbial safety and stability as well as the organoleptic and nutritional quality and the economic viability of food products. The organoleptic quality of the food refers to its sensory properties, that is its look, taste, smell, and texture.

Examples of hurdles in a food system are high temperature during processing, low temperature during storage, increasing the acidity, lowering the water activity or redox potential, and the presence of preservatives or biopreservatives. According to the type of pathogens and how risky they are, the intensity of the hurdles can be adjusted individually to meet consumer preferences in an economical way, without sacrificing the safety of the product.

Principal hurdles used for food preservation (after Leistner, 1995)		
Parameter	**Symbol**	**Application**
High temperature	F	Heating

Low temperature	T	Chilling, freezing
Reduced water activity	a_w	Drying, curing, conserving
Increased acidity	pH	Acid addition or formation
Reduced redox potential	E_h	Removal of oxygen or addition of ascorbate
Biopreservatives		Competitive flora such as microbial fermentation
Other preservatives		Sorbates, sulfites, nitrites

Food Preservation Techniques

Food Drying

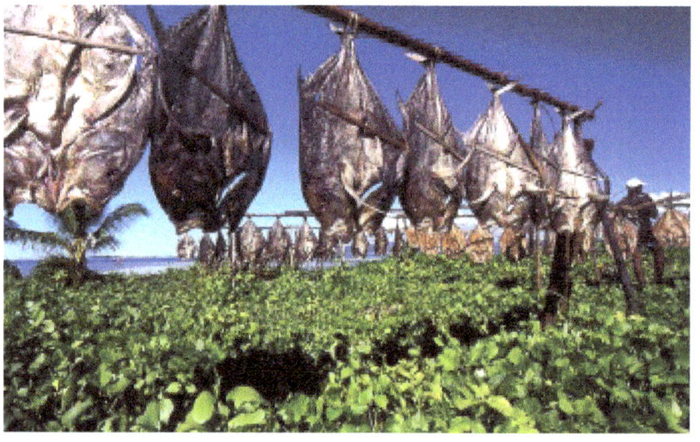

Flattened fish drying in the sun in Madagascar. Fish are preserved through such traditional methods as drying, smoking and salting.

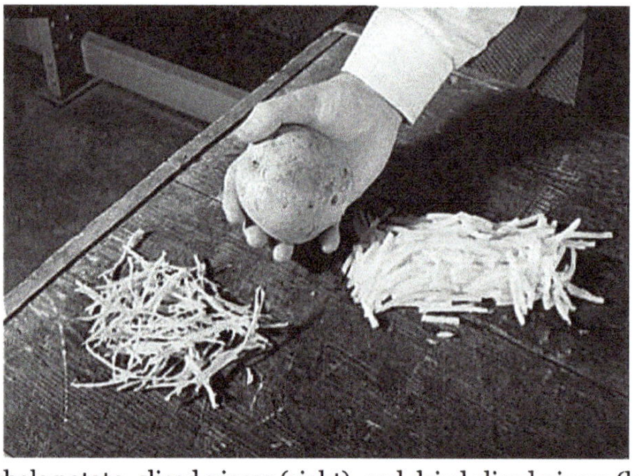

A whole potato, sliced pieces (right), and dried sliced pieces (left)

Food drying is a method of food preservation in which food is dried (dehydrated or desiccated). Drying inhibits the growth of bacteria, yeasts, and mold through the removal of water. Dehydration has been used widely for this purpose since ancient times; the earliest known practice is 12,000 B.C. by inhabitants of the modern Middle East and Asia regions. Water is traditionally removed through evaporation (air drying, sun drying, smoking or wind drying), although today electric food dehydrators or freeze-drying can be used to speed the drying process and ensure more consistent results.

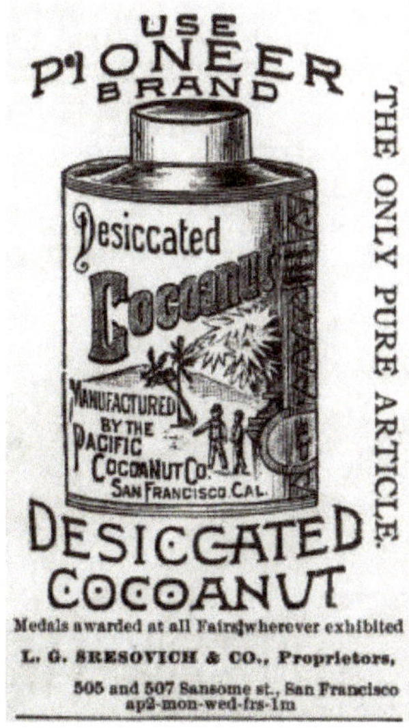

1890 newspaper advertisement showing tin of dried coconut

Food Types

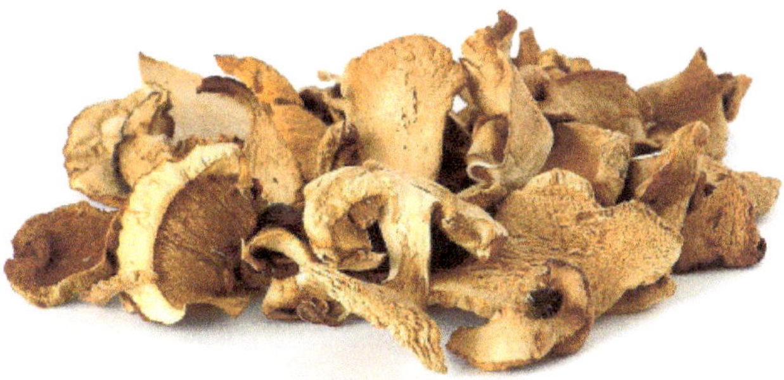

A collection of dried mushrooms

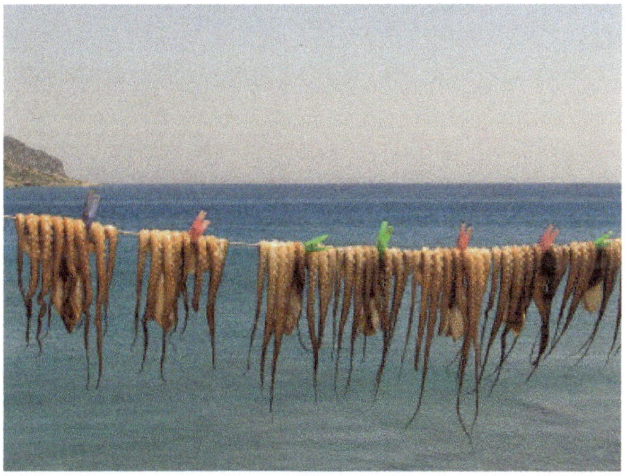

Sun-drying octopus

Many different foods can be prepared by dehydration. Meat has held an historically significant role. For centuries, much of the European diet depended on dried cod—known as salt cod, bacalhau (with salt), or stockfish (without). It formed the main protein source for the slaves on the West Indian plantations, and was a major economic force within the triangular trade. Dried shark meat, known as Hákarl, is a delicacy in Iceland, while dried reindeer meat is a traditional Sami food. Currently popular dried meats include prosciutto (a.k.a. Parma ham), bresaola, and beef jerky.

Fruits change character completely when dried. The plum becomes a prune, the grape a raisin. Figs and dates are also transformed into new, different products that can either be eaten as they are or rehydrated. However, dehydrated fruit may be nutritionally inferior to its source.

Freeze-dried vegetables are often found in food for backpackers, hunters, and the military. Garlic and onion are often dried. Edible mushrooms, as well as other fungi, are also sometimes dried for preservation purposes or to be used as seasonings.

Preparation

Home drying of vegetables, fruit and meat can be carried out with electrical dehydrators (household appliance) or by sun-drying or by wind. Preservatives such as potassium metabisulfite, BHA, or BHT may be used, but are not required. However, dried products without these preservatives may require refrigeration or freezing to ensure safe storage for a long time.

Industrial food dehydration is often accomplished by freeze-drying. In this case food is flash frozen and put into a reduced-pressure system which causes the water to sublimate directly from the solid to the gaseous phase. Although freeze-drying is more expensive than traditional dehydration techniques, it also mitigates the change in flavor, texture, and nutritional value.In addition, another widely used industrial method of drying of food is convective hot air drying. Industrial hot air dryers are simple and easy to design, construct and maintain. More so, it is very affordable and has been reported to retain most of the nutritional properties of food if dry using appropriate drying conditions.

Other Methods

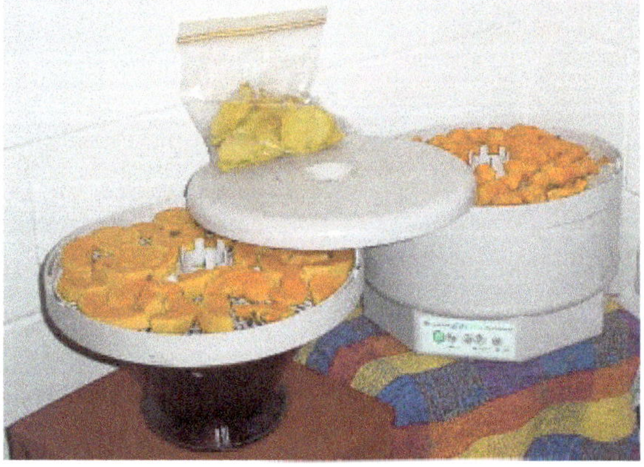

This electric food dehydrator has a hot air blower that blows air through trays with foods on them. Pictured are mango and papaya slices being dried.

There are many different methods for drying, each with their own advantages for particular applications; these include:

- Convection drying
- Bed dryers

- Drum drying
- Freeze Drying
- Microwave-vacuum drying
- Shelf dryers
- Spray drying
- Infrared radiation drying
- Sunlight
- Commercial food dehydrators
- Household oven

Refrigeration

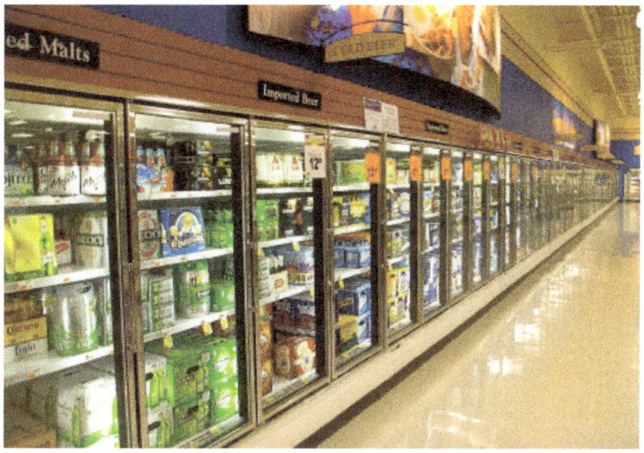

Commercial refrigeration

Refrigeration is a process of moving heat from one location to another in controlled conditions. The work of heat transport is traditionally driven by mechanical work, but can also be driven by heat, magnetism, electricity, laser, or other means. Refrigeration has many applications, including, but not limited to: household refrigerators, industrial freezers, cryogenics, and air conditioning. Heat pumps may use the heat output of the refrigeration process, and also may be designed to be reversible, but are otherwise similar to air conditioning units.

Refrigeration has had a large impact on industry, lifestyle, agriculture and settlement patterns. The idea of preserving food dates back to at least the ancient Roman and Chinese empires. However, mechanical refrigeration technology has rapidly evolved in the last century, from ice harvesting to temperature-controlled rail cars. The introduction of refrigerated rail cars contributed to the westward expansion of the United States, allowing settlement in areas that were not on main transport channels such as rivers, harbors, or valley trails. Settlements were also developing in infertile parts of the country, filled with new natural resources. These new settlement patterns sparked the building of large cities which are able to thrive in areas that were otherwise thought to be inhospitable, such as Houston, Texas and Las Vegas, Nevada. In most developed countries, cities are heavily dependent upon refrigeration in supermarkets, in order to obtain their food for daily consumption. The increase in food sources has led to a larger concentration of agricultural sales coming from a smaller percentage of existing farms. Farms today have a much larger output per person in comparison to the late 1800s. This has resulted in new food sources available to entire populations, which has had a large impact on the nutrition of society.

History

Earliest Forms of Cooling

The seasonal harvesting of snow and ice is an ancient practice estimated to have begun earlier than 1000 B.C. A Chinese collection of lyrics from this time period known as the Shih king, describes religious ceremonies for filling and emptying ice cellars. However, little is known about the construction of these ice cellars or what the ice was used for. The next ancient society to harvest ice may have been the Jews according to the book of Proverbs, which reads, "As the cold of snow in the time of harvest, so is a faithful messenger to them who sent him." Historians have interpreted this to mean that the Jews used ice to cool beverages rather than to preserve food. Other ancient cultures such as the Greeks and the Romans dug large snow pits insulated with grass, chaff, or branches of trees as cold storage. Like the Jews, the Greeks and Romans did not use ice and snow to preserve food, but primarily as a means to cool beverages. The Egyptians also developed methods to cool beverages, but in lieu of using ice to cool water, the Egyptians cooled water by putting boiling water in shallow earthen jars and placing them on the roofs of their houses at night. Slaves would moisten the outside of the jars and the resulting evaporation would cool the water. The ancient people of India used this same concept to produce ice. The Persians stored ice in a pit called a Yakhchal and may have been the first group of people to use cold storage to preserve food. In the Australian outback before a reliable electricity supply was available where the weather could be hot and dry, many farmers used a "Coolgardie safe". This consisted of a room with hessian "curtains" hanging from the ceiling soaked in water. The water would evaporate and thereby cool the hessian curtains and thereby the air circulating in the room. This would allow many perishables such as fruit, butter, and cured meats to be kept that would normally spoil in the heat.

Ice Harvesting

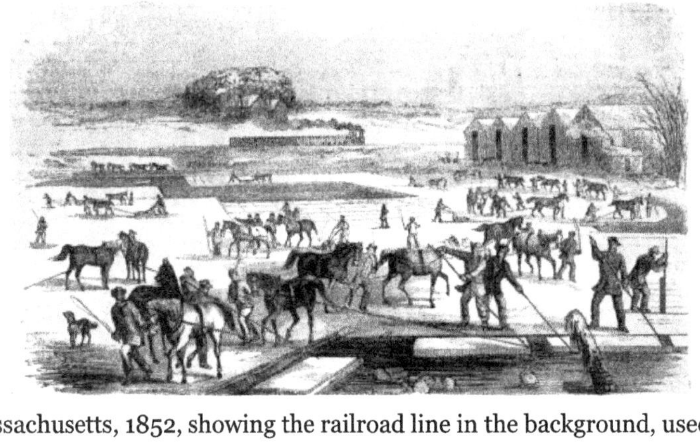

Ice harvesting in Massachusetts, 1852, showing the railroad line in the background, used to transport the ice.

Before 1830, few Americans used ice to refrigerate foods due to a lack of ice-storehouses and ice-boxes. As these two things became more widely available, individuals used axes and saws to harvest ice for their storehouses. This method proved to be difficult, dangerous, and certainly did not resemble anything that could be duplicated on a commercial scale.

Despite the difficulties of harvesting ice, Frederic Tudor thought that he could capitalize on this new commodity by harvesting ice in New England and shipping it to the Caribbean islands as well as the southern states. In the beginning, Tudor lost thousands of dollars, but eventually turned a profit as he constructed icehouses in Charleston, Virginia and in the Cuban port town of Havana. These icehouses as well as better insulated ships helped reduce ice wastage from 66% to 8%. This efficiency gain influenced Tudor to expand his ice market to other towns with icehouses such as New Orleans and Savannah. This ice market further expanded as harvesting ice became faster and cheaper after one of Tudor's suppliers, Nathaniel Wyeth, invented a horse-drawn ice cutter in 1825. This invention as well as Tudor's success inspired others to get involved in the ice trade and the ice industry grew.

Ice became a mass-market commodity by the early 1830s with the price of ice dropping from six cents per pound to a half of a cent per pound. In New York City, ice consumption increased from 12,000 tons in 1843 to 100,000 tons in 1856. Boston's consumption leapt from 6,000 tons to 85,000 tons during that same period. Ice harvesting created a "cooling culture" as majority of people used ice and iceboxes to store their dairy products, fish, meat, and even fruits and vegetables. These early cold storage practices paved the way for many Americans to accept the refrigeration technology that would soon take over the country.

Refrigeration Research

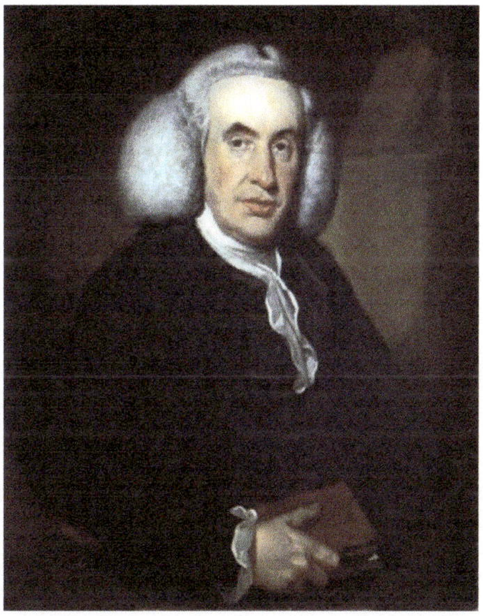

William Cullen, the first to conduct experiments into artificial refrigeration.

The history of artificial refrigeration began when Scottish professor William Cullen designed a small refrigerating machine in 1755. Cullen used a pump to create a partial vacuum over a container of diethyl ether, which then boiled, absorbing heat from the surrounding air. The experiment even created a small amount of ice, but had no practical application at that time.

In 1758, Benjamin Franklin and John Hadley, professor of chemistry, collaborated on a project investigating the principle of evaporation as a means to rapidly cool an object at Cambridge University, England. They confirmed that the evaporation of highly volatile liquids, such as alcohol and ether, could be used to drive down the temperature of an object past the freezing point of water. They conducted their experiment with the bulb of a mercury thermometer as their object and with a bellows used to "quicken" the evaporation; they lowered the temperature of the thermometer bulb down to 7 °F (−14 °C), while the ambient temperature was 65 °F (18 °C). They noted that soon after they passed the freezing point of water (32 °F), a thin film of ice formed on the surface of the thermometer's bulb and that the ice mass was about a quarter inch thick when they stopped the experiment upon reaching 7 °F (−14 °C). Franklin wrote, "From this experiment, one may see the possibility of freezing a man to death on a warm summer's day". In 1805, American inventor Oliver Evans described a closed vapor-compression refrigeration cycle for the production of ice by ether under vacuum.

In 1820, the English scientist Michael Faraday liquefied ammonia and other gases by using high pressures and low temperatures, and in 1834, an American expatriate to Great Britain, Jacob Perkins, built the first working vapor-compression refrigeration system in the world. It was a closed-cycle that could operate continuously, as he described in his patent:

> I am enabled to use volatile fluids for the purpose of producing the cooling or freezing of fluids, and yet at the same time constantly condensing such volatile fluids, and bringing them again into operation without waste.

His prototype system worked although it did not succeed commercially.

In 1842, a similar attempt was made by American physician, John Gorrie, who built a working prototype, but it was a commercial failure. Like many of the medical experts during this time, Gorrie thought too much exposure to tropical heat led to mental and physical degeneration, as well as the spread of diseases such as malaria. He conceived the idea of using his refrigeration system to cool the air for comfort in homes and hospitals to prevent disease. American engineer Alexander Twining took out a British patent in 1850 for a vapour compression system that used ether.

The first practical vapor compression refrigeration system was built by James Harrison, a British journalist who had emigrated to Australia. His 1856 patent was for a vapour compression system using ether, alcohol or ammonia. He built a mechanical ice-making machine in 1851 on the banks of the Barwon River at Rocky Point in Geelong, Victoria, and his first commercial ice-making machine followed in 1854. Harrison also introduced commercial vapour-compression refrigeration to breweries and meat packing houses, and by 1861, a dozen of his systems were in operation. He later entered the debate of how to compete against the American advantage of unrefrigerated beef sales to the United Kingdom. In 1873 he prepared the sailing ship *Norfolk* for an experimental beef shipment to the United Kingdom, which used a cold room system instead of a refrigeration system. The venture was a failure as the ice was consumed faster than expected.

The first gas absorption refrigeration system using gaseous ammonia dissolved in water (referred to as "aqua ammonia") was developed by Ferdinand Carré of France in 1859 and patented in 1860. Carl von Linde, an engineer specializing in steam locomotives and professor of engineering at the Technological University of Munich in Germany, began researching refrigeration in the 1860s and 1870s in response to demand from brewers for a technology that would allow year-round, large-scale production of lager; he patented an improved method of liquefying gases in 1876. His new process made possible using gases such as ammonia, sulfur dioxide (SO_2) and methyl chloride (CH_3Cl) as refrigerants and they were widely used for that purpose until the late 1920s.

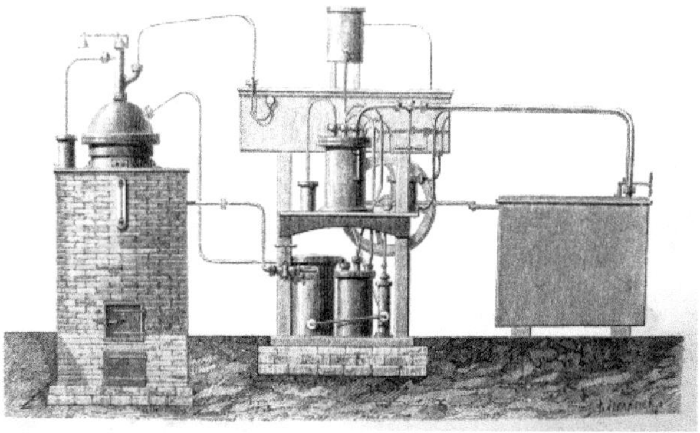

Ferdinand Carré's ice-making device

Thaddeus Lowe, an American balloonist, held several patents on ice-making machines. His "Compression Ice Machine" would revolutionize the cold-storage industry. In 1869, other investors and he purchased an old steamship onto which they loaded one of Lowe's refrigeration units and began shipping fresh fruit from New York to the Gulf Coast area, and fresh meat from Galveston, Texas back to New York, but because of Lowe's lack of knowledge about shipping, the business was a costly failure.

Commercial Use

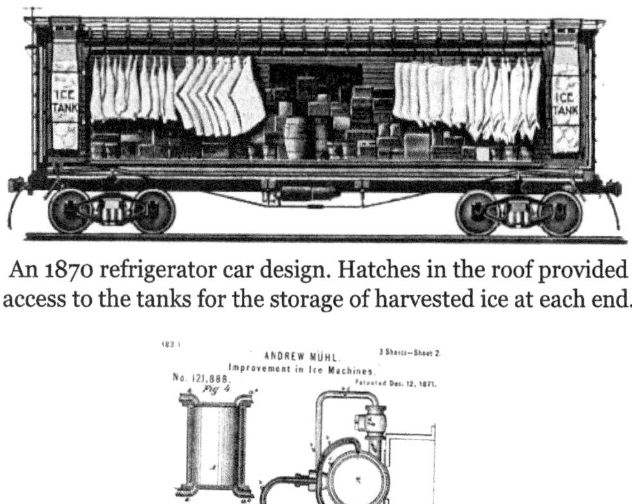

An 1870 refrigerator car design. Hatches in the roof provided access to the tanks for the storage of harvested ice at each end.

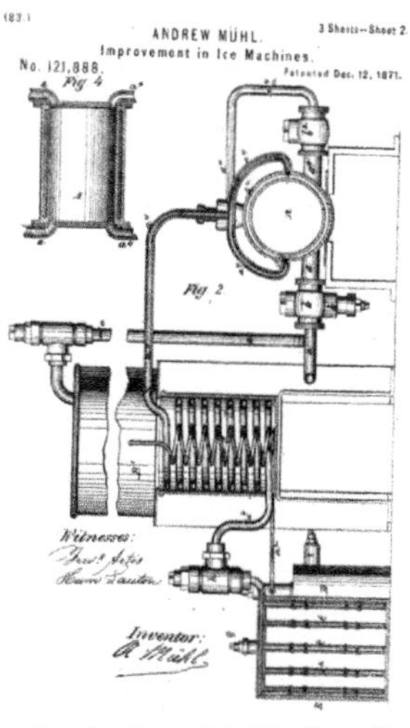

Icemaker Patent by Andrew Muhl, dated December 12, 1871.

In 1842, John Gorrie created a system capable of refrigerating water to produce ice. Although it was a commercial failure, it inspired scientists and inventors around the world. France's Ferdinand Carre was one of the inspired and he created an ice producing system that was simpler and smaller than that of Gorrie. During the Civil War, cities such as New Orleans could no longer get ice from New England via the coastal ice trade. Carre's refrigeration system became the solution to New Orleans ice problems and by 1865 the city had three of Carre's machines. In 1867, in San Antonio, Texas, a French immigrant named Andrew Muhl built an ice-making machine to help service the expanding beef industry before moving it to Waco in 1871. In 1873, the patent for this machine was contracted by the Columbus Iron Works, a company acquired by the W. C. Bradley Co., which went on to produce the first commercial ice-makers in the US.

By the 1870s, breweries had become the largest users of harvested ice. Though the ice-harvesting industry had grown immensely by the turn of the 20th century, pollution and sewage had begun to creep into natural ice, making it a problem in the metropolitan suburbs. Eventually, breweries began to complain of tainted ice. Public concern for the purity of water, from which ice was formed, began to increase in the early 1900s with the rise of germ theory. Numerous media outlets published articles connecting diseases such as typhoid fever with natural ice consumption. This caused ice harvesting to become illegal in certain areas of the country. All of these scenarios increased the demands for modern refrigeration and manufactured ice. Ice producing machines like that of Carre's and Muhl's were looked to as means of producing ice to meet the needs of grocers, farmers, and food shippers.

Refrigerated railroad cars were introduced in the US in the 1840s for short-run transport of dairy products, but these used harvested ice to maintain a cool temperature.

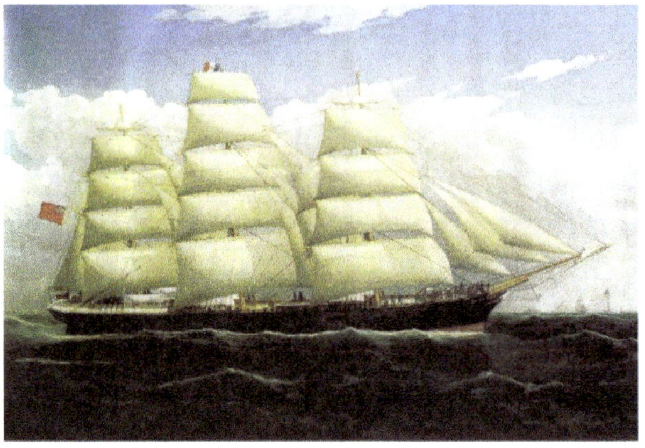

Dunedin, the first commercially successful refrigerated ship.

The new refrigerating technology first met with widespread industrial use as a means to freeze meat supplies for transport by sea from the British Dominions and other countries to the British Isles. The first to achieve this breakthrough was an entrepreneur who had emigrated to New Zealand. William Soltau Davidson thought that Britain's rising population and meat demand could mitigate the slump in world wool markets that was heavily affecting New Zealand. After extensive research, he commissioned the *Dunedin* to be refitted with a compression refrigeration unit for meat shipment in 1881. On February 15, 1882, the *Dunedin* sailed for London with what was to be the first commercially successful refrigerated shipping voyage, and the foundation of the refrigerated meat industry.

The Times commented "Today we have to record such a triumph over physical difficulties, as would have been incredible, even unimaginable, a very few days ago...". The *Marlborough*—sister ship to the *Dunedin* – was immediately converted and joined the trade the following year, along with the rival New Zealand Shipping Company vessel *Mataurua*, while the German Steamer *Marsala* began carrying frozen New Zealand lamb in December 1882. Within five years, 172 shipments of frozen meat were sent from New Zealand to the United Kingdom, of which only 9 had significant amounts of meat condemned. Refrigerated shipping also led to a broader meat and dairy boom in Australasia and South America. J & E Hall of Dartford, England outfitted the 'SS Selembria' with a vapor compression system to bring 30,000 carcasses of mutton from the Falkland Islands in 1886. In the years ahead, the industry rapidly expanded to Australia, Argentina and the United States.

By the 1890s, refrigeration played a vital role in the distribution of food. The meat-packing industry relied heavily on natural ice in the 1880s and continued to rely on manufactured ice as those technologies became available. By 1900, the meat-packing houses of Chicago had adopted ammonia-cycle commercial refrigeration. By 1914, almost every location used artificial refrigeration. The big meat-packers, Armour, Swift, and Wilson, had purchased the most expensive units which they installed on train cars and in branch houses and storage facilities in the more remote distribution areas.

By the middle of the 20th century, refrigeration units were designed for installation on trucks or lorries. Refrigerated vehicles are used to transport perishable goods, such as frozen foods, fruit and vegetables, and temperature-sensitive chemicals. Most modern refrigerators keep the temperature between −40 and −20 °C, and have a maximum payload of around 24,000 kg gross weight (in Europe).

Although commercial refrigeration quickly progressed, it had limitations that prevented it from moving into the household. First, most refrigerators were far too large. Some of the commercial units being used in 1910 weighed between five and two hundred tons. Second, commercial refrigerators were expensive to produce, purchase, and maintain. Lastly, these refrigerators were unsafe. It was not uncommon for commercial refrigerators to catch fire, explode, or leak toxic gases. Refrigeration did not become a household technology until these three challenges were overcome.

Home and Consumer Use

During the early 1800s, consumers preserved their food by storing food and ice purchased from ice harvesters in iceboxes. In 1803, Thomas Moore patented a metal-lined butter-storage tub which became the prototype for most iceboxes. These iceboxes were used until nearly 1910 and the technology did not progress. In fact, consumers that used the icebox in 1910 faced the same challenge of a moldy and stinky icebox that consumers had in the early 1800s.

General Electric (GE) was one of the first companies to overcome these challenges. In 1911, GE released a household refrigeration unit that was powered by gas. The use of gas eliminated the need for motor and decreased the size of the refrigerator. However, electric companies that were customers of GE did not benefit from a gas-powered unit. Thus, GE invested in developing an electric model. In 1927, GE released the Monitor Top, the first refrigerator to run off electricity.

In 1930, Frigidaire, one of GE's main competitors, synthesized Freon. With the invention of synthetic refrigerants based mostly on a chlorofluorocarbon (CFC) chemical, safer refrigerators were possible for home and consumer use. Freon led to the development of smaller, lighter, and cheaper refrigerators. The average price of a refrigerator dropped from $275 to $154 with the synthesis of Freon. This lower price allowed ownership of refrigerators in American households to exceed 50%. Freon is a trademark of the DuPont Corporation and refers to these CFCs, and later hydro chlorofluorocarbon (HCFC) and hydro fluorocarbon (HFC), refrigerants developed in the late 1920s. These refrigerants were considered at the time to be less harmful than the commonly-used refrigerants of the time, including methyl formate, ammonia, methyl chloride, and sulfur dioxide. The intent was to provide refrigeration equipment for home use without danger. These CFC refrigerants answered that need. In the 1970s, though, the compounds were found to be reacting with atmospheric ozone, an important protection against solar ultraviolet radiation, and their use as a refrigerant worldwide was curtailed in the Montreal Protocol of 1987.

Impact on Settlement Patterns

In the last century refrigeration allowed new settlement patterns to emerge. This new technology has allowed for new areas to be settled that are not on a natural channel of transport such as a river, valley trail or harbor that may have otherwise not been settled. Refrigeration has given opportunities to early settlers to expand westward and into rural areas that were unpopulated. These new settlers with rich and untapped soil saw opportunity to profit by sending raw goods to the eastern cities and states. In the 20th century, refrigeration has made "Galactic Cities" such as Dallas, Phoenix and Los Angeles possible.

Refrigerated Rail Cars

The refrigerated rail car, along with the dense railroad network, became an exceedingly important link between the marketplace and the farm allowing for a national opportunity rather than a just a regional one. Before the invention of the refrigerated rail car it was impossible to ship perishable food products long distances. The beef packing industry made the first demand push for refrigeration cars. The railroad companies were slow to adopt this new invention because of their heavy investments in cattle cars, stockyards, and feedlots. Refrigeration cars were also complex and costly compared to other rail cars, which also slowed the adoption of the refrigerated rail car. After the slow adoption of the refrigerated car, the beef packing industry dominated the refrigerated rail car business with their ability to control ice plants and the setting of icing fees. The United States Department of Agriculture estimated that in 1916 over sixty-nine percent of the cattle killed in the country was done in plants involved in interstate trade. The same companies that were also involved in the meat trade later implemented refrigerated transport to include vegetables and fruit. The meat packing companies had much of the expensive machinery, such as refrigerated cars, and cold storage facilities that allowed for them to effectively distribute all types of perishable goods. During World War I, a national refrigerator car pool was established by the United States Administration to deal with problem of idle cars and was later continued after the war. The idle car problem was the problem of refrigeration cars sitting pointlessly in between seasonal harvests. This meant that very expensive cars sat in rail yards for a good portion of the year while making no revenue for the car's owner. The car pool was a system where cars were distributed to areas as crops matured ensuring maximum use of the cars. Refrigerated rail cars moved eastward from vineyards, orchards, fields, and gardens in western states to satisfy Americas consuming market in the east.

The refrigerated car made it possible to transport perishable crops hundreds and even thousands of miles. The most noticeable effect the car gave was a regional specialization of vegetables and fruits. The refrigeration rail car was widely used for the transportation of perishable goods up until the 1950s. By the 1960s the nation's interstate highway system was adequately complete allowing for trucks to carry the majority of the perishable food loads and to push out the old system of the refrigerated rail cars.

Expansion west and into Rural Areas

The widespread use of refrigeration allowed for a vast amount of new agricultural opportunities to open up in the United States. New markets emerged throughout the United States in areas that were previously uninhabited and far-removed from heavily populated areas. New agricultural opportunity presented itself in areas that were considered rural such as states in the south and in the west. Shipments on a large scale from the south and California were both made around the same time although natural ice was used from the Sierras in California rather than manufactured ice in the south. Refrigeration allowed for many areas to specialize in the growing of specific fruits. California specialized in several fruits, grapes, peaches, pears, plums, and apples while Georgia became famous for specifically its peaches. In California, the acceptance of the refrigerated rail carts lead to an increase of car loads from 4,500 carloads in 1895 to between 8,000 and 10,000 carloads in 1905. The Gulf States, Arkansas, Missouri and Tennessee entered into strawberry production on a large-scale while Mississippi became the center of the tomato industry. New Mexico, Colorado, Arizona, and Nevada grew cantaloupes. Without refrigeration this would have not been possible. By 1917, well-established fruit and vegetable areas that were close to eastern markets felt the pressure of competition from these distant specialized centers. Refrigeration was not limited to meat, fruit and vegetables but it also encompassed dairy product and dairy farms. In the early twentieth century large cities got their dairy supply from farms as far as 400 miles. Dairy products were not as easily transported great distances like fruits and vegetables due to greater perishability. Refrigeration made production possible in the west far from eastern markets, so much in fact that dairy farmers could pay transportation cost and still undersell their eastern competitors. Refrigeration and the refrigerated rail gave opportunity to areas with rich soil far from natural channel of transport such as a river, valley trail or harbors.

Rise of the Galactic City

"Edge city" was a term coined by Joel Garreau, whereas the term "galactic city" was coined by Lewis Mumford. These terms refer to a concentration of business, shopping, and entertainment outside a traditional downtown or central business district in what had previously been a residential or rural area. There were several factors contributing to the growth of these cities such as Los Angeles, Las Vegas, Houston, and Phoenix. The factors that contributed to these large cities include reliable automobiles, highway systems, refrigeration, and agricultural production increases. Large cities such as the ones mentioned above have not been uncommon in history but what separates these cities from the rest are that these cities are not along some natural channel of transport, or at some crossroad of two or more channels such as a trail, harbor, mountain, river, or valley. These large cities have been developed in areas that only a few hundred years ago would have been uninhabitable. Without a cost efficient way of cooling air and transporting water and food great distances these large cities would have never developed. The rapid growth of these cities was influenced by refrigeration and an agricultural productivity increase, allowing more distant farms to effectively feed the population.

Impact on Agriculture and Food Production

Agriculture's role in developed countries has drastically changed in the last century due to many factors, including refrigeration. Statistics from the 2007 census gives information on the large concentration of agricultural sales coming from a small portion of the existing farms in the United States today. This is a partial result of the market created for the frozen meat trade by the first successful shipment of frozen sheep carcasses coming from New Zealand in the 1880s. As the market continued to grow, regulations on food processing and quality began to be enforced. Eventually, electricity was introduced into rural homes in the United States, which allowed refrigeration technology to continue to expand on the farm, increasing output per person. Today, refrigeration's use on the farm reduces humidity levels, avoids spoiling due to bacterial growth, and assists in preservation.

Demographics

The introduction of refrigeration and evolution of additional technologies drastically changed agriculture in the United States. During the beginning of the 20th century, farming was a common occupation and lifestyle for United States citizens, as most farmers actually lived on their farm. In 1935, there were 6.8 million farms in the United States and a population of 127 million. Yet, while the United States population has continued to climb, citizens pursuing agriculture continue to decline. Based on the 2007 US Census, less than one percent of a population of 310 million people claim farming as an occupation today. However, the increasing population has led to an increasing demand for agricultural products, which is met through a greater variety of crops, fertilizers, pesticides, and improved technology. Improved technology has decreased the risk and time involved if agricultural management and allows larger farms to increase their output per person to meet society's demand.

Meat packing and Trade

Prior to 1882, the South Island of New Zealand had been experimenting with sowing grass and crossbreeding sheep, which immediately gave their farmers economic potential in the exportation of meat. In 1882, the first successful shipment of sheep carcasses was sent from Port Chalmers in Dunedin, New Zealand to London. By the 1890s, the frozen meat trade became increasingly more profitable in New Zealand, especially in Canterbury, where 50% of exported sheep carcasses came from in 1900. It wasn't long before Canterbury meat was known for the highest quality, creating a demand for New Zealand meat around the world. In order to meet this new demand, the farmers improved their feed so sheep to be ready for the slaughter in only seven months. This new method of shipping lead to an economic boom in New Zealand by the mid 1890s.

In the United States, the Meat Inspection Act of 1891 was put in place in the United States because local butchers felt the refrigerated railcar system was unwholesome. When meat packing began to take off, consumers became nervous about the quality of the meat for consumption. The Jungle, a book written by Upton Sinclair, brought negative attention to the meat packing industry, by drawing to light unsanitary working conditions and processing of diseased animals. The book caught the attention of President Theodore Roosevelt, and the 1906 Meat Inspection Act was put into place as an amendment to the Meat Inspection Act of 1891. This new act focused on the quality of the meat and environment it is processed in.

Electricity in Rural Areas

In the early 1930s, 90 percent of the urban population had electric power, in comparison to only 10 percent of rural homes. At the time, power companies did not feel that extending power to rural areas would produce enough profit to make it worth their while. However, in the midst of the Great Depression, President Franklin D. Roosevelt realized that rural areas would continue to lag behind urban areas in both poverty and production if they were not electrically wired. On May 11, 1935, the president signed an executive order called the Rural Electrification Administration, also known as REA. The agency provided loans to fund electric infrastructure in the rural areas. In just a few years, 300,000 people in rural areas of the United States had received power in their homes.

While electricity dramatically improved working conditions on farms, it also had a large impact on the safety of food production. Refrigeration systems were introduced to the farming process, which helped in food preservation and kept food supplies safe. Refrigeration also allowed for production of perishable commodities, which could then be shipped throughout the United States. As a result, the United States farmers quickly became the most productive in the world.

Farm Use

In order to reduce humidity levels and spoiling due to bacterial growth, refrigeration is used for meat, produce, and dairy processing in farming today. Refrigeration systems are used the heaviest in the warmer months for farming produce, which must be cooled as soon as possible in order to meet quality standards and increase the shelf life. Meanwhile, dairy farms refrigerate milk year round to avoid spoiling.

Effects on Lifestyle and Diet

A trip to the market before refrigeration became widespread would have been different from a trip today. In the late 19th Century and into the very early 20th Century, other than staple foods (sugar, rice, and beans), your diet was affected heavily by the seasons and what could be grown relatively close to your region. Today, thanks to refrigeration, we are no longer restricted by these limitations. Refrigeration played a large part in the feasibility and then popularity of the modern supermarket. If you are willing to pay slightly more for a fruit or vegetable that is out of season in your region, your local supermarket will most likely have what you are looking for. Refrigerators have led to a huge increase in meat and dairy as a portion of overall supermarket sales. As well as changing the goods purchased at the market, the ability to store these foods for extended periods of time has led to an increase in leisure time. Prior to the advent of the household refrigerator, people would have to shop on a daily basis for the supplies needed for their meals.

Impact on Nutrition

The introduction of refrigeration allowed for the hygienic handling and storage of perishables, and as such, promoted output growth, consumption, and nutrition. The change in our method of food preservation moved us away from salts to a more manageable sodium level. The ability to move and store perishables such as meat and dairy led to a 1.7% increase in dairy consumption and overall protein intake by 1.25% annually in the US after the 1890s. People were not only consuming these perishables because it became easier for they themselves to store them, but because the innovations in refrigerated transportation and storage led to less spoilage and waste, and drove the prices of these products down. Refrigeration accounts for at least 5.1% of the increase in adult stature (in the US) through improved nutrition including the indirect effects associated with improvements in the quality of nutrients and the reduction in illness, the overall impact was considerably larger. Recent studies have also shown a negative relationship between the number of refrigerators in a household and the rate of gastric cancer mortality.

Current Applications of Refrigeration

Probably the most widely used current applications of refrigeration are for air conditioning of private homes and public buildings, and refrigerating foodstuffs in homes, restaurants and large storage warehouses. The use of refrigerators in kitchens for storing fruits and vegetables has allowed adding fresh salads to the modern diet year round, and storing fish and meats safely for long periods. Optimum temperature range for perishable food storage is 3 to 5 °C (37 to 41 °F).

In commerce and manufacturing, there are many uses for refrigeration. Refrigeration is used to liquify gases - oxygen, nitrogen, propane and methane, for example. In compressed air purification, it is used to condense water vapor from compressed air to reduce its moisture content. In oil refineries, chemical plants, and petrochemical plants, refrigeration is used to maintain certain processes at their needed low temperatures (for example, in alkylation of butenes and butane to produce a high octane gasoline component). Metal workers use refrigeration to temper steel and cutlery. In transporting temperature-sensitive foodstuffs and other materials by trucks, trains, airplanes and seagoing vessels, refrigeration is a necessity.

Dairy products are constantly in need of refrigeration, and it was only discovered in the past few decades that eggs needed to be refrigerated during shipment rather than waiting to be refrigerated after arrival at the grocery store. Meats, poultry and fish all must be kept in climate-controlled environments before being sold. Refrigeration also helps keep fruits and vegetables edible longer.

One of the most influential uses of refrigeration was in the development of the sushi/sashimi industry in Japan. Before the discovery of refrigeration, many sushi connoisseurs were at risk of contracting diseases. The dangers of unrefrigerated sashimi were not brought to light for decades due to the lack of research and healthcare distribution across rural Japan. Around mid-century, the Zojirushi corporation, based in Kyoto, made breakthroughs in refrigerator designs, making refrigerators cheaper and more accessible for restaurant proprietors and the general public.

Methods of Refrigeration

Methods of refrigeration can be classified as *non-cyclic, cyclic, thermoelectric* and *magnetic.*

Non-cyclic Refrigeration

This refrigeration method cools a contained area by melting ice, or by sublimating dry ice. Perhaps the simplest example of this is a portable cooler, where items are put in it, then ice is poured over the top. Regular ice can maintain temperatures near, but not below the freezing point, unless salt is used to cool the ice down further (as in a traditional ice-cream maker). Dry ice can reliably bring the temperature well below freezing.

Cyclic Refrigeration

This consists of a refrigeration cycle, where heat is removed from a low-temperature space or source and rejected to a high-temperature sink with the help of external work, and its inverse, the thermodynamic power cycle. In the power cycle, heat is supplied from a high-temperature source to the engine, part of the heat being used to produce work and the rest being rejected to a low-temperature sink. This satisfies the second law of thermodynamics.

A *refrigeration cycle* describes the changes that take place in the refrigerant as it alternately absorbs and rejects heat as it circulates through a refrigerator. It is also applied to heating, ventilation, and air conditioning HVACR work, when describing the "process" of refrigerant flow through an HVACR unit, whether it is a packaged or split system.

Heat naturally flows from hot to cold. Work is applied to cool a living space or storage volume by pumping heat from a lower temperature heat source into a higher temperature heat sink. Insulation is used to reduce the work and energy needed to achieve and maintain a lower temperature in the cooled space. The operating principle of the refrigeration cycle was described mathematically by Sadi Carnot in 1824 as a heat engine.

The most common types of refrigeration systems use the reverse-Rankine vapor-compression refrigeration cycle, although absorption heat pumps are used in a minority of applications.

Cyclic refrigeration can be classified as:

1. Vapor cycle, and
2. Gas cycle

Vapor cycle refrigeration can further be classified as:

1. Vapor-compression refrigeration
2. Vapor-absorption refrigeration

Vapor-compression Cycle

The vapor-compression cycle is used in most household refrigerators as well as in many large commercial and industrial refrigeration systems. Figure 1 provides a schematic diagram of the components of a typical vapor-compression refrigeration system.

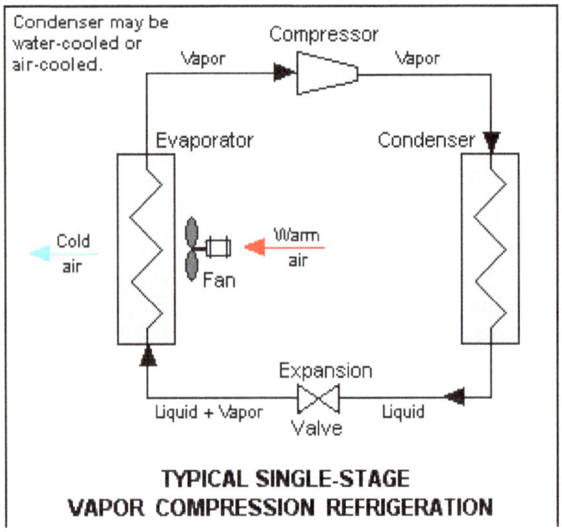

Figure 1: Vapor compression refrigeration

The thermodynamics of the cycle can be analyzed on a diagram as shown in Figure 2. In this cycle, a circulating refrigerant such as Freon enters the compressor as a vapor. From point 1 to point 2, the vapor is compressed at constant entropy and exits the compressor as a vapor at a higher temperature, but still below the vapor pressure at that temperature. From point 2 to point 3 and on to point 4, the vapor travels through the condenser which cools the vapor until it starts condensing, and then condenses the vapor into a liquid by removing additional heat at constant pressure and temperature. Between points 4 and 5, the liquid refrigerant goes through the expansion valve (also called a throttle valve) where its pressure abruptly decreases, causing flash evaporation and auto-refrigeration of, typically, less than half of the liquid.

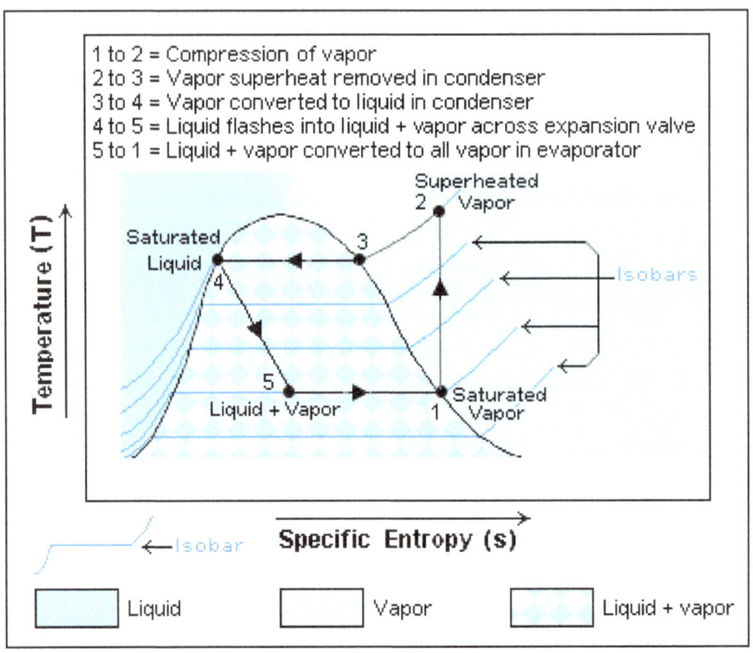

Figure 2: Temperature–Entropy diagram

That results in a mixture of liquid and vapor at a lower temperature and pressure as shown at point 5. The cold liquid-vapor mixture then travels through the evaporator coil or tubes and is completely vaporized by cooling the warm air (from the space being refrigerated) being blown by a fan across the evaporator coil or tubes. The resulting refrigerant vapor returns to the compressor inlet at point 1 to complete the thermodynamic cycle.

The above discussion is based on the ideal vapor-compression refrigeration cycle, and does not take into account real-world effects like frictional pressure drop in the system, slight thermodynamic irreversibility during the compression of the refrigerant vapor, or non-ideal gas behavior, if any.

More information about the design and performance of vapor-compression refrigeration systems is available in the classic *Perry's Chemical Engineers' Handbook*.

Vapor Absorption Cycle

In the early years of the twentieth century, the vapor absorption cycle using water-ammonia systems was popular and widely used. After the development of the vapor compression cycle, the vapor absorption cycle lost much of its importance because of its low coefficient of performance (about one fifth of that of the vapor compression cycle). Today, the vapor absorption cycle is used mainly where fuel for heating is available but electricity is not, such as in recreational vehicles that carry LP gas. It is also used in industrial environments where plentiful waste heat overcomes its inefficiency.

The absorption cycle is similar to the compression cycle, except for the method of raising the pressure of the refrigerant vapor. In the absorption system, the compressor is replaced by an absorber which dissolves the refrigerant in a suitable liquid, a liquid pump which raises the pressure and a generator which, on heat addition, drives off the refrigerant vapor from the high-pressure liquid. Some work is needed by the liquid pump but, for a given quantity of refrigerant, it is much smaller than needed by the compressor in the vapor compression cycle. In an absorption refrigerator, a suitable combination of refrigerant and absorbent is used. The most common combinations are ammonia (refrigerant) with water (absorbent), and water (refrigerant) with lithium bromide (absorbent).

Gas Cycle

When the working fluid is a gas that is compressed and expanded but doesn't change phase, the refrigeration cycle is called a *gas cycle*. Air is most often this working fluid. As there is no condensation and evaporation intended in a gas cycle, components corresponding to the condenser and evaporator in a vapor compression cycle are the hot and cold gas-to-gas heat exchangers in gas cycles.

The gas cycle is less efficient than the vapor compression cycle because the gas cycle works on the reverse Brayton cycle instead of the reverse Rankine cycle. As such the working fluid does not receive and reject heat at constant temperature. In the gas cycle, the refrigeration effect is equal to the product of the specific heat of the gas and the rise in temperature of the gas in the low temperature side. Therefore, for the same cooling load, a gas refrigeration cycle needs a large mass flow rate and is bulky.

Because of their lower efficiency and larger bulk, *air cycle* coolers are not often used nowadays in terrestrial cooling devices. However, the air cycle machine is very common on gas turbine-powered jet aircraft as cooling and ventilation units, because compressed air is readily available from the engines' compressor sections. Such units also serve the purpose of pressurizing the aircraft.

Thermoelectric Refrigeration

Thermoelectric cooling uses the Peltier effect to create a heat flux between the junction of two types of material. This effect is commonly used in camping and portable coolers and for cooling electronic components and small instruments.

Magnetic Refrigeration

Magnetic refrigeration, or adiabatic demagnetization, is a cooling technology based on the magnetocaloric effect, an intrinsic property of magnetic solids. The refrigerant is often a paramagnetic salt, such as cerium magnesium nitrate. The active magnetic dipoles in this case are those of the electron shells of the paramagnetic atoms.

A strong magnetic field is applied to the refrigerant, forcing its various magnetic dipoles to align and putting these degrees of freedom of the refrigerant into a state of lowered entropy. A heat sink then absorbs the heat released by the refrigerant due to its loss of entropy. Thermal contact with the heat sink is then broken so that the system is insulated, and the magnetic field is switched off. This increases the heat capacity of the refrigerant, thus decreasing its temperature below the temperature of the heat sink.

Because few materials exhibit the needed properties at room temperature, applications have so far been limited to cryogenics and research.

Other Methods

Other methods of refrigeration include the air cycle machine used in aircraft; the vortex tube used for spot cooling, when compressed air is available; and thermoacoustic refrigeration using sound waves in a pressurized gas to drive heat transfer and heat exchange; steam jet cooling popular in the early 1930s for air conditioning large buildings; thermoelastic cooling using a smart metal alloy stretching and relaxing. Many Stirling cycle heat engines can be run backwards to act as a refrigerator, and therefore these engines have a niche use in cryogenics. In addition there are other types of cryocoolers such as Gifford-McMahon coolers, Joule-Thomson coolers, pulse-tube refrigerators and, for temperatures between 2 mK and 500 mK, dilution refrigerators.

Fridge Gate

The Fridge Gate method is a theoretical application of using a single logic gate to drive a refrigerator in the most energy efficient way possible without violating the laws of thermodynamics. It operates on the fact that there are two energy states in which a particle can exist: the ground state and the excited state. The excited state carries a little more energy than the ground state, small enough so that the transition occurs with high probability. There are three components or particle types associated with the fridge gate. The first is on the interior of the fridge, the second on the outside and the third is connected to a power supply which heats up every so often that it can reach the E state and replenish the source. In the cooling step on the inside of the fridge, the g state particle absorbs energy from ambient particles, cooling them, and itself jumping to the e state. In the second step, on the outside of the fridge where the particles are also at an e state, the particle falls to the g state, releasing energy and heating the outside particles. In the third and final step, the power supply moves a particle at the e state, and when it falls to the g state it induces an energy-neutral swap where the interior e particle is replaced by a new g particle, restarting the cycle.

Capacity Ratings

The measured capacity of refrigeration is always dimensioned in units of power. Domestic and commercial refrigerators may be rated in kJ/s, or Btu/h of cooling. For commercial and industrial refrigeration systems, most of the world uses the kilowatt (kW) as the basic unit of refrigeration. Typically, commercial and industrial refrigeration systems in North America are rated in tons of refrigeration (TR). Historically, one TR was defined as the energy removal rate that will freeze one short ton of water at 0 °C (32 °F) in one day. This was very important because many early refrigeration systems were in ice houses. The simple unit allowed owners of these early refrigeration systems to measure a day's output of ice against energy consumption, and to compare their plant to one down the street. While ice houses make up a much smaller part of the refrigeration industry than they once did, the unit TR has remained in North America. The unit's value as historically defined was approximately 11,958 Btu/hr (3.505 kW), and has now been conventionally redefined as exactly 12,000 Btu/hr (3.517 kW).

A refrigeration system's coefficient of performance (CoP) is very important in determining a system's overall efficiency. It is defined as refrigeration capacity in kW divided by the energy input in kW. While CoP is a very simple measure of performance, it is typically not used for industrial refrigeration in North America. Owners and manufacturers of these systems typically use performance factor (PF). A system's PF is defined as a system's energy input in horsepower divided by its refrigeration capacity in TR. Both CoP and PF can be applied to either the entire system or to system components. For example, an individual compressor can be rated by comparing the energy needed to run the compressor versus the expected refrigeration capacity based on inlet volume flow rate. It is important to note that both CoP and PF for a refrigeration system are only defined at specific operating conditions, including temperatures and thermal loads. Moving away from the specified operating conditions can dramatically change a system's performance.

Frozen Food

Freezing food preserves it from the time it is prepared to the time it is eaten. Since early times, farmers, fishermen, and trappers have preserved their grains and produce in unheated buildings during the winter season. Freezing food slows down decomposition by turning residual moisture into ice, inhibiting the growth of most bacterial species. In the food commodity industry, there are two processes: mechanical and cryogenic (or flash freezing). The freezing kinetics is important to preserve the food quality and texture. Quicker freezing generates smaller ice crystals and maintains cellular structure. Cryogenic freezing is the quickest freezing technology available due to the ultra low liquid nitrogen temperature −196 °C (−320 °F).

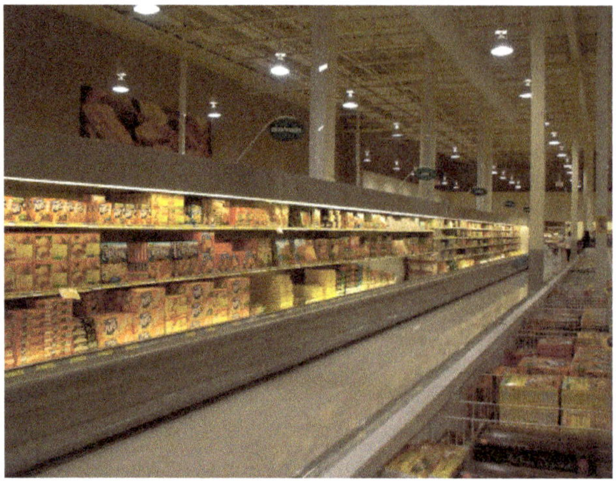

A frozen processed foods aisle at a supermarket in Canada

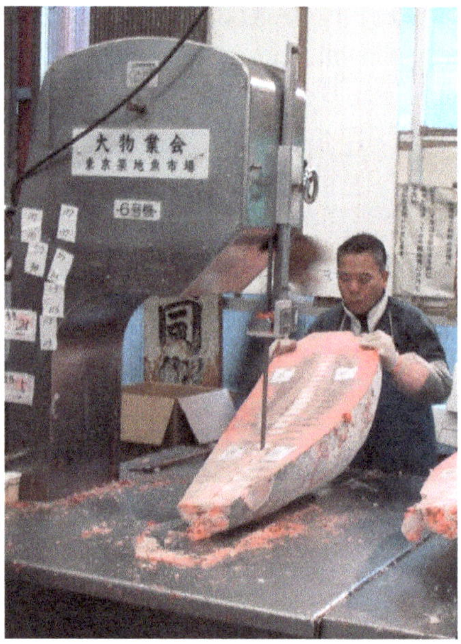

Cutting frozen tuna using a bandsaw in the Tsukiji fish market in Tokyo, Japan (2002)

Preserving food in domestic kitchens during the 20th and 21st centuries is achieved using household freezers. Accepted advice to householders was to freeze food on the day of purchase. An initiative by a supermarket group in 2012 (backed by the UK's Waste & Resources Action Programme) promotes advising the freezing of food "as soon as possible up to the product's 'use by' date". The Food Standards Agency was reported as supporting the change, providing the food had been stored correctly up to that time.

Preservatives

Frozen products do not require any added preservatives because microorganisms do not grow when the temperature of the food is below −9.5 °C (15 °F), which is sufficient on its own in preventing food spoilage. Long-term preservation of food may call for food storage at even lower temperatures. Carboxymethylcellulose (CMC), a tasteless and odorless stabilizer, is typically added to frozen food because it does not adulterate the quality of the product.

History

Natural food freezing (using winter frosts) had been in use by tribes in cold climates for centuries. By 1885 a small number of chicken and geese were being shipped from Russia to London in insulated cases using this technique. By March 1899, the "British Refrigeration and Allied Interests" reported that a food importing business, "Baerselman Bros", was shipping some 200,000 frozen geese and chickens per week from three Russian depots to New Star Wharf, Lower Shadwell, London over three or four winter months. This trade in frozen food was enabled by the introduction of Linde cold air freezing plants in three Russian depots and the London warehouse. The Shadwell warehouse stored the frozen goods until they were shipped to markets in London, Birmingham, Liverpool and Manchester. The techniques were later expanded into the meat packing industry.

From 1929, Clarence Birdseye introduced "flash freezing" to the American public. Birdseye first became interested in food freezing during fur-trapping expeditions to Labrador in 1912 and 1916, where he saw the natives use natural freezing to preserve foods. More advanced attempts include food frozen for Eleanor Roosevelt on her trip to Russia. Other experiments, involving orange juice, ice cream and vegetables were conducted by the military near the end of World War II.

Technology

The freezing technique itself, just like the frozen food market, is developing to become faster, more efficient and more cost-effective.

Mechanical freezers were the first to be used in the food industry and are used in the vast majority of freezing / refrigerating lines. They function by circulating a refrigerant, normally ammonia, around the system, which withdraws heat from the food product. This heat is then transferred to a condenser and dissipated into air or water. The refrigerant itself, now a high pressure, hot liquid, is directed into an evaporator. As it passes through an expansion valve, it is cooled and then vaporises into a gaseous state. Now a low pressure, low temperature gas again, it can be reintroduced into the system.

Cryogenic or (flash freezing) of food is a more recent development, but is used by many leading food manufacturers all over the world. Cryogenic equipment uses very low temperature gases – usually liquid nitrogen or solid carbon dioxide – which are applied directly to the food product.

Packaging

Frozen food packaging must maintain its integrity throughout machine filling, sealing, freezing, storage, transportation, thawing, and often cooking. As many frozen foods are cooked in a microwave oven, manufacturers have developed packaging that can go straight from freezer to the microwave.

In 1974, the first differential heating container (DHC) was sold to the public. A DHC is a sleeve of metal designed to allow frozen foods to receive the correct amount of heat. Various sized apertures were positioned around the sleeve. The consumer would put the frozen dinner into the sleeve according to what needed the most heat. This ensured proper cooking.

Today there are multiple options for packaging frozen foods. Boxes, cartons, bags, pouches, Boil-in-Bags, lidded trays and pans, crystallized PET trays, and composite and plastic cans.

Scientists are continually researching new aspects of frozen food packaging. Active packaging offers a host of new technologies that can actively sense and then neutralize the presence of bacteria or other harmful species. Active packaging can extend shelf-life, maintain product safety, and help preserve the food over a longer period of time. Several functions of active packaging are being researched:

- Oxygen scavengers
- Time Temperature Indicators and digital temperature data loggers
- Antimicrobials
- Carbon Dioxide controllers
- Microwave susceptors
- Moisture control: Water activity, Moisture vapor transmission rate, etc.
- Flavor enhancers
- Odor generators
- Oxygen-permeable films
- Oxygen generators
- Validation of cold chain

Effects on Nutrients

Vitamin Content of Frozen Foods

- Vitamin C: Usually lost in a higher concentration than any other vitamin. A study was performed on peas to determine the cause of vitamin C loss. A vitamin loss of ten percent occurred during the blanching phase with the rest of the loss occurring during the cooling and washing stages. The vitamin loss was not actually accredited to the freezing process. Another experiment was performed involving peas and lima beans. Frozen and canned vegetables were both used in the experiment. The frozen vegetables were stored at −23 °C (−10 °F) and the canned vegetables were stored at room temperature 24 °C (75 °F). After 0, 3, 6, and 12 months of storage, the vegetables were analyzed with and without cooking. O'Hara, the scientist performing the experiment said, "From the view point of the vitamin content of the two vegetables when they were ready for the plate of the consumer, there did not appear to be any marked advantages attributable to method of preservation, frozen storage, processed in a tin, or processed in glass."
- Vitamin B_1 (Thiamin): A vitamin loss of 25 percent is normal. Thiamin is easily soluble in water and is destroyed by heat.
- Vitamin B_2 (Riboflavin): Not much research has been done to see how much freezing af-

fects Riboflavin levels. Studies that have been performed are inconclusive; one study found an 18 percent vitamin loss in green vegetables, while another determined a 4 percent loss. It is commonly accepted that the loss of Riboflavin has to do with the preparation for freezing rather than the actual freezing process itself.

- Vitamin A (Carotene): There is little loss of carotene during preparation for freezing and freezing of most vegetables. Much of the vitamin loss is incurred during the extended storage period.

Effectiveness

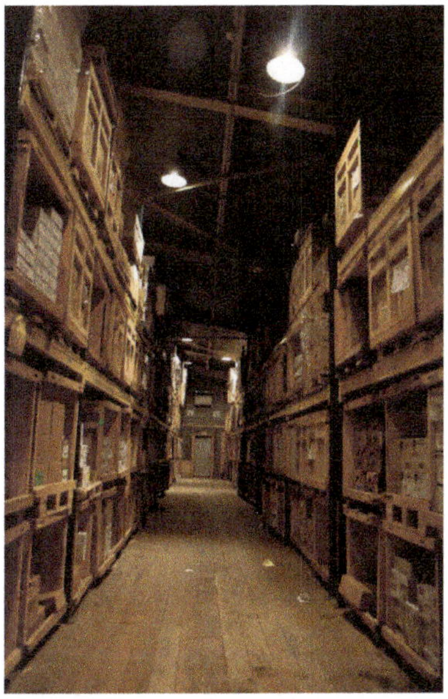

A frozen food warehouse at McMurdo Station, Antarctica

Freezing is an effective form of food preservation because the pathogens that cause food spoilage are killed or do not grow very rapidly at reduced temperatures. The process is less effective in food preservation than are thermal techniques, such as boiling, because pathogens are more likely to be able to survive cold temperatures rather than hot temperatures. One of the problems surrounding the use of freezing as a method of food preservation is the danger that pathogens deactivated (but not killed) by the process will once again become active when the frozen food thaws.

Foods may be preserved for several months by freezing. Long-term frozen storage requires a constant temperature of –18 °C (0 °F) or less.

Quality

The speed of the freezing has a direct impact on the size and the number of ice crystals formed within a food product's cells and extracellular space. Slow freezing leads to fewer but larger ice crystals while fast freezing leads to smaller but more numerous ice crystals. Large ice crystals can puncture the walls of the cells of the food product which will cause a degradation of the texture of the product as well as the loss of its natural juices during thawing. That is why there will be a qualitative difference observed between food products frozen by ventilated mechanical freezing, non-ventilated mechanical freezing or cryogenic freezing with liquid nitrogen.

Reaction

According to a study, an American consumes on average 71 frozen foods a year, most of which are pre-cooked frozen meals. Many food critics host shows are dedicated to the tasting and reviewing of frozen foods.

Curing (Food Preservation)

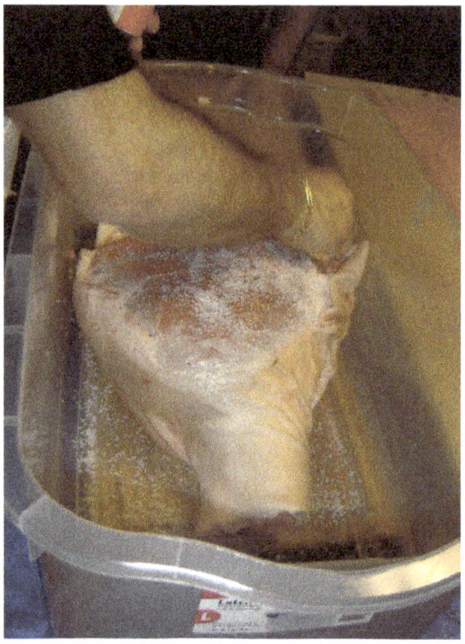

Sea salt being added to raw ham to make prosciutto

Curing is any of various food preservation and flavoring processes of foods such as meat, fish and vegetables, by the addition of combinations of salt, nitrates, nitrites, or sugar, with the aim of drawing moisture out of the food by the process of osmosis. Many curing processes also involve smoking, spicing, or cooking. Dehydration was the earliest form of food curing. Because curing increases the solute concentration in the food and hence decreases its water potential, the food becomes inhospitable for the microbe growth that causes food spoilage. Curing can be traced back to antiquity, and was the primary way of preserving meat and fish until the late 19th century.

Nitrates and nitrites, in conjunction with salt, are one of the most common agents in curing meat because they further inhibit the growth of *Clostridium botulinum*. They also contribute to the characteristic pink color of cured meats like ham.

Meat preservation in general (of meat from livestock, game, and poultry) is the set of all treatment processes for preserving the nutritious properties, taste, texture, and color of raw, partially cooked, or cooked meats while keeping them edible and safe to consume. Curing has been the dominant method of meat preservation for thousands of years, although modern developments like refrigeration and synthetic preservatives are now beginning to complement and supplant it.

While meat preservation processes like curing were mainly developed in order to prevent disease and increase food security, the advent of modern preservation methods mean that in most developed countries today, curing is instead mainly practised for its cultural value and desirable impact on the texture and taste of food. For lesser-developed countries, curing remains a key process in ensuring the viability of meat production, transport and access.

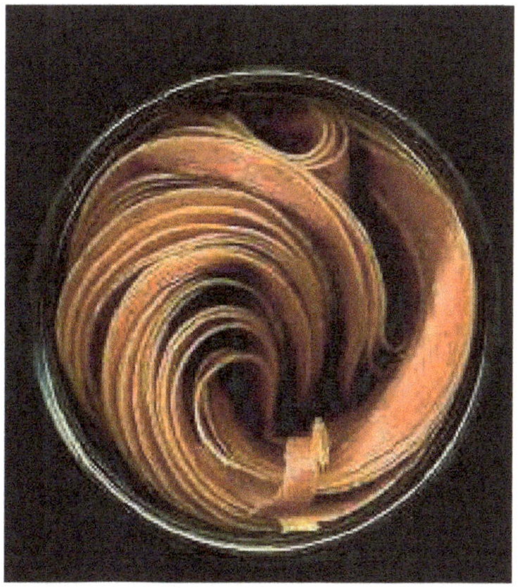

Slices of beef in a can.

Necessity of Curing

Untreated meat decomposes rapidly if it is not preserved, at a speed that depends on several factors, including ambient humidity, temperature, and the presence of pathogens. Most meats cannot be kept at room temperature in excess of a few days without spoiling, even in winter.

If kept in excess of this time, meat begins to change colour and exude a foul odour, indicating the decomposition of the food. Ingestion of such spoiled meat can cause serious food poisonings, like botulism.

While the short shelf life of fresh meat does not pose a significant problem when access to it is easy and supply is abundant, in times of scarcity and famine, or when the meat must be carried over long voyages, it spoils very quickly. In such circumstances the usefulness of preserving foods containing nutritional value for transport and storage is obvious.

Curing is able to significantly extend the life of meat before it spoils, by making it inhospitable to the growth of spoilage microbes.

History

A survival technique since prehistory, the conservation of meat has become, over the centuries, a topic of political, economic, and social importance worldwide.

Traditional Methods

Food curing dates back to ancient times, both in the form of smoked meat and salt-cured meat.

Several sources describe the salting of meat in the ancient Mediterranean world. Diodore of Sicily in his *Bibliotheca historica* wrote that the Cosséens in the mountains of Persia salted the flesh of carnivorous animals. Strabo indicates that people at Borsippa were catching bats and salting them to eat. The Romans called this dish *salsamentum* – which term later included salted fat, the sauces and spices used for its preparation. Also evidence of ancient sausage production exists. The Roman gourmet Apicius speaks of a sausage-making technique involving *œnogaros* (a mixture of the fermented fish sauce garum with oil or wine). Preserved meats were furthermore a part of religious traditions: resulting meat for offerings to the gods was salted before being given to priests, after which it could be picked up again by the offerer, or even sold in the butcher's.

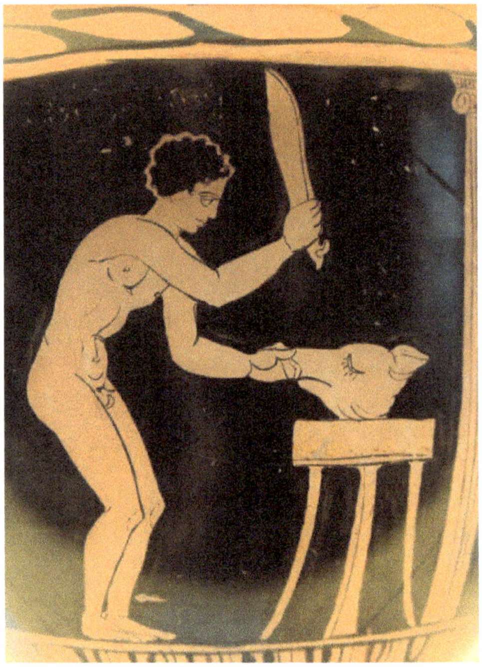

Young man preparing a pig's head after a sacrifice. Vase v. 360-340 BC, National Archaeological Museum of Spain

A trade in salt meat occurred across ancient Europe. In Polybius's time, the Gauls exported salt pork each year to Rome in large quantities, where it was sold in different cuts: rear cuts, middle cuts, hams, and sausages. This meat, after having been salted with the greatest care, was sometime smoked. These goods had to have been considerably important, since they fed part of the Roman people and the armies. The Belgians were celebrated above all for the care which they gave to the fattening of their pigs. Their herds of sheep and pigs were so many, they could provide skins and salt meat not only for Rome, but also for most of Italy. The Ceretani of Spain drew a large export income from their hams, which were so succulent, they were in no way inferior to those of Cantabria. These *tarichos* of pig would become especially sought, to the point that the ancients considered this meat the most nourishing of all and the easiest to digest.

In Ethiopia, according to Pliny, and in Libya according to Saint Jerome, the Acridophages (literally, the locust-eaters) salted and smoked the crickets which arrived at their settlements in the spring in great swarms and which constituted, it was said, their sole food.

The smoking of meat was a traditional practice in North America, where Plains Indians hung their meat at the top of their tipis to increase the amount of smoke coming into contact with the food.

Middle Ages

In Europe, medieval cuisine made great use of meat and vegetables, and the guild of butchers was amongst the most powerful. During the 12th century, salt beef was consumed by all social classes. Smoked meat was called *carbouclée* in Romance tongues and *bacon* if it was pork.

The Middle Ages made pâté a masterpiece: that which is, in the 21st century, merely spiced minced meat (or fish), baked in a terrine and eaten cold, was at that time composed of a dough envelope stuffed with varied meats and superbly decorated for ceremonial feasts. The first French recipe, written in verse by Gace de La Bigne, mentions in the same pâté three great partridges, six fat quail, and a dozen larks. *Le Ménagier de Paris* mentions pâtés of fish, game, young rabbit, fresh venison, beef, pigeons, mutton, veal, and pork, and even pâtés of lark, turtledove, cow, baby bird, goose, and hen. Bartolomeo Sacchi, called Platine, prefect of the Vatican Library, gives the recipe for a pâté of wild beasts: the flesh, after being boiled with salt and vinegar, was larded and placed inside an envelope of spiced fat, with a *mélange* of pepper, cinnamon and pounded lard; one studded the fat with cloves until it was entirely covered, then placed it inside a pâte.

In the 16th century, the most fashionable pâtés were of woodcock, au bec doré, chapon, beef tongue, cow feet, sheep feet, chicken, veal, and venison. In the same era, Pierre Belon notes that the inhabitants of Crete and Chios lightly salted then oven-dried entire hares, sheep, and roe deer cut into pieces, and that in Turkey, cattle and sheep, cut and minced rouelles, salted then dried, were eaten on voyages with onions and no other preparation.

Early Modern Era

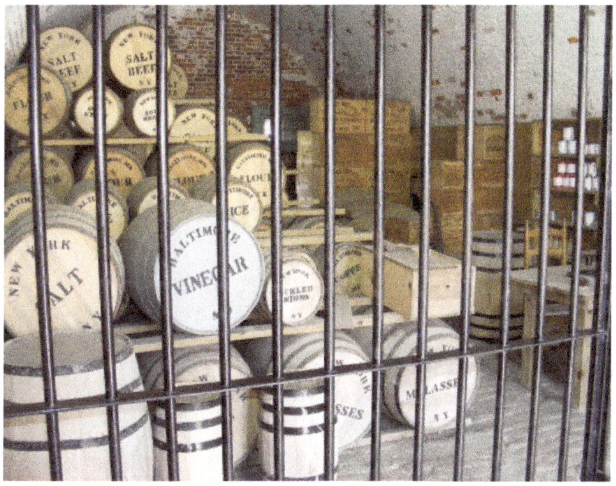

Barrels of salt beef in a reconstruction of an American Civil War stockpile, at Fort Macon State Park, North Carolina

During the Age of Discovery, salt meat was one of the main foods for sailors on long voyages, for instance in the merchant marine or the navy. In the 18th century, salted Irish beef, transported in barrels, was considered finest.

Scientific research on meat by chemists and pharmacists led to the creation of a new, extremely practical product: meat extract, which could appear in different forms. The need to properly feed soldiers during long campaigns outside the country, such as the Napoleonic Wars, and to nourish a constantly growing population often living in appalling conditions drove scientific research, but a confectioner, Nicolas Appert, in 1795 developed through experimentation a method which would become universal and in one language bears his name: airtight storage, called *appertisation* in French.

With the spread of *appertisation*, the 19th-century world entered the era of the "food industry", which developed new products such as canned salt meat (for example corned beef), but also led to lowered standards of food quality and hygiene – such as those Upton Sinclair described in *The Jungle*. These bad practices led to the creation of the Pure Food and Drug Act in 1906, followed by the national agencies for health security and the establishment of food traceability over the course of the 20th century. It also led to continuing technological innovation.

In France, the summer of 1857 was so hot that most butchers refused to slaughter animals and charcutiers lost considerable amounts of meat, due to inadequate conservation methods. A member of the Academy of Medicine and his son issued a 34-page summary of works printed between 1663 and 1857, which proposed some solutions: not less than 91 texts exist, of which 64 edited for only the years between 1851 and 1857.

Chemical Actions

Salt

Table salt (sodium chloride) is the primary ingredient used in meat curing. Removal of water and addition of salt to meat creates a solute-rich environment where osmotic pressure draws water out of microorganisms, slowing down their growth. Doing this requires a concentration of salt of nearly 20%. In addition, salt causes the soluble meat proteins to come to the surface of the meat particles within sausages. These proteins coagulate when the sausage is heated, helping to hold the sausage together.

Sugar

The sugar added to meat for the purpose of curing it comes in many forms, including honey, corn syrup solids, and maple syrup. However, with the exception of bacon, it does not contribute much to the flavor, but it does alleviate the harsh flavor of the salt. Sugar also contributes to the growth of beneficial bacteria such as *Lactobacillus* by feeding them.

Nitrates and Nitrites

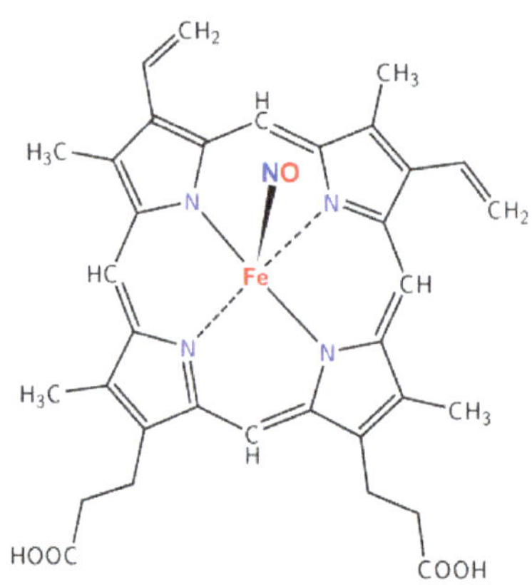

Nitrosyl-heme

Nitrates and nitrites not only help kill bacteria, but also produce a characteristic flavor and give meat a pink or red color. Nitrite ($NO-2$) is generally supplied by sodium nitrite or (indirectly) by potassium nitrate. Nitrite salts are most often used in curing. Nitrate is specifically used only in a few curing conditions and products where nitrite (which may be generated from nitrate) must be generated in the product over long periods of time.

Nitrite further breaks down in the meat into nitric oxide (NO), which then binds to the iron atom in the center of myoglobin's heme group, reducing oxidation and causing a reddish-brown color (nitrosomyoglobin) when raw, and the characteristic cooked-ham pink color (nitrosohemochrome or nitrosyl-heme) when cooked. The addition of ascorbate to cured meat reduces formation of nitrosamines, but increases the nitrosylation of iron.

The use of nitrite and nitrate salts for meat curing goes back to the Middle Ages, and in the US has been formally used since 1925. Because of the relatively high toxicity of nitrite (the lethal dose in humans is about 22 mg/kg of body weight), the maximum allowed nitrite concentration in meat products is 200 ppm. Plasma nitrite is reduced in persons with endothelial dysfunction.

The use of nitrites in food preservation is controversial due to the potential for the formation of nitrosamines when nitrites are present in high concentrations and the product is cooked at high temperatures. The effect is seen for red or processed meat, but not for white meat or fish. The production of carcinogenic nitrosamines can be potently inhibited by the use of the antioxidants Vitamin C and the alpha-tocopherol form of Vitamin E during curing. Under simulated gastric conditions, nitrosothiols rather than nitrosamines are the main nitroso species being formed. The use of either compound is therefore regulated; for example, in the United States, the concentration of nitrates and nitrites is generally limited to 200 ppm or lower. They are considered irreplaceable in the prevention of botulism from consumption of cured dry sausages by preventing spore germination.

Smoke

Meat can also be preserved by "smoking", which means exposing it to smoke from burning or smoldering plant materials, usually wood. If the smoke is hot enough to slow-cook the meat, it will also keep it tender. One method of smoking calls for a smokehouse with damp wood chips or sawdust. In North America, hardwoods such as hickory, mesquite, and maple are commonly used for smoking, as are the wood from fruit trees such as apple, cherry, and plum, and even corncobs.

Smoking helps seal the outer layer of the food being cured, making it more difficult for bacteria to enter. It can be done in combination with other curing methods such as salting. Common smoking styles include hot smoking, smoke roasting (pit barbecuing) and cold smoking. Smoke roasting and hot smoking cook the meat while cold smoking does not. If the meat is cold smoked, it should be dried quickly to limit bacterial growth during the critical period where the meat is not yet dry. This can be achieved, as with jerky, by slicing the meat thinly.

Effect of Meat Preservation

On Health

The preservation of meat has allowed safe and plentiful access to this nutrient-rich food for thousands of years. It has therefore prevented countless cases of malnutrition and of food poisoning.

Since the 20th century, with respect to the relationship between diet and human disease (e.g. cardiovascular, etc.), scientists have conducted studies on the effects of lipolysis on vacuum-packed or frozen meat. In particular, by analyzing entrecôtes of frozen beef during 270 days at −20 °C (−4 °F), scientists found an important phospholipase that accompanies the loss of some unsaturated fat n-3 and n-6, which are already low in the flesh of ruminants.

In 2015, the International Agency for Research on Cancer of the World Health Organization classified processed meat, that is, meat that has undergone salting, curing, fermenting, and smoking, as "carcinogenic to humans".

On Trade

The improvement of methods of meat preservation, and of the means of transport of preserved products, has notably permitted the separation of areas of production and areas of consumption, which can now be distant without it posing a problem, permitting the exportation of meats.

For example, the appearance in the 1980s of preservation techniques under controlled atmosphere sparked a small revolution in the world's market for sheep meat: the lamb of New Zealand, one of the world's largest exporters of lamb, could henceforth be sold as fresh meat, since it could be preserved from 12 to 16 weeks, which would be a sufficient duration for it to reach Europe by boat. Before, meat from New Zealand was frozen, thus had a much lower value on European shelves. With the arrival of the new "chilled" meats, New Zealand could compete even more strongly with local producers of fresh meat. The use of controlled atmosphere to avoid the depreciation which affects frozen meat is equally useful in other meat markets, such as that for pork, which now also enjoys an international trade.

Smoking (Cooking)

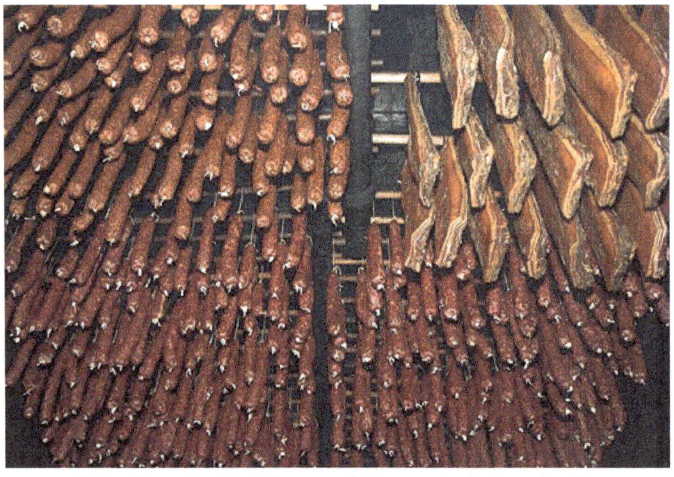
Meat hanging inside a smokehouse in Switzerland.

Smoking is the process of flavoring, cooking, or preserving food by exposing it to smoke from burning or smoldering material, most often wood. Meats and fish are the most common smoked foods, though cheeses, vegetables, and ingredients used to make beverages such as whisky, smoked beer, and *lapsang souchong* tea are also smoked.

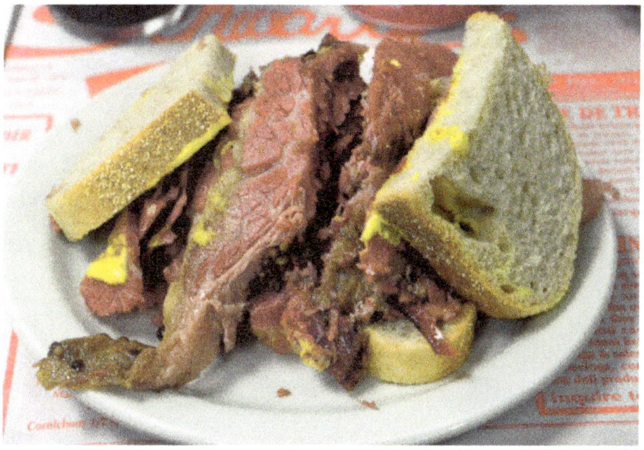

A Montreal Smoked Meat Sandwich, a well-known Canadian dish.

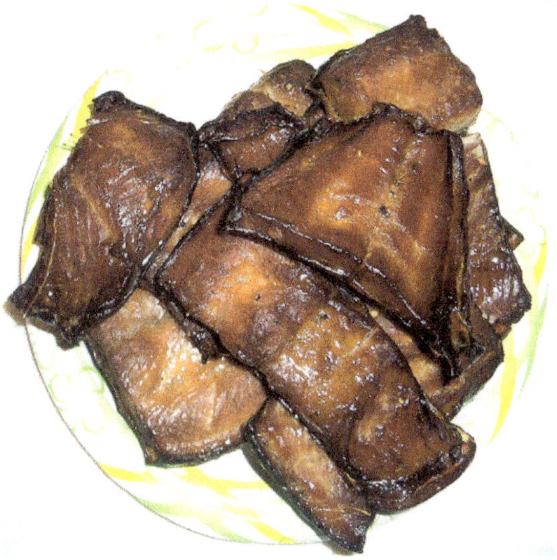

Hot-smoked chum salmon

In Europe, alder is the traditional smoking wood, but oak is more often used now, and beech to a lesser extent. In North America, hickory, mesquite, oak, pecan, alder, maple, and fruit-tree woods, such as apple, cherry, and plum, are commonly used for smoking. Other fuels besides wood can also be employed, sometimes with the addition of flavoring ingredients. Chinese tea-smoking uses a mixture of uncooked rice, sugar, and tea, heated at the base of a wok.

Some North American ham and bacon makers smoke their products over burning corncobs. Peat is burned to dry and smoke the barley malt used to make whisky and some beers. In New Zealand, sawdust from the native manuka (tea tree) is commonly used for hot smoking fish. In Iceland, dried sheep dung is used to cold-smoke fish, lamb, mutton and whale.

Historically, farms in the Western world included a small building termed the *smokehouse*, where meats could be smoked and stored. This was generally well-separated from other buildings both because of the fire danger and because of the smoke emanations.

The smoking of food is known to contaminate the food with carcinogenic polycyclic aromatic hydrocarbons.

History

The smoking of food dates back to the time of primitive cavemen. As caves or simple huts lacked chimneys, these dwellings could become very smoky. The early men would often hang meat up to dry, and they soon became aware that meat that was stored in smoky areas acquired a different flavor and was better preserved than meat that simply dried out. Over time this process was combined with pre-curing the food in salt or salty brines, resulting in a remarkably effective preservation process that was adapted and developed by numerous cultures around the world. Until the modern era, smoking was of a more "heavy duty" nature as the main goal was to preserve the food. Large quantities of salt were used in the curing process and smoking times were quite long, sometimes involving days of exposure.

The advent of modern transportation made it easier to transport food products over long distances and the need for the time and material intensive heavy salting and smoking declined. Smoking became more of a way to flavor than to preserve food. In 1939 a device called the Torry Kiln was invented at the Torry Research Station in Scotland. The kiln allowed for uniform mass-smoking and is considered the prototype for all modern large-scale commercial smokers. Although refinements in technique and advancements in technology have made smoking much easier, the basic steps involved remain essentially the same today as they were hundreds if not thousands of years ago.

Types

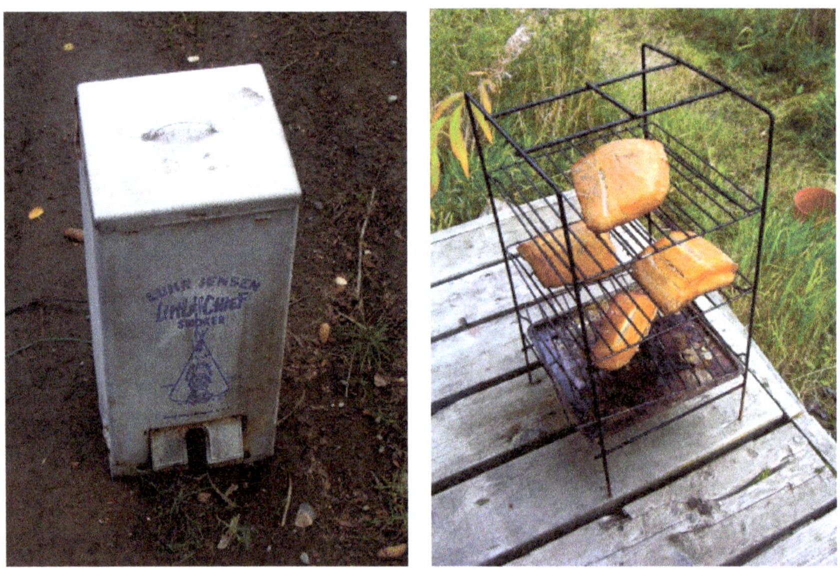

A "Little Chief" home smoker and racks with hot smoked Pacific halibut

- Cold smoking can be used as a flavor enhancer for items such as chicken breasts, beef, pork chops, salmon, scallops, and steak. The item is hung first to develop a pellicle, then can be cold smoked for just long enough to give some flavor. Some cold smoked foods are baked, grilled, steamed, roasted, or sautéed before eating. Smokehouse temperatures for cold smoking are typically done between 20 to 30 °C (68 to 86 °F). In this temperature range, foods take on a smoked flavor, but remain relatively moist. Cold smoking does not cook foods. Meats should be fully cured before cold smoking.

- Hot smoking exposes the foods to smoke and heat in a controlled environment. Like cold smoking, the item is hung first to develop a pellicle, then smoked. Although foods that have been hot smoked are often reheated or cooked, they are typically safe to eat without further cooking. Hams and ham hocks are fully cooked once they are properly smoked. Hot smoking occurs within the range of 52 to 80 °C (126 to 176 °F). Within this temperature range, foods are fully cooked, moist, and flavorful. If the smoker is allowed to get hotter than 185 °F (85 °C), the foods will shrink excessively, buckle, or even split. Smoking at high temperatures also reduces yield, as both moisture and fat are "cooked" away.

- Smoke roasting or smoke baking refers to any process that has the attributes of smoking combined with either roasting or baking. In North America, this smoking method is commonly referred to as "barbecuing", "pit baking", or "pit roasting". It may be done in a smoke roaster, closed wood-fired masonry oven or barbecue pit, any smoker that can reach above 250 °F (121 °C), or in a conventional oven by placing a pan filled with hardwood chips on the floor of the oven so the chips smolder and produce a smoke bath. However, this should only be done in a well-ventilated area to prevent carbon monoxide poisoning.

Wood Smoke

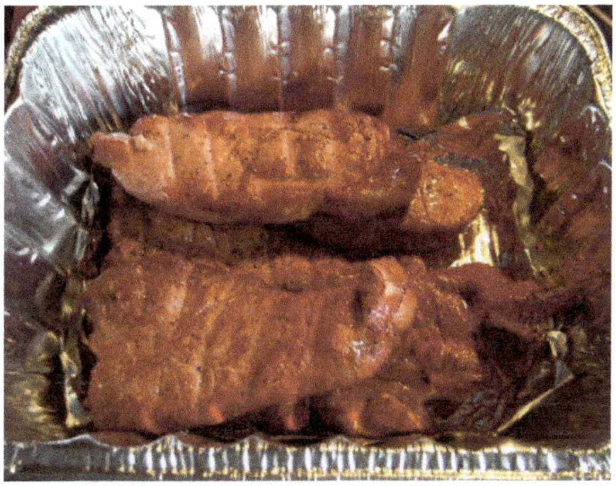

Hickory-smoked country-style ribs.

Hardwoods are made up mostly of three materials: cellulose, hemicellulose, and lignin. Cellulose and hemicellulose are the basic structural material of the wood cells; lignin acts as a kind of cell-bonding glue. Some softwoods, especially pines and firs, hold significant quantities of resin, which produces a harsh-tasting soot when burned; these woods are not often used for smoking.

Cellulose and hemicellulose are aggregate sugar molecules; when burnt, they effectively caramelize, producing carbonyls, which provide most of the color components and sweet, flowery, and fruity aromas. Lignin, a highly complex arrangement of interlocked phenolic molecules, also produces a number of distinctive aromatic elements when burnt, including smoky, spicy, and pungent compounds such as guaiacol, phenol, and syringol, and sweeter scents such as the vanilla-scented vanillin and clove-like isoeugenol. Guaiacol is the phenolic compound most responsible for the "smokey" taste, while syringol is the primary contributor to smokey aroma. Wood also contains small quantities of proteins, which contribute roasted flavors. Many of the odor compounds in wood smoke, especially the phenolic compounds, are unstable, dissipating after a few weeks or months.

A number of wood smoke compounds act as preservatives. Phenol and other phenolic compounds in wood smoke are both antioxidants, which slow rancidification of animal fats, and antimicrobials, which slow bacterial growth. Other antimicrobials in wood smoke include formaldehyde, acetic acid, and other organic acids, which give wood smoke a low pH—about 2.5. Some of these compounds are toxic to people as well, and may have health effects in the quantities found in cooking applications.

Since different species of trees have different ratios of components, various types of wood do impart a different flavor to food. Another important factor is the temperature at which the wood burns. High-temperature fires see the flavor molecules broken down further into unpleasant or flavorless compounds. The optimal conditions for smoke flavor are low, smoldering temperatures between 570 and 750 °F (299 and 399 °C). This is the temperature of the burning wood itself, not of the smoking environment, which uses much lower temperatures. Woods that are high in lignin content tend to burn hot; to keep them smoldering requires restricted oxygen supplies or a high moisture content. When smoking using wood chips or chunks, the combustion temperature is often raised by soaking the pieces in water before placing them on a fire.

Types of Smokers

There are a few basic types of smoker designs, each with their own advantages and disadvantages.

Offset Smokers

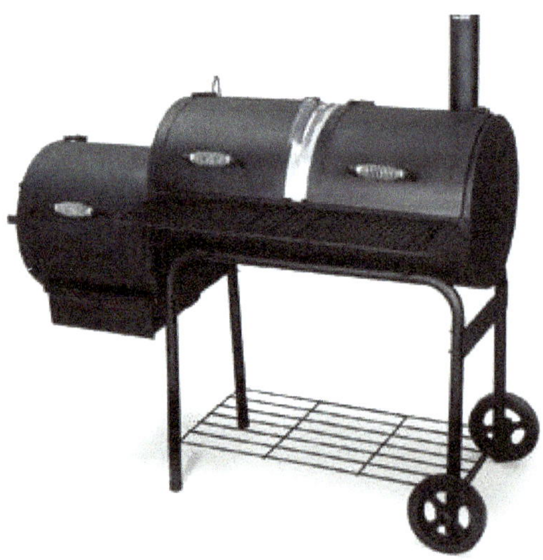

An example of a common offset smoker.

The main characteristics of the offset smoker are that the cooking chamber is usually cylindrical in shape, with a shorter, smaller diameter cylinder attached to the bottom of one end for a firebox. To cook the meat, a small fire is lit in the firebox, where airflow is tightly controlled. The heat and smoke from the fire is drawn through a connecting pipe or opening into the cooking chamber.

The heat and smoke cook and flavor the meat before escaping through an exhaust vent at the opposite end of the cooking chamber. Most manufacturers' models are based on this simple but effective design, and this is what most people picture when they think of a "BBQ smoker." Even large capacity commercial units use this same basic design of a separate, smaller fire box and a larger cooking chamber.

Upright Drum Smoker

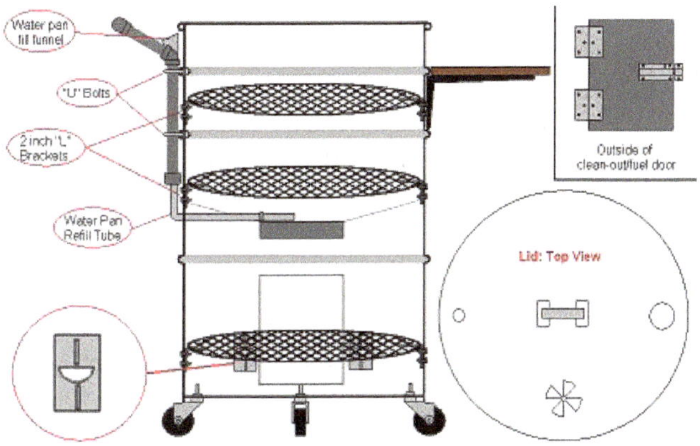

A diagram of a typical upright drum smoker

The upright drum smoker (also referred to as an ugly drum smoker or UDS) is exactly what its name suggests; an upright steel drum that has been modified for the purpose of pseudo-indirect hot smoking. There are many ways to accomplish this, but the basics include the use of a complete steel drum, a basket to hold charcoal near the bottom, and cooking rack (or racks) near the top; all covered by a vented lid of some sort. They have been built using many different sizes of steel drums, such as 30 US gallons (110 l; 25 imp gal), 55 US gallons (210 l; 46 imp gal), and 85 US gallons (320 l; 71 imp gal) for example, but the most popular size is the common 55 gallon drum.

This design is similar to smoking with indirect heat due to the distance from the coals and the racks (typically 24 inches (61 cm)). The temperatures used for smoking are controlled by limiting the amount of air intake at the bottom of the drum, and allowing a similar amount of exhaust out of vents in the lid. UDSs are very efficient with fuel consumption and flexible in their abilities to produce proper smoking conditions, with or without the use of a water pan or drip pan. Most UDS builders/users would say a water pan defeats the true pit BBQ nature of the UDS, as the drippings from the smoked meat should land on the coals, burning up, and imparting a unique flavor one cannot get with a water pan.

Vertical Water Smoker

A vertical water smoker (also referred to as a bullet smoker because of its shape) is a variation of the upright drum smoker. It uses charcoal or wood to generate smoke and heat, and contains a water bowl between the fire and the cooking grates. The water bowl serves to maintain optimal smoking temperatures and also adds humidity to the smoke chamber. It also creates an effect in which the water vapor and smoke condense together, which adds flavor to smoked foods. In addition, the bowl catches any drippings from the meat that may cause a flare-up. Vertical water smokers are extremely temperature stable and require very little adjustment once the desired temperature has been reached. Because of their relatively low cost and stable temperature, they are sometimes used in barbecue competitions where propane and electric smokers are not allowed.

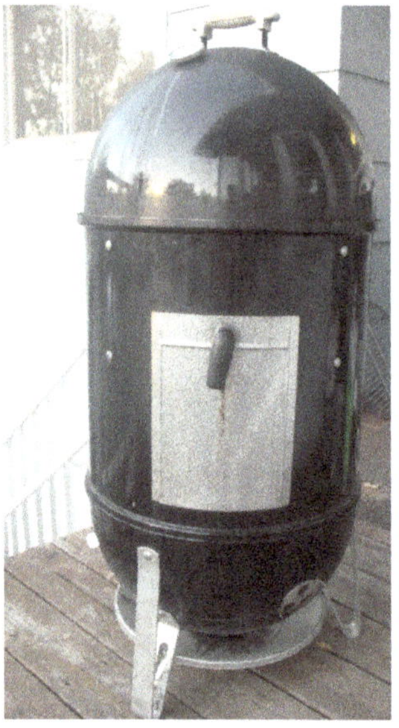

A typical vertical water smoker

Propane Smoker

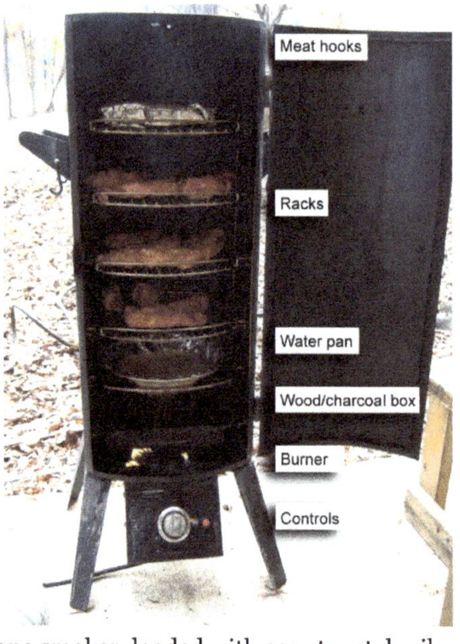

A diagram of a propane smoker, loaded with country style ribs and pork loin in foil.

A propane smoker is designed to allow the smoking of meat in a somewhat more controlled environment. The primary differences are the sources of heat and of the smoke. In a propane smoker, the heat is generated by a gas burner directly under a steel or iron box containing the wood or charcoal that provides the smoke. The steel box has few vent holes, on the top of the box only. By starving the heated wood of oxygen, it smokes instead of burning. Any combination of woods and charcoal may used. This method uses less wood.

Smoke Box Method

This more traditional method uses a two-box system: a fire box and a food box. The fire box is typically adjacent or under the cooking box, and can be controlled to a finer degree. The heat and smoke from the fire box exhausts into the food box, where it is used to cook and smoke the meat. These may be as simple as an electric heating element with a pan of wood chips placed on it, although more advanced models have finer temperature controls.

Commercial Smoke House

Commercial smokehouses, mostly made from stainless steel, have independent systems for smoke generation and cooking. Smoke generators use friction, an electric coil or a small flame to ignite sawdust on demand. Heat from steam coils or gas flames is balanced with live steam or water sprays to control the temperature and humidity. Elaborate air handling systems reduce hot or cold spots, to reduce variation in the finished product. Racks on wheels or rails are used to hold the product and facilitate movement.

Preservation

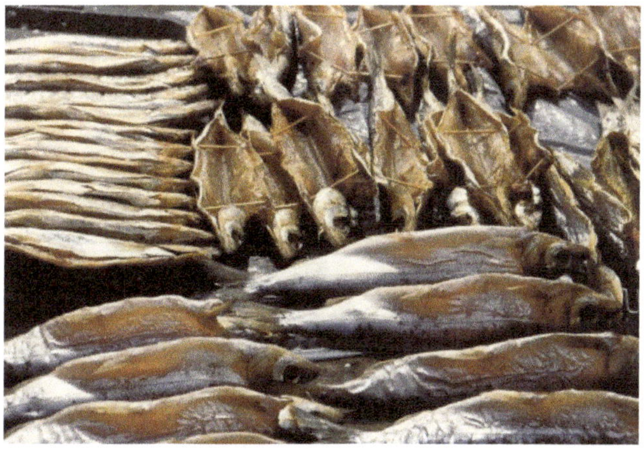

Smoked omul fish, endemic to Lake Baikal in Russia, on sale at Listyanka market.

Smoke is an antimicrobial and antioxidant, but smoke alone is insufficient for preserving food in practice, unless combined with another preservation method. The main problem is the smoke compounds adhere only to the outer surfaces of the food; smoke does not actually penetrate far into meat or fish. In modern times, almost all smoking is carried out for its flavor. Artificial smoke flavoring can be purchased as a liquid to mimic the flavor of smoking, but not its preservative qualities.

In the past, smoking was a useful preservation tool, in combination with other techniques, most commonly salt-curing or drying. In some cases, particularly in climates without much hot sunshine, smoking was simply an unavoidable side effect of drying over a fire. For some long-smoked foods, the smoking time also served to dry the food. Drying, curing, or other techniques can render the interior of foods inhospitable to bacterial life, while the smoking gives the vulnerable exterior surfaces an extra layer of protection.

Smoking is especially useful for oily fish, as its antioxidant properties delay surface fat rancidification. (Interior fat is not as exposed to oxygen, which is what causes rancidity.) Some heavily-salted, long-smoked fish can keep without refrigeration for weeks or months. Such heavily-preserved foods usually require a treatment such as boiling in fresh water to make them palatable before eating.

Some Smoked Foods

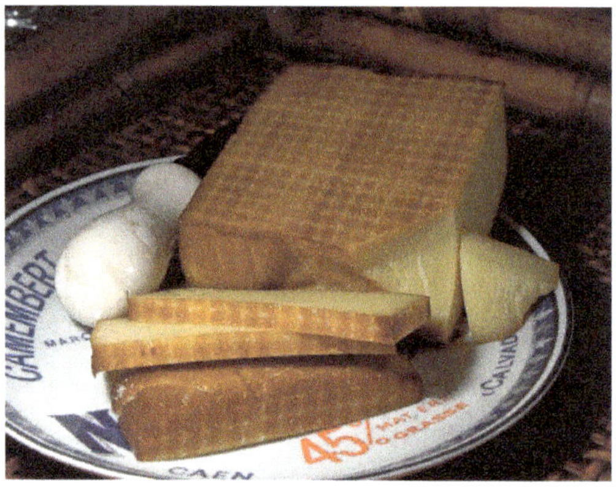

Smoked Gruyère cheese

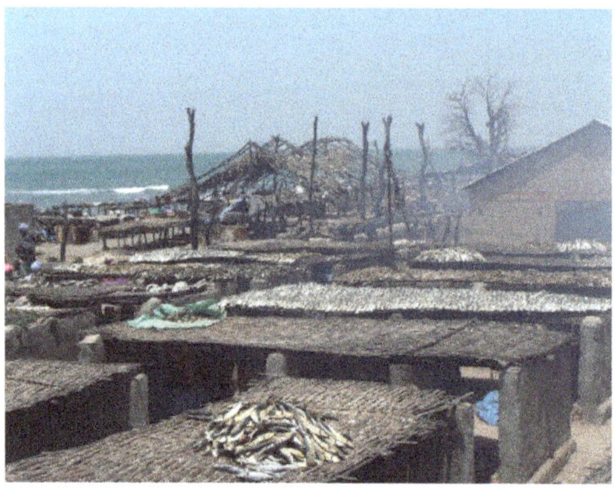
Fish being smoked in Tanji, The Gambia

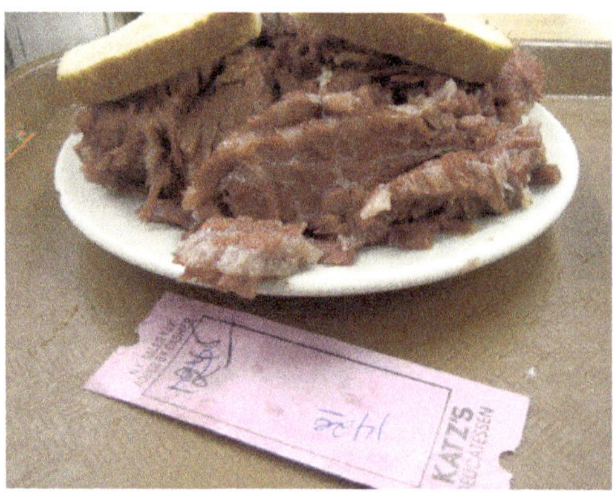

Pastrami, a smoked and cured beef product

Many foods can be smoked. Some of the more common are listed here.

Beverages

- *Lapsang souchong* tea leaves are smoked and dried over pine or cedar fires

- Malt beverages
    - The malt used to make whisky
    - Rauchbier (smoked beer)

Fruit and vegetables

- Capsicums: chipotles (smoked, ripe jalapeños), paprika
- Prunes (dried plums) can be smoked while drying
- *Wumei* are smoked plum fruits
- *Iburi-gakko* are a smoked daikon pickle from Akita Prefecture, Japan

Protein

- Cheeses
- Egg (eggs and fish eggs)
- Fish
    - Eel popular in eastern/northern Europe
    - Traditional Grimsby smoked fish (cod and haddock)
    - Haddock and Arbroath Smokies (haddock)
    - Buckling, kippers and bloater (herring)
    - Salmon
    - Mackerel
- Beef
    - Traditionally-prepared jerky
    - Pastrami (pickled, spiced and smoked beef brisket)
- Pork
    - Bacon
    - Ham
    - Bakkwa
    - Various sausages
- Tofu
- Turkey

- Various kinds of nuts

Spices

- Paprika
- Salt

Pickling

Pickling is the process of preserving or expanding the lifespan of food by either anaerobic fermentation in brine or immersion in vinegar. The resulting food is called a *pickle*, or, to prevent ambiguity, prefaced with the adjective *pickled*. The pickling procedure will typically affect the food's texture and flavor. In East Asia, vinaigrette (vegetable oil and vinegar) is also used as a pickling medium. Foods that are pickled include meats, fruits, eggs, and vegetables.

Another distinguishing characteristic is a pH 4.6 or lower, which is sufficient to kill most bacteria. Pickling can preserve perishable foods for months. Antimicrobial herbs and spices, such as mustard seed, garlic, cinnamon or cloves, are often added. If the food contains sufficient moisture, a pickling brine may be produced simply by adding dry salt. For example, German sauerkraut and Korean kimchi are produced by salting the vegetables to draw out excess water. Natural fermentation at room temperature, by lactic acid bacteria, produces the required acidity. Other pickles are made by placing vegetables in vinegar. Unlike the canning process, pickling (which includes fermentation) does not require that the food be completely sterile before it is sealed. The acidity or salinity of the solution, the temperature of fermentation, and the exclusion of oxygen determine which microorganisms dominate, and determine the flavor of the end product.

When both salt concentration and temperature are low, *Leuconostoc mesenteroides* dominates, producing a mix of acids, alcohol, and aroma compounds. At higher temperatures *Lactobacillus plantarum* dominates, which produces primarily lactic acid. Many pickles start with *Leuconostoc*, and change to *Lactobacillus* with higher acidity.

History

Pickling began 4000 years ago using cucumbers native to India. This was used as a way to preserve food for out-of-season use and for long journeys, especially by sea. Salt pork and salt beef were common staples for sailors before the days of steam engines. Although the process was invented to preserve foods, pickles are also made and eaten because people enjoy the resulting flavors. Pickling may also improve the nutritional value of food by introducing B vitamins produced by bacteria.

Etymology

The term *pickle* is derived from the Dutch word *pekel*, meaning *brine*. In the U.S. and Canada, and sometimes Australia and New Zealand, the word *pickle* alone almost always refers to a pickled cucumber, except when it is used figuratively. It may also refer to other types of pickles such as "pickled onion", "pickled cauliflower", etc. In the UK, pickle, as in a "cheese and pickle sandwich", may also refer to Ploughman's pickle, a kind of chutney.

Popularity of Pickles Around the World

South Asia

South Asia has a large variety of pickles (known as *achar* in Assamese, Punjabi, Hindi, Bengali, *uppinakaayi* in Kannada, *lonacha* in Marathi, *uppilittathu* or *achar* in Malayalam *oorukai* in Tamil, *ooragaya* in Telugu), which are mainly made from varieties of mango, lemon, lime, goongura(a sour leafy shrub), tamarind and Indian gooseberry (amla), chilli. Vegetables such as brinjal, carrots, cauliflower, tomato, bitter gourd, green tamarind, ginger, garlic, onion, and citron are also occasionally used. These fruits and vegetables are generally mixed with ingredients like salt, spices, and vegetable oils and are set to mature in a moistureless medium.

In Pakistan, pickles are known locally as *achaar* (in Urdu) and come in a variety of flavors. A popular item is the traditional mixed Hyderabadi pickle, a common delicacy prepared from an assortment of fruits (most notably mangoes) and vegetables blended with selected spices.

In Sri Lanka, *achcharu* is traditionally prepared from carrots, onions, and ground dates that are mixed with mustard powder, ground pepper, crushed ginger, garlic, and vinegar, and left to sit in a clay pot.

Southeast Asia

Singapore, Indonesian and Malaysian pickles, called *acar*, are typically made out of cucumber, carrot, bird's eye chilies, and shallots, these items being seasoned with vinegar, sugar and salt. Fruits, such as papaya and pineapple, are also sometimes pickled.

In the Philippines, *achara* is primarily made out of green papaya, carrots, and shallots, with cloves of garlic and vinegar. Other versions could include ginger, bell peppers, daikon, cucumbers or bamboo shoots. Separately, in some provinces, unripe mangoes or *burong mangga*, unripe tomatoes, green apple guavas, jicama turnips, bitter gourd and other fruit and vegetables are also pickled. Siling labuyo, sometimes with garlic and red onions, are also pickled in bottled vinegar. The spiced vinegar itself is a staple condiment in Filipino cuisine.

In Vietnam, vegetable pickles are called *dưa muối* ("salted vegetables") or *dưa chua* ("sour vegetables"). In Burma, tea leaves are pickled to produce lahpet, which has strong social and cultural importance.

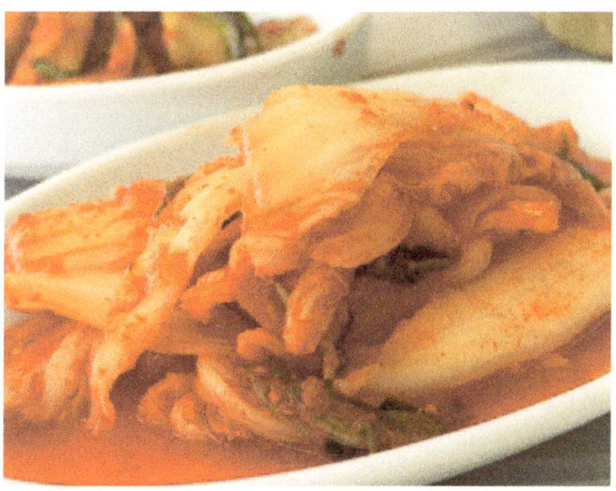

Kimchi is a very common side dish in Korea.

East Asia

China is home to a huge variety of pickled vegetables, including radish, *baicai* (Chinese cabbage, notably *suan cai*, *la bai cai*, *pao cai*, and Tianjin preserved vegetable), *zha cai*, chili pepper, and cucumbers, among many others.

Japanese *tsukemono* (pickled foods) include *takuan* (daikon), *umeboshi* (ume plum), *gari* & *beni shoga* (ginger), turnip, cucumber, and Chinese cabbage.

The Korean staple kimchi is usually made from pickled napa cabbage and radish, but is also made from green onions, garlic stems, chives and a host of other vegetables. Kimchi is popular throughout East Asia. Jangajji is another example of pickled vegetables.

Western Asia

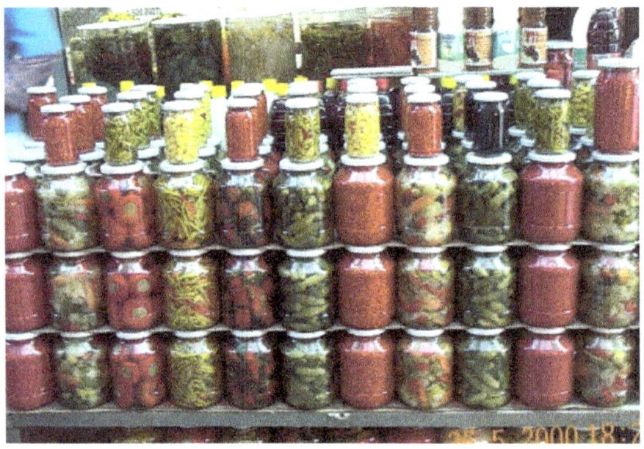

Torshi, traditional pickles in Southeast Europe, Western Asia and the Caucasus

In Iran, Turkey, Arab countries, the Balkans, and the Caucasus, pickles (called torshi in Persian, *turşu* in Turkish language and *mekhallel* in Arabic) are commonly made from turnips, peppers, carrots, green olives, cucumbers, cabbage, green tomatoes, lemons, and cauliflower.

Europe

Central and Eastern Europe

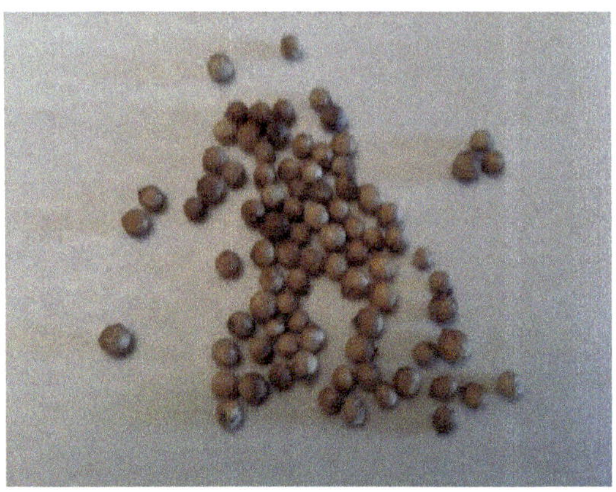

Coriander seeds are one of the spices popularly added to pickled vegetables in Europe.

In Hungary the main meal *(lunch)* usually goes with some kind of pickles *(savanyúság)* but they are commonly consumed at other times of the day too. The most commonly consumed pickles are sauerkraut *(savanyú káposzta)*, the different kinds of pickled cucumbers and peppers and *csalamádé* but tomatoes, carrots, beetroot, baby corn, onions, garlic, certain squashes and melons and a few fruits like plums and apples are used to make pickles too. Stuffed pickles are specialties usually made of peppers or melons pickled after being stuffed with a cabbage filling. Pickled plum stuffed with garlic is a unique Hungarian type of pickle just like *csalamádé* and leavened cucumber *(kovászos uborka)*. *Csalamádé* a type of mixed pickle made of cabbage, cucumber, paprika, onion, carrot, tomatoes and bay leaf mixed up with vinegar as the fermenting agent. Leavened cucumber, unlike other types of pickled cucumbers that are around all year long, is rather a seasonal pickle produced in the summer. Cucumbers, spices, herbs and slices of bread are put in a glass jar with salt water and kept in direct sunlight for a few days. The yeast from the bread, along with other pickling agents and spices fermented under the hot sun, give the cucumbers a unique flavor, texture and slight carbonation. Its juice can be used to make a special type of spritzer *('Újházy fröccs')* instead of carbonated water. It is common for Hungarian households to produce their own pickles. Different regions or towns have their special recipes unique to them. Among them all the Vecsési Sauerkraut *(Vecsési savanyú káposzta)* is the most famous.

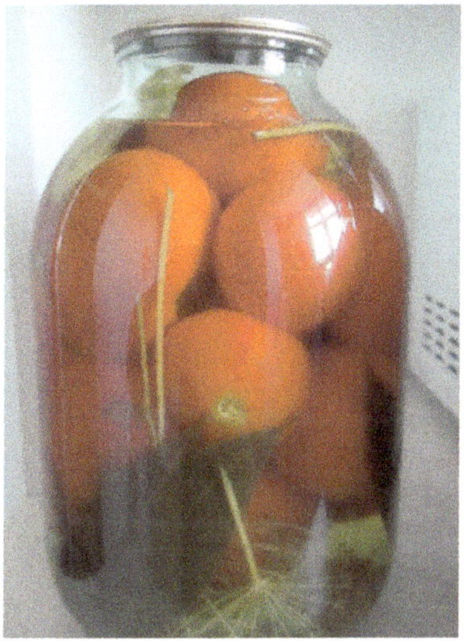

Pickled tomatoes are common in CIS

Romanian pickles (murături) are made out of beetroot, cucumbers, green tomatoes (*gogonele*), carrots, cabbage, garlic , sauerkraut (bell peppers stuffed with cabbage), bell peppers, melons, mushrooms, turnips, celery and cauliflower. Meat, like pork, can also be preserved in salt and lard.

Polish and Czech traditional pickles are cucumbers and sauerkraut, but other pickled fruits and vegetables, including plums, pumpkins and mushrooms are also common.

Russian, Ukrainian and Belarusian pickled items include beets, mushrooms, tomatoes, sauerkraut, cucumbers, ramsons, garlic, eggplant (which is typically stuffed with julienned carrots), custard squash, and watermelon. In these countries countries garden produce is commonly pickled using salt, dill, blackcurrant leaves, bay leaves and garlic and is stored in a cool, dark place.

Southern Europe

An Italian pickled vegetable dish is giardiniera, which includes onions, carrots, celery and cauliflower. Many places in southern Italy, particularly in Sicily, pickle eggplants and hot peppers.

In Albania, Bulgaria, Serbia, Macedonia and Turkey, mixed pickles, known as *turshi* or *turshu* form popular appetizers, which are typically eaten with *rakia*. Pickled green tomatoes, cucumbers, carrots, bell peppers, peppers, eggplants, and sauerkraut are also popular.

Turkish pickles, called *turşu*, are made out of vegetables, roots, and fruits such as peppers, cucumber, Armenian cucumber, cabbage, tomato, eggplant (aubergine), carrot, turnip, beetroot, green almond, baby watermelon, baby cantaloupe, garlic, cauliflower, bean and green plum. A mixture of spices flavor the pickles.

In Greece, pickles, called *τουρσί(α)*, are made out of carrots, celery, eggplants stuffed with diced carrots, cauliflower, tomatoes, and peppers.

Northern Europe

In Britain, pickled onions and pickled eggs are often sold in pubs and fish and chip shops. Pickled beetroot, walnuts, and gherkins, and condiments such as Branston Pickle and piccalilli are typically eaten as an accompaniment to pork pies and cold meats, sandwiches or a ploughman's lunch. Other popular pickles in the UK are pickled mussels, cockles, red cabbage, mango chutney, sauerkraut, and olives. Rollmops are also quite widely available under a range of names from various producers both within and out of the UK.

Pickled herring, rollmops, and salmon are popular in Scandinavia. Pickled cucumbers and red garden beets are important as condiments for several traditional dishes. Pickled capers are also common in Scandinavian cuisine.

United States and Canada

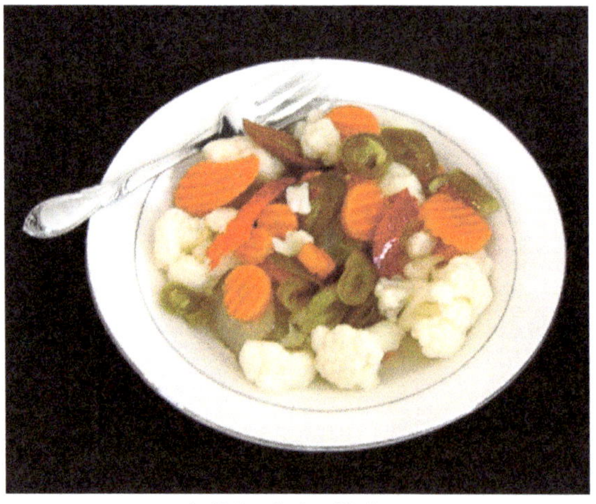

A dish of giardiniera

In the United States and Canada, pickled cucumbers (most often referred to simply as "pickles" in Canada and the United States), olives, and sauerkraut are most popular, although pickles popular in other nations are also available.

Canadian pickling is similar to that of Britain. Through the winter, pickling is an important method of food preservation. Pickled cucumbers, onions, and eggs are very popular. Chow Chow is a tart vegetable mix popular in the Maritime Provinces and the Southern United States, similar to picalily. Pickled fish is very popular, as in Scotland. Meat is often also pickled or preserved in different brines throughout the winter, most prominently in the harsh climate of Newfoundland.

Giardiniera, a mixture of pickled peppers, celery and olives, is a popular condiment in Chicago and other cities with large Italian-American populations, and is often consumed with Italian beef sandwiches. Pickled eggs are common in the Upper Peninsula of Michigan. Pickled herring is available in the Upper Midwest. Pennsylvania Dutch Country has a strong tradition of pickled foods, including chow-chow and red beet eggs. In the Southern United States, pickled okra and watermelon rind are popular, as are deep-fried pickles and pickled pig's feet, pickled chicken eggs, pickled quail eggs, pickled Garden vegetables and pickled sausage. In Mexico, chili peppers, particularly of the Jalapeño and serrano varieties, pickled with onions, carrots and herbs form common condiments. Various pickled vegetables, fish, or eggs may make a side dish to a Canadian lunch or dinner.

In the United States, National Pickle Day is a popular food holiday every year on November 14.

Mexico, Central America, and South America

In the Mesoamerican region pickling is known as "encurtido" or "curtido" for short. The pickles or "curtidos" as known in Latin America are served cold, as an appetizer, as a side dish or as a tapas dish in Spain. In several Central American countries it is prepared with cabbage, onions, carrots, lemon, vinegar, oregano, and salt. In Mexico, "curtido" consists of carrots, onions, and jalapeño peppers and used to accompany meals still common in taquerias and restaurants. In order to prepare a carrot "curtido" simply add carrots to vinegar and other ingredients that are common to the region such as chilli, tomato, and onions. Varies depending on the food, in the case of sour. Another example of a type of pickling which involves the pickling of meats or seafood is the "escabeche" or "ceviches" popular in Peru, Ecuador, and throughout Latin America and the Caribbean. These dishes include the pickling of pig's feet, pig's ears, and gizzards prepared as an "escabeche" with spices and seasonings to flavor it. The ceviches consists of shrimp, octopus, and various fishes seasoned and served cold.

Process

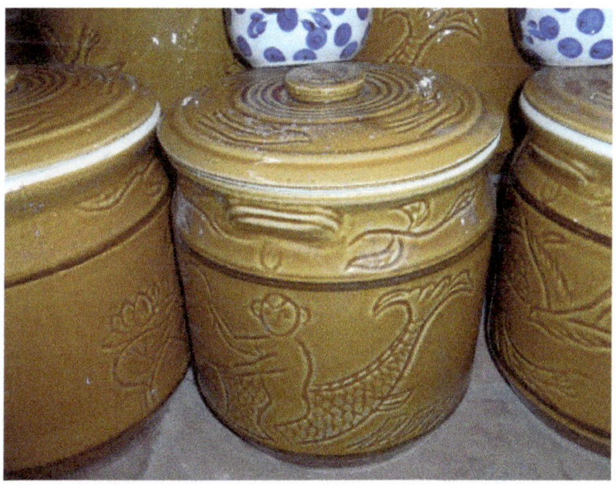

Vase by Bát Tràng porcelain for pickling

In traditional pickling fruit or vegetables are submerged in a brine (20-40 grams/L of salt (3.2–6.4 oz/imp gal or 2.7–5.3 oz/US gal)) or shredded and salted as in sauerkraut preparation and held underwater by flat stones layered on top. Alternatively a lid with an airtrap or a tight lid could be used if the lid is able to release pressure which might result from carbon dioxide build up. When using an open container it should be covered with cloth to keep insects away. Mold or (white) kahm yeast may form on the surface and should be removed. Kahm yeast is mostly harmless but can impart an off-taste.

In chemical pickling, the jar and lid are first boiled in order to sterilize them. The fruits or vegetables to be pickled are then added to the jar along with brine, vinegar, or both, as well as spices, and are then allowed to mature until the desired taste is obtained.

The food can be pre-soaked in brine before transferring to vinegar. This reduces the water content of the food which would otherwise dilute the vinegar. This method is particularly useful for fruit and vegetables with a high natural water content.

In commercial pickling, a preservative like sodium benzoate or EDTA may also be added to enhance shelf life. In fermentation pickling, the food itself produces the preservation agent, typically by a process involving Lactobacillus bacteria that produce lactic acid as the preservative agent.

Alum is used in pickling to promote crisp texture and approved as a food additive by the United States Food and Drug Administration.

“Refrigerator pickles” are unfermented pickles made by marinating fruit or vegetables in a seasoned vinegar solution. They must be stored under refrigeration or undergo canning to achieve long-term storage.

Possible Health Hazards of Pickled Vegetables

The *British Journal of Cancer* released an online 2009 meta-analysis of research on pickles as increasing the risks of esophageal cancer. The report, citing limited data in a statistical meta analysis, indicates a potential two-fold increased risk of oesophageal cancer associated with Asian pickled vegetable consumption. Results from the research are described as having “high heterogeneity” and the study said that further well-designed prospective studies were warranted.

Some common fungi can facilitate the formation of N-nitroso compounds, which are strong oesophageal carcinogens in several animal models. Roussin red methyl ester, a non-alkylating nitroso compound with tumour-promoting effect in vitro, was identified in pickles from Linxian in much higher concentrations than in samples from low-incidence areas. Fumonisin mycotoxins have been shown to cause liver and kidney tumours in rodents.

Food Storage

Food logistics is both a traditional domestic skill and is important industrially. The transport and storing of food as well as timely delivery to consumers is important in order to secure the procurement of food. Food is stored by almost every human society and by many animals. Storing of food has several main purposes:

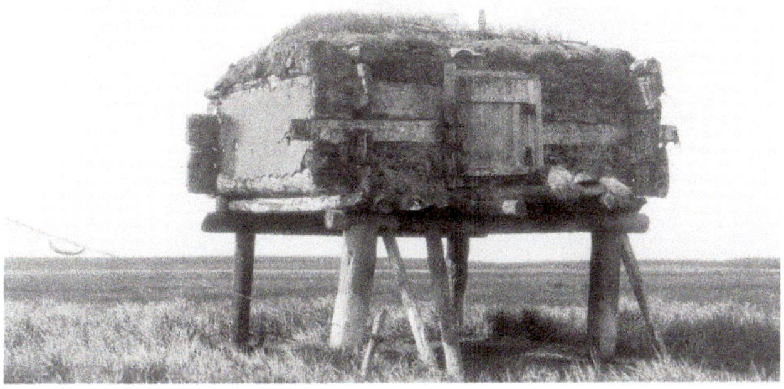

Yup'ik elevated food cache (*qulvarvik*), Hooper Bay, Alaska, 1929. Photograph by Edward S. Curtis

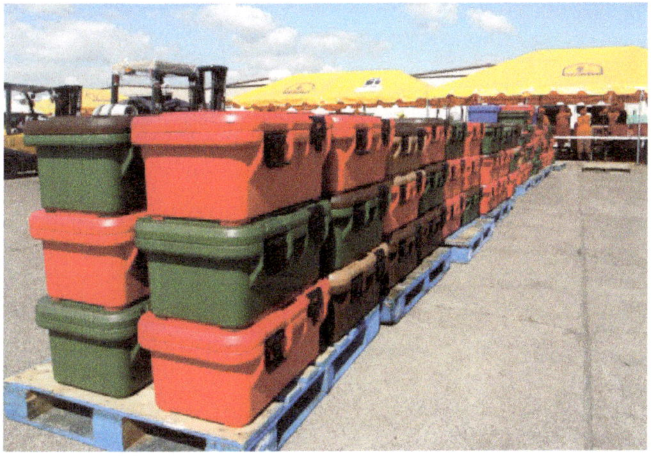

U.S. Federal Emergency Management Agency (FEMA) food storage containers stacked on shipping pallets in Texas, 2008.

- Storage of harvested and processed plant and animal food products for distribution to consumers
- Enabling a better balanced diet throughout the year
- Reducing kitchen waste by preserving unused or uneaten food for later use
- Preserving pantry food, such as spices or dry ingredients like rice and flour, for eventual use in cooking
- Preparedness for catastrophes, emergencies and periods of food scarcity or famine
- Religious reasons (Example: LDS Church leaders instruct church members to store food)
- Protection from animals or theft

Domestic Food Storage

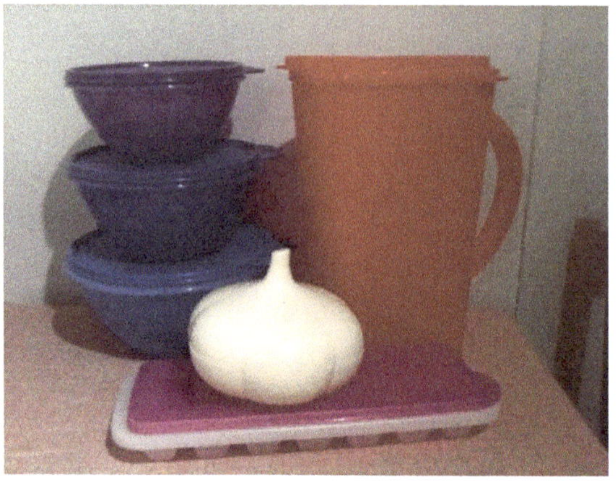

Tupperware kitchen storage containers designed for a variety of uses.

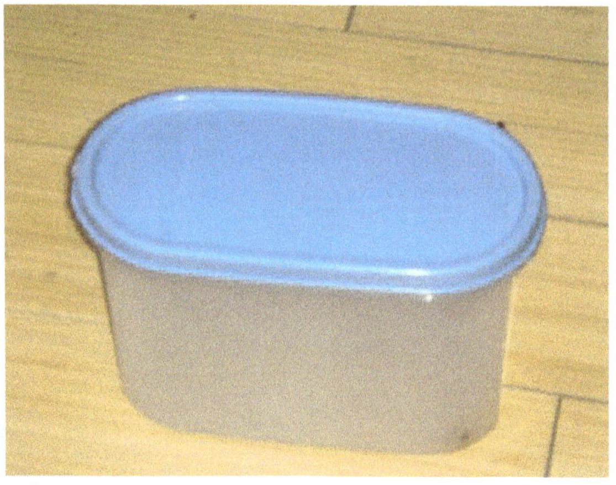

Plastic storage containers can be used to store food.

The safe storage of food for home use should strictly adhere to guidelines set out by reliable sources, such as the United States Department of Agriculture. These guidelines have been thoroughly researched by scientists to determine the best methods for reducing the real threat of food poisoning from unsafe food storage. It is also important to maintain proper kitchen hygiene, to reduce risks of bacteria or virus growth and food poisoning. The common food poisoning illnesses include Listeriosis, Mycotoxicosis, Salmonellosis, E. coli, Staphylococcal food poisoning and Botulism. There are many other organisms that can also cause food poisoning.

There are also safety guidelines available for the correct methods of home canning of food. For example, there are specific boiling times that apply depending upon whether pressure canning or waterbath canning is being used in the process. These safety guidelines are intended to reduce the growth of mold and bacteria and the threat of potentially-fatal food poisoning.

Food Storage safety

Freezers and Thawing Food

Freezer temperature should be maintained below 0 °F. Food should never be thawed at room temperature, this increases the risk of bacterial and fungal growth and accordingly the risk of food poisoning. Once thawed, food should be used and never refrozen. Frozen food should be thawed using the following methods:

- Microwave oven
- During cooking
- In cold water (place food in watertight, plastic bag; change water every 30 minutes)
- In the refrigerator

Throw out foods that have been warmer than 40 °F for more than 2 hours. If there is any doubt at all about the length of time the food has been defrosted at room temperature, it should be thrown out. Freezing does not destroy microbes present in food. Freezing at 0 °F does inactivate microbes (bacteria, yeasts and molds). However, once food has been thawed, these microbes can again become active. Microbes in thawed food can multiply to levels that can lead to foodborne illness. Thawed food should be handled according to the same guidelines as perishable fresh food.

Food frozen at 0 °F and below is preserved indefinitely. However, the quality of the food will deteriorate if it is frozen over a lengthy period. The United States Department of Agriculture, Food Safety and Inspection Service publishes a chart showing the suggested freezer storage time for common foods.

Refrigeration

It is important to note that safe food storage using refrigeration requires adhering to temperature guidelines:

For safety, it is important to verify the temperature of the refrigerator. Refrigerators should be set to maintain a temperature of 40 °F or below. Some refrigerators have built-in thermometers to measure their internal temperature. For those refrigerators without this feature, keep an appliance thermometer in the refrigerator to monitor the temperature. This can be critical in the event of a power outage. When the power goes back on, if the refrigerator is still 40 °F, the food is safe. Foods held at temperatures above 40 °F for more than 2 hours should not be consumed. Appliance thermometers are specifically designed to provide accuracy at cold temperatures. Be sure refrigerator/freezer doors are closed tightly at all times. Don't open refrigerator/freezer doors more often than necessary and close them as soon as possible.

Storage Times for Refrigerated Food

The United States Department of Agriculture, Food Safety and Inspection Service publishes recommended storage times for refrigerated food.

Storing Oils and Fats

Oils and fats can begin to go rancid quickly when not stored safely. Rancid cooking oils and fats do not often smell rancid until well after they have spoiled. Oxygen, light and heat all contribute to cooking oils becoming rancid. The higher the level of polyunsaturated fat that an oil contains, the faster it spoils. The percentage of polyunsaturated fat in some common cooking oils is: safflower (74%); sunflower (66%); corn (60%); soybean (37%); peanut (32%); canola (29%); olive (8%).

To help preserve oils from rancidification, they should be refrigerated once opened. Opened, refrigerated cooking oils should be used within a few weeks, when some types begin to go rancid. Unopened oils can have a storage life of up to one year, but some types have a shorter shelf-life even when unopened (such as sesame and flaxseed).

Dry Storage of Foods

Vegetables

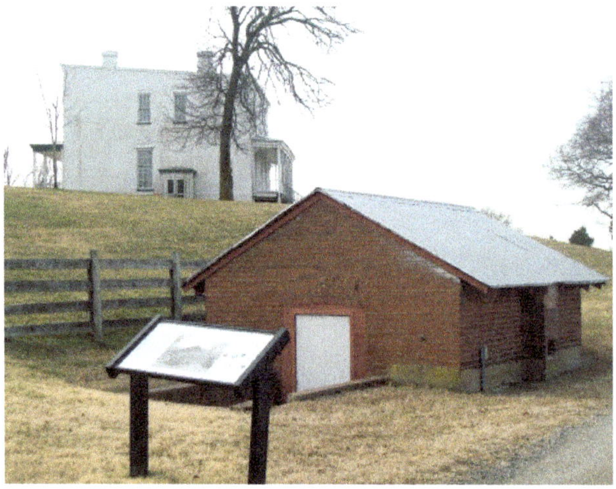

A large root cellar at the Oxon Hill Manor farm in Maryland

The guidelines vary for safe storage of vegetables under dry conditions (without refrigerating or freezing). This is because different vegetables have different characteristics, for example, tomatoes contain a lot of water, while root vegetables such as carrots and potatoes contain less. These factors, and many others, affect the amount of time that a vegetable can be kept in dry storage, as well as the temperature needed to preserve its usefulness. The following guideline shows the required dry storage conditions:

- Cool and dry: onion
- Cool and moist: root vegetable, potato, cabbage
- Warm and dry: winter squash, pumpkin, sweet potatoes, dried hot peppers

Many cultures have developed innovative ways of preserving vegetables so that they can be stored for several months between harvest seasons. Techniques include pickling, home canning, food dehydration, or storage in a root cellar.

Grain

Grain, which includes dry kitchen ingredients such as flour, rice, millet, couscous, cornmeal, and so on, can be stored in rigid sealed containers to prevent moisture contamination or insect or rodent infestation. For kitchen use, glass containers are the most traditional method. During the

20th century plastic containers were introduced for kitchen use. They are now sold in a vast variety of sizes and designs.

Metal cans are used (in the United States the smallest practical grain storage uses closed-top #10 metal cans). Storage in grain sacks is ineffective; mold and pests destroy a 25 kg cloth sack of grain in a year, even if stored off the ground in a dry area. On the ground or damp concrete, grain can spoil in as little as three days, and the grain might have to be dried before it can be milled. Food stored under unsuitable conditions should not be purchased or used because of risk of spoilage. To test whether grain is still good, it can be sprouted. If it sprouts, it is still good, but if not, it should not be eaten. It may take up to a week for grains to sprout. When in doubt about the safety of the food, throw it out as quickly as possible.

Spices and Herbs

Spices and herbs are today often sold prepackaged in a way that is convenient for pantry storage. The packaging has dual purposes of both storing and dispensing the spices or herbs. They are sold in small glass or plastic containers or resealable plastic packaging. When spices or herbs are homegrown or bought in bulk, they can be stored at home in glass or plastic containers. They can be stored for extended periods, in some cases for years. However, after 6 months to a year, spices and herbs will gradually lose their flavour as oils they contain will slowly evaporate during storage.

Spices and herbs can be preserved in vinegar for short periods of up to a month, creating a flavoured vinegar.

Alternative methods for preserving herbs include freezing in water or unsalted butter. Herbs can be chopped and added to water in an ice cube tray. After freezing, the ice cubes are emptied into a plastic freezer bag for storing in the freezer. Herbs also can be stirred into a bowl with unsalted butter, then spread on wax paper and rolled into a cylinder shape. The wax paper roll containing the butter and herbs is then stored in a freezer, and can be cut off in the desired amount for cooking. Using either of these techniques, the herbs should be used within a year.

Meat

Unpreserved meat has only a relatively short life in storage. Perishable meats should be refrigerated, frozen, dried promptly or cured. Storage of fresh meats is a complex discipline that affects the costs, storage life and eating quality of the meat, and the appropriate techniques vary with the kind of meat and the particular requirements. For example, dry ageing techniques are sometimes used to tenderize gourmet meats by hanging them in carefully controlled environments for up to 21 days, while game animals of various kinds may be hung after shooting. Details depend on personal tastes and local traditions. Modern techniques of preparing meat for storage vary with the type of meat and special requirements of tenderness, flavour, hygiene, and economy.

Semi-dried meats like salamis and country style hams are processed first with salt, smoke, sugar, acid, or other "cures" then hung in cool dry storage for extended periods, sometimes exceeding a year. Some of the materials added during the curing of meats serve to reduce the risks of food poisoning from anaerobic bacteria such as species of Clostridium that release botulinum toxin that can cause botulism. Typical ingredients of curing agents that inhibit anaerobic bacteria include nitrates. Such salts are dangerously poisonous in their own right and must be added in carefully controlled quantities and according to proper techniques. Their proper use has however saved many lives and much food spoilage.

Like the semi-dried meats, most salted, smoked, and simply-dried meats of different kinds that once were staples in particular regions, now are largely luxury snacks or garnishes; examples include jerky, biltong, and varieties of pemmican, but ham and bacon for instance, still are staples in many communities.

Food Rotation

Food rotation is important to preserve freshness. When food is rotated, the food that has been in storage the longest is used first. As food is used, new food is added to the pantry to replace it; the essential rationale is to use the oldest food as soon as possible so that nothing is in storage too long and becomes unsafe to eat. Labelling food with paper labels on the storage container, marking the date that the container is placed in storage, can make this practice simpler. The best way to rotate food storage is to prepare meals with stored food on a daily basis.

For emergency Preparation

Guides for surviving emergency conditions in many parts of the world recommend maintaining a store of essential foods; typically water, cereals, oil, dried milk, and protein rich foods such as beans, lentils, tinned meat and fish. A food storage calculator can be used to help determine how much of these staple foods a person would need to store in order to sustain life for one full year. In addition to storing the basic food items many people choose to supplement their food storage with frozen or preserved garden-grown fruits and vegetables and freeze-dried or canned produce. An unvarying diet of staple foods prepared in the same manner can cause appetite exhaustion, leading to less caloric intake. Another benefit to having a basic supply of food storage in the home is for the potential cost savings. Costs of dry bulk foods (before preparation) are often considerably less than convenience and fresh foods purchased at local markets or supermarkets. There is a significant market in convenience foods for campers, such as dehydrated food products.

Commercial Food Logistics

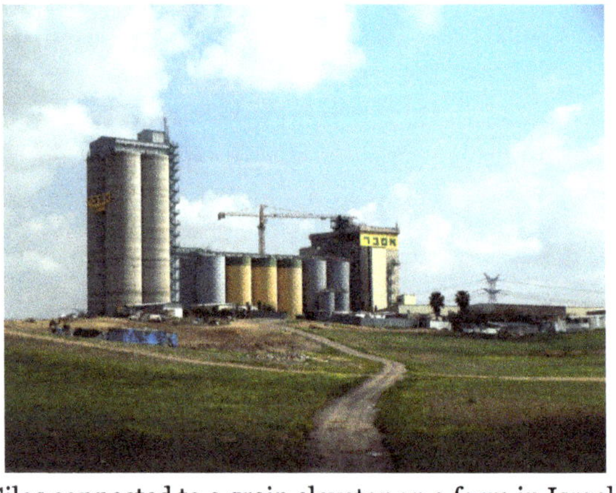

Silos connected to a grain elevator on a farm in Israel.

Grain and beans are stored in tall grain elevators, almost always at a rail head near the point of production. The grain is shipped to a final user in hopper cars. In the former Soviet Union, where harvest was poorly controlled, grain was often irradiated at the point of production to suppress mold and insects. In the U.S., threshing and drying is performed in the field, and transport is nearly sterile and in large containers that effectively suppresses pest access, which eliminates the need for irradiation. At any given time, the U.S. usually has about two weeks worth of stored grains for the population.

Fresh fruits and vegetables are sometimes packed in plastic packages and cups for fresh premium markets, or placed in large plastic tubs for sauce and soup processors. Fruits and vegetables are usually refrigerated at the earliest possible moment, and even so have a shelf life of two weeks or less.

In the United States, livestock is usually transported live, slaughtered at a major distribution point, hung and transported for two days to a week in refrigerated rail cars, and then butchered and sold locally. Before refrigerated rail cars, meat had to be transported live, and this placed its cost so high that only farmers and the wealthy could afford it every day. In Europe much meat is transported live and slaughtered close to the point of sale. In much of Africa and Asia most meat is for local populations is raised, slaughtered and eaten locally, which is believed to be less stressful for the animals involved and minimizes meat storage needs. In Australia and New Zealand, where a large proportion of meat production is for export, meat enters the cold chain early, being stored in large freezer plants before being shipped overseas in freezer ships.

Calcium Propanoate

Calcium propanoate or calcium propionate has the formula $Ca(C_2H_5COO)_2$. It is the calcium salt of propanoic acid.

Uses

As a food additive, it is listed as E number 282 in the Codex Alimentarius. Calcium propanoate is used as a preservative in a wide variety of products, including but not limited to: bread, other baked goods, processed meat, whey, and other dairy products. In agriculture, it is used, amongst other things, to prevent milk fever in cows and as a feed supplement Propanoates prevent microbes from producing the energy they need, like benzoates do. However, unlike benzoates, propanoates do not require an acidic environment.

Calcium propanoate is used in bakery products as a mold inhibitor, typically at 0.1-0.4% (though animal feed may contain up to 1%). Mold contamination is considered a serious problem amongst bakers, and conditions commonly found in baking present near-optimal conditions for mold growth.

A few decades ago, *Bacillus mesentericus* (rope), was a serious problem, but today's improved sanitary practices in the bakery, combined with rapid turnover of the finished product, have virtually eliminated this form of spoilage. Calcium propanoate and sodium propanoate are effective against both *B. mesentericus* rope and mold.

Metabolism of propanoate begins with its conversion to propionyl coenzyme A (propionyl-CoA), the usual first step in the metabolism of carboxylic acids. Since propanoic acid has three carbons, propionyl-CoA can directly enter neither beta oxidation nor the citric acid cycles. In most vertebrates, propionyl-CoA is carboxylated to D-methylmalonyl-CoA, which is isomerised to L-methylmalonyl-CoA. A vitamin B_{12}-dependent enzyme catalyzes rearrangement of L-methylmalonyl-CoA to succinyl-CoA, which is an intermediate of the citric acid cycle and can be readily incorporated there.

When propanoic acid is infused directly into rodents' brains, it produces reversible behavior changes (e.g. hyperactivity, dystonia, social impairment, perseveration) and brain changes (e.g. innate neuroinflammation, glutathione depletion) that may be used as a model of human autism in rats.

According to the Pesticide Action Network North America, calcium propionate is slightly toxic. This rating is not uncommon for food products; vitamin C is also rated by the same standards as being slightly toxic. Calcium propanoate can be used as a fungicide on fruit.

Polylysine

Polylysine refers to several types of lysine homopolymers, which may differ from each other in terms of stereochemistry and link position.

Chemical Structure and Function

The precursor amino acid lysine contains two amino groups, one at the α-carbon and one at the ε-carbon. Either can be the location of polymerization, resulting in α-polylysine or ε-polylysine. Polylysine is a homopolypeptide belonging to the group of cationic polymers: at pH 7, polylysine contains a positively charged hydrophilic amino group.

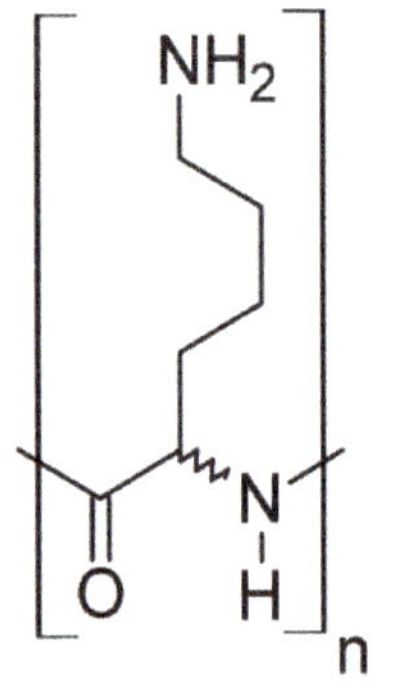

Structure of α-polylysine

α-Polylysine is a synthetic polymer, which can be composed of either L-lysine or D-lysine. "L" and "D" refer to the chirality at lysine's central carbon. This results in poly-L-lysine (PLL) and poly-D-lysine (PDL) respectively.

ε-Polylysine (ε-poly-L-lysine, EPL) is typically produced as a homopolypeptide of approximately 25–30 L-lysine residues. According to research, ε-polylysine is adsorbed electrostatically to the cell surface of the bacteria, followed by a stripping of the outer membrane. This eventually leads to the abnormal distribution of the cytoplasm causing damage to the bacterial cell that is produced by bacterial fermentation. ε-Poly-L-lysine is used as a natural preservative in food products.

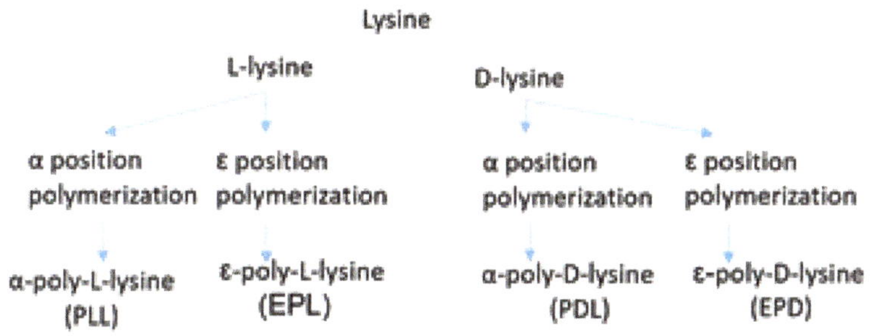

Production

Production of polylysine by natural fermentation is only observed in strains of bacteria in the genus *Streptomyces*. *Streptomyces albulus* is most often used in scientific studies and is also used for the commercial production of ε-polylysine.

α-Polylysine is synthetically produced by a basic polycondensation reaction.

History

The production of ε-polylysine by natural fermentation was first described by researchers Shoji Shima and Heiichi Sakai in 1977. Since the late 1980s, polylysine has been approved by the Japanese Ministry of Health, Labour and Welfare as a preservative in food. In January 2004, polylysine became generally recognized as safe (GRAS) certified in the United States.

Polylysine in Food

ε-Polylysine is used commercially as a food preservative in Japan, Korea and in imported items sold in the United States. Food products containing polylysine are mainly found in Japan. The use of polylysine is common in food applications such as boiled rice, cooked vegetables, soups, noodles and sliced fish (sushi).

Literature studies have reported an antimicrobial effect of ε-polylysine against yeast, fungi, Gram-positive bacteria and Gram-negative bacteria.

Polylysine has a light yellow appearance and is slightly bitter in taste whether in powder or liquid form.

Polylysine in Tissue Culture

α-Polylysine is commonly used to coat tissue cultureware as an attachment factor which improves cell adherence. This phenomenon is based on the interaction between the positively charged polymer and negatively charged cells or proteins. While the poly-L-lysine (PLL) precursor amino acid occurs naturally, the poly-D-lysine (PDL) precursor is an artificial product. The latter is therefore thought to be resistant to enzymatic degradation and so may prolong cell adherence.

Polylysine in Drug Delivery

Polylysine is featured by high positive charge density which allows them to form soluble complexes with negatively charged macromolecules. Polylysine homopolymers or block copolymers have been widely used for delivery of DNA and proteins. Polylysine-based nanoparticles have also been shown to passively accumulate in the injured sites of blood vessle after stroke due to incorporation into newly formed thrombus, which offers a new way to deliver therapeutic agents specifically to the sites of injury after vascular damage.

Chemical Modification

In 2010, hydrophobically modified ε-polylysine was synthesized by reacting EPL with octenyl succinic anhydride (OSA). It was found that OSA-g-EPLs had glass transition temperatures lower than EPL. They were able to form polymer micelles in water and to lower the surface tension of water, confirming their amphiphilic properties. The antimicrobial activities of OSA-g-EPLs were also examined, and the minimum inhibitory concentrations of OSA-g-EPLs against *Escherichia coli* O157:H7 remained the same as that of EPL. Therefore, modified EPLs have the potential of becoming bifunctional molecules, which can be used either as surfactants or emulsifiers in the encapsulation of water-insoluble drugs or as antimicrobial agents.

References

- Neuburger, Albert (2003). The technical arts and sciences of the ancients. London: Kegan Paul. pp. 122–124. ISBN 0710307551.
- Anderson, Oscar Edward (1953). Refrigeration in America; a history of a new technology and its impact. [Princeton]: Published for the University of Cincinnati by Princeton University Press. pp. 5–6. ISBN 0804616213.
- Freidberg, Susanne (2010). Fresh : a perishable history (1st Harvard University Press pbk. ed.). Cambridge, Mass.: Belknap. pp. 20–23. ISBN 0674057228.
- Arora, Ramesh Chandra. "Mechanical vapour compression refrigeration". Refrigeration and Air Conditioning. New Delhi, India: PHI Learning. p. 3. ISBN 81-203-3915-0.
- Freidberg, Susanne (2010). Fresh : a perishable history (1st Harvard University Press pbk. ed.). Cambridge, Mass.: Belknap. p. 23. ISBN 0674057228.
- Freidberg, Susanne (2010). Fresh : a perishable history (1st Harvard University Press pbk. ed.). Cambridge, Mass.: Belknap. p. 45. ISBN 0674057228.
- Rockoff, Gary M. Walton, Hugh (2010). History of the American Economy (11th ed.). Mason, Ohio: South-Western/Cengage Learning. pp. 336–368. ISBN 0324786611.
- Perry, R.H. & Green, D.W. (1984). Perry's Chemical Engineers' Handbook (6th ed.). McGraw Hill, Inc. ISBN 0-07-049479-7. (see pages 12-27 through 12-38)
- McGee, Harold (2004). On Food and Cooking: The Science and Lore of the Kitchen. New York: Scribner, pp. 291–296. ISBN 0-684-80001-2.
- Marotz, Lynn R. (2008). Health, Safety, and Nutrition for the Young Child. Wadsworth Publishing. p. 482. ISBN 978-1-4283-2070-3.
- Mitchell, Deborah (2004). Safe foods: the A-to-Z guide to the most wholesome foods for you and your family. Penguin. pp. Ch. 15. ISBN 978-1-101-21015-4.
- Editors of Creative Publishing. Dressing & Cooking Wild Game. Publisher: Creative Publishing international 1999 ISBN 978-0865731080

Permissions

All chapters in this book are published with permission under the Creative Commons Attribution Share Alike License or equivalent. Every chapter published in this book has been scrutinized by our experts. Their significance has been extensively debated. The topics covered herein carry significant information for a comprehensive understanding. They may even be implemented as practical applications or may be referred to as a beginning point for further studies.

We would like to thank the editorial team for lending their expertise to make the book truly unique. They have played a crucial role in the development of this book. Without their invaluable contributions this book wouldn't have been possible. They have made vital efforts to compile up to date information on the varied aspects of this subject to make this book a valuable addition to the collection of many professionals and students.

This book was conceptualized with the vision of imparting up-to-date and integrated information in this field. To ensure the same, a matchless editorial board was set up. Every individual on the board went through rigorous rounds of assessment to prove their worth. After which they invested a large part of their time researching and compiling the most relevant data for our readers.

The editorial board has been involved in producing this book since its inception. They have spent rigorous hours researching and exploring the diverse topics which have resulted in the successful publishing of this book. They have passed on their knowledge of decades through this book. To expedite this challenging task, the publisher supported the team at every step. A small team of assistant editors was also appointed to further simplify the editing procedure and attain best results for the readers.

Apart from the editorial board, the designing team has also invested a significant amount of their time in understanding the subject and creating the most relevant covers. They scrutinized every image to scout for the most suitable representation of the subject and create an appropriate cover for the book.

The publishing team has been an ardent support to the editorial, designing and production team. Their endless efforts to recruit the best for this project, has resulted in the accomplishment of this book. They are a veteran in the field of academics and their pool of knowledge is as vast as their experience in printing. Their expertise and guidance has proved useful at every step. Their uncompromising quality standards have made this book an exceptional effort. Their encouragement from time to time has been an inspiration for everyone.

The publisher and the editorial board hope that this book will prove to be a valuable piece of knowledge for students, practitioners and scholars across the globe.

Index